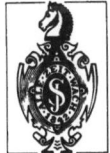

M. Nishi · H. Ichikawa · T. Nakajima
K. Maruyama · E. Tahara (Eds.)

Gastric Cancer

With 196 Figures, Including 13 in Color

Springer Japan KK

Mitsumasa Nishi, M.D.
Cancer Institute Hospital, 1-37-1 Kami-Ikebukuro, Toshima-ku, Tokyo, 170 Japan

Heizaburo Ichikawa, M.D.
National Cancer Center Hospital, 5-1-1 Tsukiji, Chuo-ku, Tokyo, 104 Japan

Toshifusa Nakajima, M.D.
Department of Surgery, Cancer Institute Hospital, 1-37-1 Kami-Ikebukuro, Toshima-ku, Tokyo, 170 Japan

Keiichi Maruyama, M.D.
Gastric Surgery Division, National Cancer Center Hospital, 5-1-1 Tsukiji, Chuo-ku, Tokyo, 104 Japan

Eiichi Tahara, M.D.
Department of Pathology, Hiroshima University School of Medicine, 1-2-3 Kasumi, Minami-ku, Hiroshima, 734 Japan

On the frontcover: Well differentiated ardenocarcinoma (*see p. 60*).

ISBN 978-4-431-68330-8

Library of Congress Cataloging-in-Publication Data
Gastric cancer / M. Nishi . . . [et al.] (eds.).   p.   cm.   Includes bibliographical references and index.
ISBN 978-4-431-68330-8   ISBN 978-4-431-68328-5 (eBook)
DOI 10.1007/978-4-431-68328-5
1. Stomach—Cancer.   I. Nishi, Mitsumasa. [DNLM:
1. Stomach   Neoplasms.   WI   320   G2555   1993]   RC280.S8G373   1993.   616.99'433—dc20.
DNLM/DLC.   for Library of Congress.   93-31369

Printed on acid-free paper

Preface

Gastric cancer is still the most common cause of cancer death in the world, although in most countries, with the notable exception of the United States, its incidence is slowly declining. In statistical terms, gastric cancer is therefore the most formidable of cancer types, and its control is a pressing issue.

Recent evidence indicates that the conversion of normal cells to so-called "clinical cancer" is the prerequisite for a multistage process which is intimately associated with an accumulation of multiple gene alterations including both oncogenes and tumor-suppressor genes. Gastric cancer is no exception, in that it reveals multiple gene changes whose scenario differs, depending on their occurrence in intestinal-type or diffuse-type gastric cancers.

This book was planned for publication by the Japanese Research Society for Gastric Cancer in order to shed light on basic research and clinical practice in gastric cancer. The individual chapters, written by a variety of experts, contain numerous new topics related to all aspects of the disease, including epidemiology, experimental carcinogenesis, pathology, biology, diagnosis, and treatment. It is hoped that this book will be of use in basic research, pathological diagnosis, early detection, and therapy of gastric cancer. We would like to thank the staff of Springer-Verlag Tokyo for the excellent technical production.

June, 1993

M. Nishi
H. Ichikawa
T. Nakajima
K. Maruyama
E. Tahara

Table of Contents

Part 4. Biology

Part 5. Diagnosis

Part 6. Treatment

List of Contributors

Part 1
Epidemiology and Prevention

Epidemiology of Stomach Cancer

Kunio Aoki[1]

Key words. Stomach cancer—Epidemiology—Mortality Trend—Familial cancer —International differences—Causative factors

Worldwide Declining Trends in Mortality Rates for Stomach Cancer

Age-adjusted stomach cancer death rates [1] have been steadily decreasing in most countries since World War II, although in Japan the highest mortality has been shown after 1950.

Figure 1 shows the observed and estimated mortality rates of stomach cancer in selected countries in the period 1950 to 2000.

Differences in the levels of mortality rates between countries do not seem to become reduced until the year 2000. Females show more remarkable down slopes of the declining curves than males.

The declining trend in the United States was estimated to have started before 1900 and the death rate had already been recorded at as low a level as 30 per 100 000 in 1920 [1–4]. However, the age-adjusted rate of stomach cancer mortality in Japan has increased after World War II, reaching 70 per 100 000, and then declining after around 1960. The declining slope of the trend curve in Japan does not seem to be steeper than that in other counties. Similar temporary rises in stomach cancer death rates were observed in Poland and Italy, both of which showed gradually decreasing trends in the 1960s. In Portugal (not shown in Fig. 1) an increasing trend continued until 1975 and then levelled off, although the peak of mortality was not as high as that in Japan.

The temporary increase in stomach cancer mortality was estimated to be due, in part, to an increase in the number of people who survived tuberculosis and other infections diseases and who thus reached an age when stomach cancer could develop. The rapid increase in the aged populations has elevated the incidence of stomach cancer. On the other hand, a steadily declining trend has been observed

---

[1] Aichi Cancer Center, 1-1 Kanokoden, Chikusa-ku, Nagoya, 464 Japan

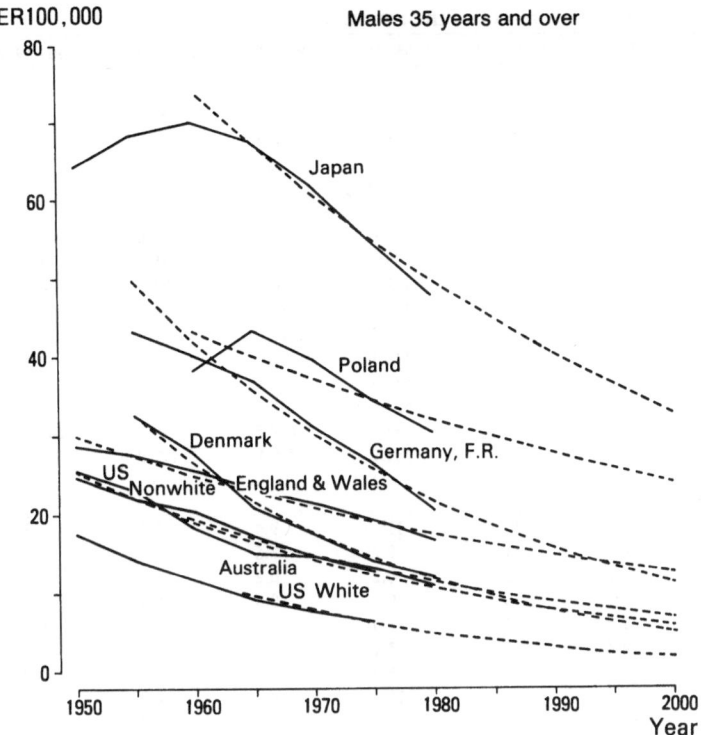

PER100,000   Males 35 years and over

Fig. 1. Observed (*solid lines*) and estimated (*dashed lines*) age-adjusted stomach cancer death rates in selected countries for the period 1950–2000

in stomach cancer in the younger birth cohorts [5]. The inverse trends were offset by a temporary rise and have since shifted to a gradual decrease over the last two decades.

Trends in Age-Specific Stomach Cancer Death Rate by Birth Cohort [5]

The trend curves in age-specific death rates for males, by birth cohort, of US whites and Japan were similar, although the levels of frequency were different. The age-specific death rate of the age group 80–84 in the 1878–1882 birth cohort of the US-white was about 100 per 100 000, which was lower than that of the 1928–1932 birth cohort in Japan. Table 1 [5] shows trends in age-specific death rates for stomach cancer per 100 000 since 1953–1957 in Japan and in US-whites. The rate of decline of the death rate in each age cohort seemed to be much faster in the US-whites than in Japan. The level of the death rates for stomach cancer in England-Wales was in between that of the US-whites and Japan.

4 K. Aoki

Table 1. Malignant neoplasm of the stomach.

All ages	1953–1957	1958–1962	1963–1967	1968–1972	1973–1977	1978–1982	1983–1987
Japan (Male)							
Crude	52.2	56.7	59.1	59.2	55.9	53.1	51.4
Adjusted	69.5	70.3	68.3	63.6	55.8	47.8	40.8
25–29	3.1	3.2	3.8	3.5	3.0	2.5	2.0
30–34	7.3	7.5	7.9	7.7	6.4	5.5	4.4
35–39	17.1	16.1	16.1	15.1	13.0	10.8	8.8
40–44	34.8	33.3	30.0	28.0	24.6	19.8	16.2
45–49	69.8	65.9	59.8	51.2	45.3	38.2	30.1
50–54	129.4	119.5	108.8	94.2	76.0	67.3	57.3
55–59	213.2	207.9	188.1	164.0	138.3	109.5	96.3
60–64	333.3	319.2	305.3	267.3	221.6	183.7	148.1
65–69	455.0	460.1	444.1	406.2	340.2	280.8	233.6
70–74	552.9	581.6	575.4	554.9	490.1	406.2	333.2
75–79	524.9	601.1	637.6	655.7	613.0	550.9	466.3
80–84	368.9	493.6	562.5	624.8	648.5	619.6	597.6
85 & +	246.6	322.0	364.9	429.9	499.9	558.7	618.1
United States, white (Male)							
Crude	17.3	14.1	11.2	9.4	8.3	7.5	6.9
Adjusted	14.7	11.8	9.2	7.6	6.5	5.6	5.0
25–29	0.4	0.2	0.2	0.2	0.2	0.2	0.2
30–34	0.9	0.8	0.6	0.5	0.4	0.4	0.4
35–39	2.2	1.8	1.5	1.1	1.1	0.9	0.9
40–44	4.4	3.5	3.1	2.5	2.4	1.9	1.9
45–49	8.9	7.5	5.9	5.2	4.6	4.2	3.7
50–54	17.6	14.5	11.1	9.2	8.2	7.6	7.0
55–59	30.8	24.2	19.3	16.8	14.3	12.4	12.2
60–64	54.9	42.0	32.3	27.8	24.0	21.3	18.3
65–69	92.3	71.5	53.7	42.5	34.9	31.4	27.3
70–74	131.4	105.9	81.6	63.7	52.5	45.3	39.7
75–79	177.5	143.0	111.5	93.5	79.1	63.9	55.3
80–84	222.7	185.5	147.4	118.6	104.0	86.1	70.9
85 & +	222.9	195.6	168.3	137.1	121.7	106.7	93.1

Per 100 000

Differences in Stomach Cancer Death Rates Between Japan and US Whites and England-Wales

Age adjusted stomach cancer death rates for males in the US-white population, England-Wales, Canada, and Japan in selected years since 1920 are shown in Table 2 [1–3, 6]. The rate of reduction was slow before World War II. Since 1950, the duration for halving the mortality of stomach cancer was about 30 years in England-Wales, about 25 years in Canada, and 16 years in US-whites. The decreasing trend in Japan became steeper after 1980 and the reduction rate in Japan between 1960–1961 and 1984–1985 was about 40% for males and 46% for females. If this reduction rate, shown for the last 25 years in Japan, continues in the future, the year in which the rate of 25 per 100 000 will be recorded for males will be the year 2010, and that of a rate of 9 per 100 000 be 2060. It will take almost 100 years to reach the level of the rate of the US-whites in 1964–1965.

Table 2. Trends in reduction of mortality due to stomach cancer (males).

	1920	1930	1940	1950–1951	1960–1961	1970–1971	1980–1981
U.S. white	30			17	11	7	6
England-Wales		40		29	25	21	16
Canada		50		26	19	15	10
Japan			50–55	64	70	62	50

Per 100 000

The speed of reduction in Canada was rather faster than England-Wales. Such regional differences in the speed of reduction may suggest effective preventive methods. The main causes of differences in frequency between the US-whites and England-Wales might be due to diet and to other socioeconomic conditions, although the lifestyle was similar in many respects. The rate of population growth and changes in age-groups over the last 100 years in the two countries may be other factors contributing to the differences in mortality from stomach cancer.

Figure 2 shows the trends in the proportions of various age groups to the total population in the United States and England-Wales from 1950 to 1989 [7, 8] (T. Kuroishi and K. Aoki; unpublished data). The proportion of age-groups less than 40 years old was more than 60% in the United States and about 50% for England-Wales in 1989. Between 1800 and 1980 population growth in the United States was remarkable; this was due to a higher birth rate and to the inflow of millions of young migrants between the years 1840 and 1920. Younger birth cohorts, in general, have a lower incidence of stomach cancer. England-Wales had fewer migrants in that period; the increase in the aged population might slow down the decreasing trends for stomach cancer.

The population in Japan increased very rapidly, from 34.5 million in 1865 to 83.2 million in 1950. After World War II, the rate of population growth slowed due to decreased birth rates, i.e., the rate dropped from 28.1 per 1000 in 1950 to 10.9 in 1989; however, the death rate has gradually decreased over this period. As a consequence, the proportion of the aged population 65 years and over to the total population has increased from 4.9% to 11.6% over the last four decades [10], and the number of deaths from stomach cancer in the aged group have increased year by year.

Considering the rapidly increasing aged population in Japan, the declining trend in stomach cancer mortality rate might be slowed down in the near future.

Causative Factors and Web of Causation

Many risk factors have been reported world wide, and combinations of risk factors have been found to differ depending on specific lifestyles with respect to region and time. In Japan, the following have been shown to be risk or protective factors [11–38].

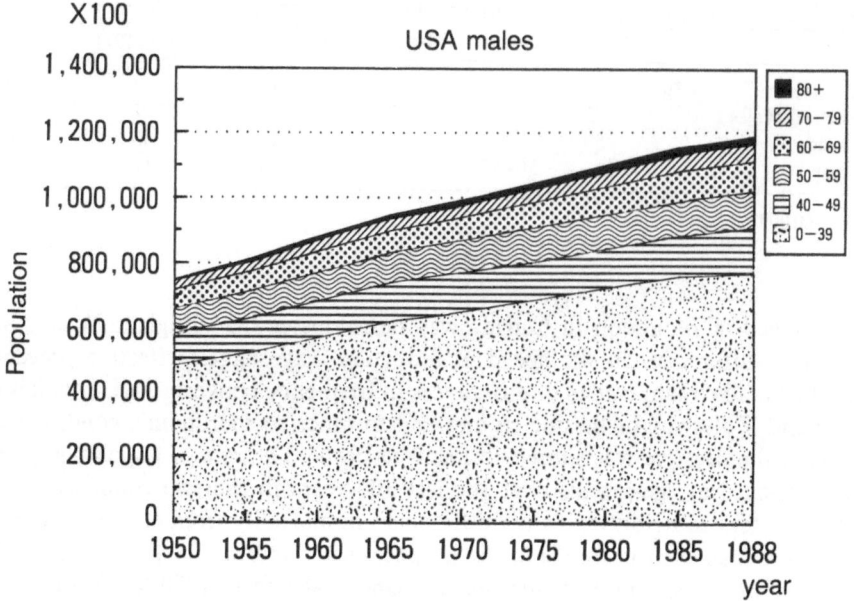

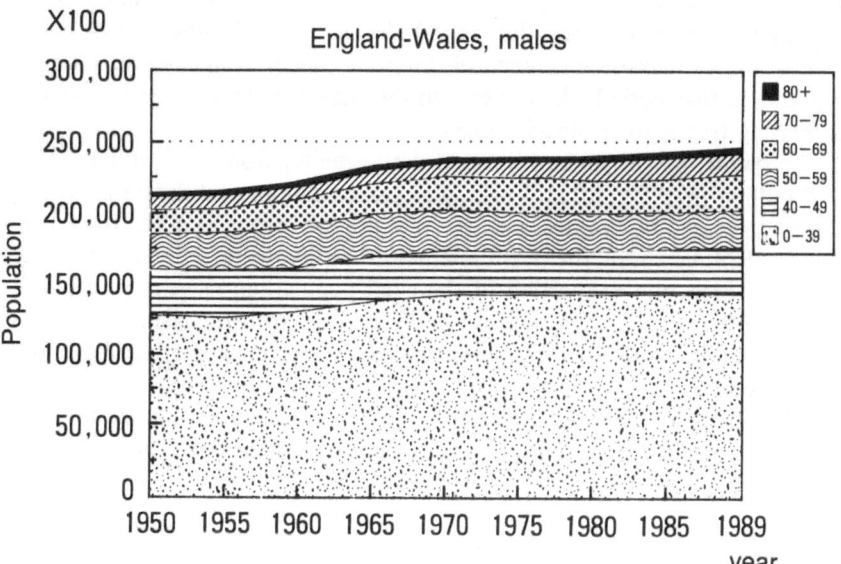

Fig. 2. Trends of increases in population by age (based on data in [9])

Risk factors are: salty foods (pickles, salty fish, dried fish, etc.), large intake of unrefined cereals, low intake of milk/milk products and animal-derived food, hot food/drinks, low intake of fruit, smoking (only in Japanese, not in Caucasians), high alcohol intake, irregular meal times, shorter duration of schooling, low socio-economic class, hard physical labor, and mental stress.

Protective factors were: intake of food derived from animals, milk/milk products, green-yellow vegetables, fruit and bean-curd, and daily intake of miso soup. (Miso is made from fermented bean curd).

It should be noted that changes in lifestyles among Japanese Americans in Hawaii showed a drastic reduction in stomach cancer after 1930 [36, 37] and that, in a recent study performed in Shandong, People's Republic of China [38], Chinese males who were heavy smokers (more than 20 cigarettes a day) showed a 50% increased risk of stomach cancer.

A brief historical review of the Japanese diet follows.

Figure 3 shows the food supply per person per year (kg) from 1911–1915 to 1970–1974 in Japan [39]. The Japanese diet was radically changed immediately after the Meiji Restoration (1868), being affecting by the rapid inflow of Western knowledge and cultures [40–43]. Meat, milk and milk products, and new types of vegetables and fruits were introduced to the public and new habits gradually became prevalent throughout the country. The consumption of meat, milk and milk products, eggs, fish and shellfish, and sea weed increased gradually year by year, while the consumption of beans and some cereals was reduced. In 1905, a private Institute of Nutrition was founded in Tokyo; this changed to the National Institute of Nutrition in 1920. Both of these institutions promoted a better diet for Japanese.

High salt consumption has been a big problem in the Japanese diet. Trends in supplies of salt, miso, and soy sauce per person per year have been stable for the 60-year period referred to in Fig. 3, except at the end of World War II [15, 39, 44]. There were, however, large regional differences in the amount of salt consumed in Japan, this amount ranging from 10–28 g per day, although the differences have been diminishing since World War II. The salt intake of 12.0–12.5 g per day per person noted in the 1980s still seems to be high, considering the incidence of stomach cancer in Japan [44]. A new type of Japanese diet, modified by Western dishes seems to have become prevalent throughout Japan since around 1965, and the changes in diet may alter stomach cancer patterns in the future.

A higher incidence of intestinal metaplasia, chronic gastritis, and/or repeated gastric ulcers has been observed in groups that were at high risk of developing gastric cancer [45–52]. A previous history of gastric diseases has often been recorded in patients with gastric cancer. Familial aggregations of gastric cancer suggest that both genetic and environmental factors are involved in carcinogenesis in this disease [53, 54].

Dietary factors are believed to play a major role in gastric cancer, but diet is affected by many environmental conditions. Figure 4 shows a web of causation for stomach cancer. The diet of a community depends to a great extent on the food supply and the sales system, on methods of food storage, on cultural back-

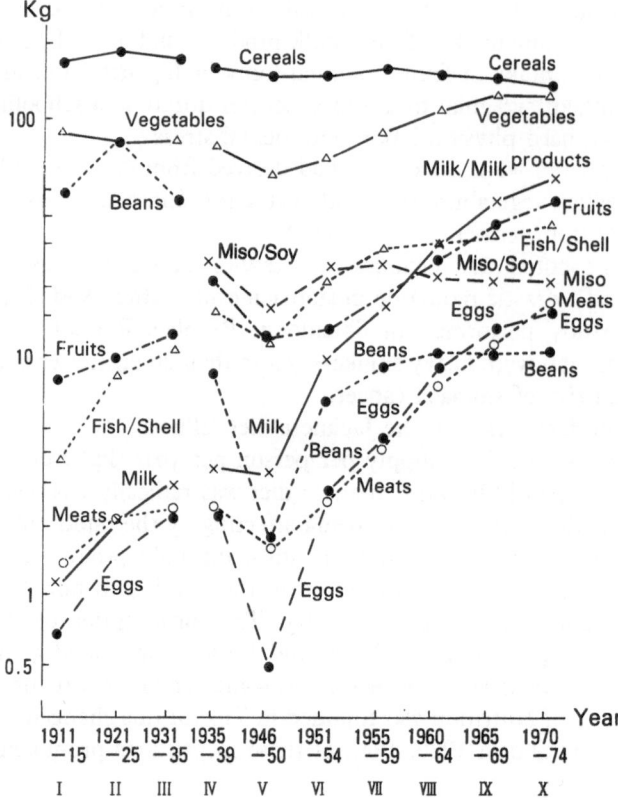

Fig. 3. Food supply per person per year; average values for 5-year periods (based on data in [39])

ground, and on knowledge of cooking methods, and knowledge of a healthy diet. Social and economic factors, i.e., types of industries in which people work, labor conditions, transportation networks, and the geographic and meteorological environment also seem to be closely related to the diet. These factors are also mutually related. The web of causation suggests various methods of preventing stomach cancer, since removing one or two factors may reduce the incidence of stomach cancer remarkably; there are also many combinations of preventive measures that can be taken. A high prevalence of stomach cancer has been reported in populations with a low socioeconomic level; such populations have a poor diet and shorter duration of schooling [30, 55]. Indices of physical development such as height and weight in primary age school children were shown to be lower and age at menarche was later in low socioeconomic classes [56, 57]. Regressive changes of stomach mucosa with lower function, occurring at earlier ages seem to be related largely to nurture and to duration of schooling.

Schooling in childhood and adolescence protects children from physical labor, risky events, and also from malnutrition. Education, including physical training,

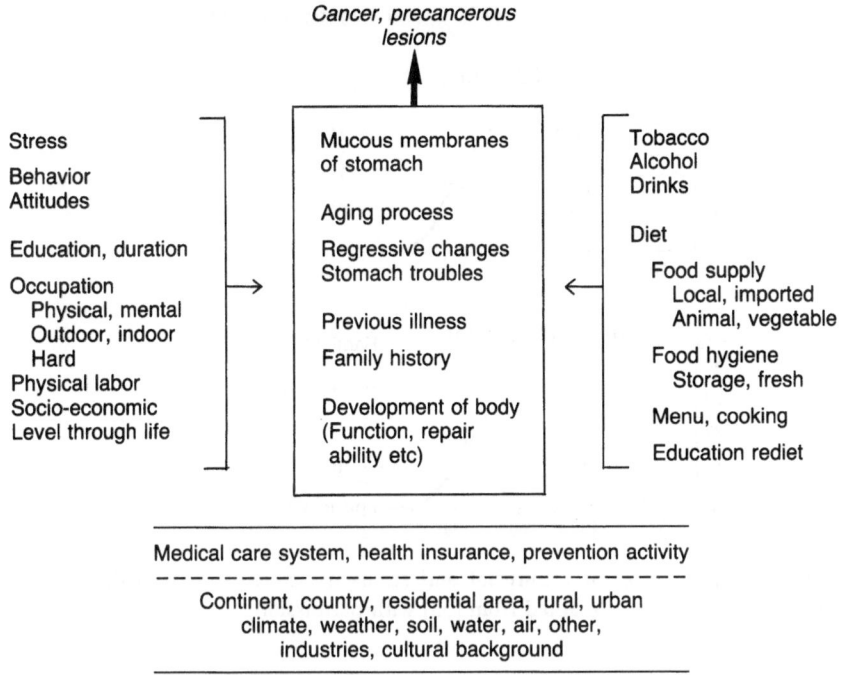

Fig. 4. Web of causation in stomach cancer

leads to a well matured body and provides adequate knowlege on how to live safely. In Japan the rate of schooling for children increased rapidly, accompanying the rapid growth in the economy from 1890; around 1920, about 80% of children had graduated from primary school [43]. Schooling might affect the later incidence of stomach cancer.

In the United States and England-Wales, compulsory schooling laws were promulgated before 1850 [58, 59], although they were not observed on a nationwide scale at that time. A decline in stomach cancer mortality was clearly observed in the 1878–1882 birth cohorts. In Japan, a similar declining trend was seen in the cohorts born after 1900.

Familial Aggregation of Stomach Cancer

Most cancers in adulthood seem to occur in the context of host and environmental interaction. The role of familial factors is briefly discussed here. Ogawa [53] analyzed 9131 cancer patients registered in the Aichi Cancer Registry in 1978–1981. The proportion of stomach cancer patients with a family history of the disease was high, at 12.2%, while this proportion for other sites ranged from 1.2% to 2.9%. These rates, however, should be adjusted by the cumulative rate of

10   K. Aoki

Aichi Cancer Registry (Ogawa)

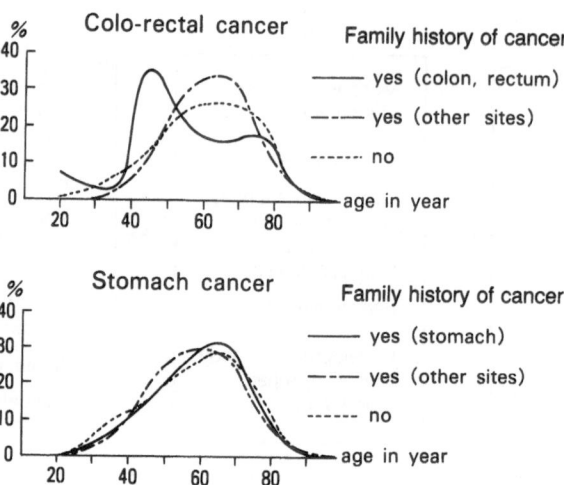

Fig. 5. Age distribution of colo-rectal and stomach cancer patients with and without family history of cancer. (Adapted from [53] with permission)

cancer patients by site, since the incidence and prevalence have differed remarkably by site for the last few decades. When the percentages of registered cancer patients showing familial cancer were grouped by site and divided by the average annual death rate for cancer by site in the last three decades, the ratio in each cancer group was similar, except for colon cancer. This rough calculation indicated that there was little difference in genetic influence in cancer sites, except for the colon. The age distribution of stomach and colorectal cancer patients with and without a family history of cancer is shown in Fig. 5. Colorectal cancer showed a bimodal distribution with younger and older peaks. The distribution with the younger peak suggested highly susceptible groups, and the older one seemed to be due largely to environmental factors. In contrast, no significant differences were observed in the age distribution of stomach cancer patients with or without family histories of cancer. These results indicate that environmental factors may have a substantial effect on stomach cancer.

The relative risks of stomach cancer by family history, smoking, alcohol intake, and occupation were examined by case-control analysis [54]. Family history elevated the relative risk by a factor of around 2, while smoking and alcohol intake had no influence on the relative risk. In this series, such occupational groups as farmers, fishermen, forest workers, and other physical laborers showed an elevated relative risk of stomach cancer, although the extent of this elevation was not great. No such effect was observed in other occupational groups. With regard to the diffuse type of stomach cancer, information on risk factors of environmental origin is poor at present.

Prevention of Stomach Cancer

Adequate diet and a clean living environment are essential for cancer prevention. The effect of improved diet and other lifestyle factors during the period of growth appears first as a lower mortality rate for cancer in the age group around 40 compared with birth cohorts in which there is no intervention. The birth cohort that has lower rates in middle age never fails to show lower rates as they become older; that is, cumulative mortality until 80 years of age is low. If such primary prevention is continued over a long period, cancer mortality will be reduced year by year, as is shown in the US-white population. These findings suggest that the lifestyle in childhood and adolescence is one of the most important determinants for the effective prevention of stomach cancer. Nurture in childhood and length of schooling seem to be very important indicators of the incidence of stomach cancer in later life. Strategy for the prevention of stomach cancer should begin in childhood and in adolescence. Of course, ongoing control programs for adults must be improved. Prevention activities should be promoted at the workplace, since labor conditions are closely associated with diet and with the incidence of gastric diseases and mental discorders related to cancer.

Considering the nature of individualized life in modern developed societies, various means of prevention may be prepared in accordance with age-sex groups. These would include periodic check-ups, education for a better lifestyle, and cancer education.

Living conditions change with time. Cancer education programs based on modern scientific knowledge, should be provided; these should correspond to changes in society.

We believe that advanced medical technology and improved medical care delivery systems will accelerate the reduction in stomach cancer mortality. It is obvious that proper medical treatment and care are indispensable for identifying and treating patients with precancerous lesions, which lesions should be removed. Chronic stomach illnesses should be treated carefully. Mass screening programs for stomach cancer should be performed. Such programs are now considered to be effective, as they identify a high percentage of early cancers, and there is thus the possibility of a high cure rate. The diffuse type of stomach cancer in which genetic factors play a major role should be subject to careful epidemiological study so that and controllable causative factors can be detected.

Finally, it should be mentioned that mental stress should not be overlooked as a factor in stomach cancer; the role played by mental stress in carcinogenesis would be clarified in the near future.

Conclusion. Declining trends in death rates for stomach cancer in Japan and other countries were reviewed and compared. The current level of the mortality rate for a country or area may be determined by identifying the year in which the death rate began to decline; the earlier that year, the lower the mortality rates in the 1980s. Socioeconomic developments may play a key role in the level of stomach cancer mortality. The difference in mortality levels between Japan and the US-white population seems to be nearly 100 years.

Familial aggregation of stomach cancer suggests that environmental factors play a large role in the incidence of stomach cancer.

Historical changes in the Japanese diet may partly explain the changes in the mortality rate for stomach cancer over the last few decades. The influence of nurture and schooling on the incidence of stomach cancer is also important.

Considering modern life in developed societies, various strategies for the prevention of stomach cancer, in accordance with age and sex, should be created, although specific control programs for children may be the first priority.

References

1. Kurihara M, Aoki K, Hisamichi S (eds) (1989) Cancer mortality statistics in the world 1950–1985. University of Nagoya Press, Nagoya
2. US Department of Health and Human Services, Public Health Service, NIH (1982) Cancer mortality in the United States: 1850–1877, NCI monograph 59. NCI, Washington
3. Cancer Facts and Figures—1992. American Cancer Society, Atlanta
4. Haenszel W (1958) Variation in incidence of and mortality from stomach cancer, with particular reference to United States. J Natl Cancer Inst 21:213–262
5. Aoki K, Kurihara M, Hayakawa N, Suzuki S (eds) (1992) Death rates for malignant neoplasms for selected sites by sex and 5-year age group in 33 countries, 1953–1957 to 1983–1987. International union against cancer. Nagoya University Coop Press, Nagoya
6. Office of Population Censuses and Surveys (1978) Trends in mortality 1951–1975. A Publication of the Government Statistical Services, London, 1978
7. Madden TA, Turner IR, Eckenfels EJ (1982) The Health Almanac, Raven
9. WHO Global Health Situation Assessment and Projections (Statistician, Lopez AD) (1991) Data base of cancer mortality statistics and mid-year population estimates for calculation of rates in the countries of the world, 1950 onward. Magnetic tape T00460, WHO
10. Health and Welfare Statistics Association (ed) (1992) Trends in national health, 1991 (in Japanese). Kosei No Shihyo [Suppl] 38(9)
11. Segi M, Fukushima I, Fujisaku S, Kurihara M, Sato S, Asano K, Kamoi M (1957) An epidemiological study on cancer in Japan. The report of the committee for epidemiological study on cancer, sponsored by the Ministry of Welfare and Public Health. Gann [Suppl] 48:1–63
12. Sato T, Fukuyama T, Suzuki T, Murakami T, Shitosugi N, Tanaka R, Tsuji R, (1959) Studies of the causation of gastric cancer, 2. The relation between gastric cancer mortality rate and salted food intake in several places in Japan. Bull Inst Publ Health 8:187–198
13. Insull W Jr, Oiso T, Tuschiya K (1968) Diet and nutritional status of Japanese. Am J Clin Nutr 21:753–777
14. Hirayama T (1971) Epidemiology of stomach cancer. Gann Monograph 11:3–19
15. Oiso T (1975) Incidence of stomach cancer and its relation to dietary habits and nutrition in Japan between 1900 and 1975. Cancer Res 35:3254–3258

16. Kono S, Ikeda M, Tokudome S, et al (1975) Cigarette smoking, alcohol and cancer mortality: A cohort study of male Japanese physicians. Jpn J Cancer Res (Gann) 35:3460–3463

17. Hirayama T (1975) Epidemiology of cancer of the stomach with special reference to its recent decrease in Japan. Cancer Res 3:3460–3463

18. Haenszel W, Kurihara M, Locke FB, Shimizu K, Segi M (1976) Stomach cancer in Japan. J Natl Cancer Inst 56:265–274

19. Kurita H (1980) Clinical epidemiology of stomach cancer (in Japanese). Kanehara, Tokyo

20. Shimizu T, Uejima I, Masuda C (1980) Tea gruel and death from gastric cancer—10 year follow up study. Jpn J Publ Health 27:237–243

21. Doll R, Peto R (1981) The cause of cancer. Quantitative estimates of avoidable risk of cancer in the United States today. Oxford Univensity Press, New York

22. Weisburger JH, Wynder EL, Horn CL (1982) Nutritional factors and etiologic mechanisms in the causation of gastrointestinal causes. Cancer 50:2541–2549

23. Hirayama T (1982) Relationship of soy-bean paste soup intake to gastric cancer risk. Nutr Cancer 3:223–233

24. Tominaga S, Ogawa H, Kuroishi T (1982) Usefulness of correlation analysis in the epidemiology of stomach cancer. In: Henderson BE (ed) Third symposium on epidemiology and cancer registries in the Pacific basin. NCI Monograph 62:135–140

25. Kamiyama S, Michioka O (1983) Mutagenic components of diets in high and low risk areas for stomach cancer. In: Stich HF (ed) Carcinogens and mutagens in the environment, vol III, naturally occurring compounds: Epidemiology and distribution. CRS, Boca Raton, pp 29–42

26. Ikeda M, Yoshimoto K, Kono S, Kato H, Kuratusne M (1983) A cohort study on the possible association between broiled fish intake and cancer. Gann 74:640–648

27. Kono S, Ikeda M, Tokudome S, et al (1984) A case-control study of gastric cancer and diet in northern Kyushu, Japan. Jpn J Cancer Res (Gann) 79:1067–1074

28. Tajima K, Tominaga S (1985) Dietary habits and gastrointestinal cancers: A comparative case-control study of stomach cancer and large intestinal cancers in Nagoya, Japan. Jpn J Cancer Res 76:705–711

29. Shimizu H, Mack TM, Ross RK, Henderson BE (1987) Cancer of the gastrointestinal tract among Japanese and white immigrants in Los Angeles County. JNCI 78:223–228

30. Hirayama T (1990) Life-Style and mortality. A large-scale census-based cohort study in Japan. Karger, Basel

31. Ogawa II, Tajima K (1990) A case-control study of psychological stress and cancer. Gan No Rinsho [Suppl] 36:391–400

32. Mettlin CJ, Aoki K (eds) (1990) Recent progress in research on nutrition and cancer. Wiley-Liss, New York

33. Tominaga S, Kato I (1990) Changing patterns of cancer and diet in Japan. In: Mettlin CJ, Aoki K (eds) Recent Progress in Research on Nutrition and cancer. Wiley-Liss, New York, pp 1–10

34. Ohno Y (1990) Methodology and evaluation of dietary factors in Japan. In: Mettlin CJ, Aoki K (eds) Recent progress in research on nutrition and cancer. Wiley-Liss, New York

35. Hirayama T (1990) Nutrition and cancer with special reference to the role of alcohol drinking. In: Mettlin CJ, Aoki K (eds) Recent progress in nutrition and cancer. Wiley-Liss, New York, pp 179–187

36. Hirohata T (ed) (1992) Cancer and lifestyle: Way to cancer prevention (in Japanese). Japanese Association of Public Health, Tokyo

37. Nomura A, Grove JS, Stemmenmann GN, Severson RK (1990) A prospective study of stomach cancer and its relation to diet, cigarettes, and alcohol consumption. Cancer Res 50:627–631

38. You W-C, Blot WJ, Chang Y-S, Ershow AG, Yang Z-T, An Q, Henderson B, Xu G-W, Fraumenin JF Jr, Wang TG (1988) Diet and the high risk of stomach cancer in Shandong, China. Cancer Res 48:3518–3523

39. Shimazono Y (1978) History of nutrition (in Japanese). Asakura Shoten, Todyo

40. Hagihara H (1960) History of nutrition in Japan (in Japanese). Kokumin Eiyo Kyokai, Tokyo

41. Saito A (1983) Chronology of dietary life in Japan (in Japanese). Yuraku Shobo, Tokyo

42. Margaret P, Anesaki M (1990) Health care in Japan. Routledge, London

43. Aoki K (1986) The changing health spectrum in Japan: Facts and implications. In: Hansluwka H, Lopez AD, Porapakkham Y, Prasartkul P (eds) New developments in the analysis of mortality and causes of death. WHO/Mahidol University, Bangkok

44. Japan Monopoly Corporation: An outline of statistics of Monopoly Corp. Senbai Kosai Kai, annually, 1960–1985 (in Japanese). Japan Monopoly Corporation, Tokyo.

45. Lauren P (1965) The two main histological types of gastric carcinoma: Diffuse and so-called intestinal type carcinoma. An attempt at a histo-clinical classification. Acta Pathol Microbiol Scand [A] 64:31–49

46. Stemmermann GN (1977) Gastric cancer in the Hawaii Japanese. Gann 68:525–535

47. Kubo T, Imai T (1971) Intestinal metaplasia of gastric mucosa in autopsy materials in Hiroshima and Yamaguchi Districts. Gann 62:49–53

48. Correa P, Cuello C, Haenszel W (1979) Epidemiologic pathology of precursor lesions and pathogenesis of gastric carcinoma in Colombia. In: Pfeiffer CJ (ed) Gastric cancer. Gerhard Witzstrock, New York, pp 112–127

49. Kimura T (1978) Aging and mucous membrane of the stomach. Rinsho Seijinbyo 3:1813–1819

50. Sugano H, Nakamura K, Kato Y (1982) Pathological studies of human gastric cancer. Acta Pathol Jpn 32(2):329–347

51. Nagayo T (1986) Histogenesis and precursors of human gastric cancer. Research and Practice. Springer, Tokyo

52. Hiyama T (1991) Tsuguma H, Fujimoto I, Takita M, Taniguchi H, Oshima A Analysis of epidemiological studies on stomach cancer and liver cancer. Study of intestinalization and stomach cancer; 1990 Report of Research Committee on Analytic Epidemiological Study on Environmental Factors and Carcinogenesis Department of Public Health, Kyushu University, Fukuoka, pp 27–30

53. Ogawa H, Kato I, Tominaga S (1985) Family history of cancer among cancer patients. Jpn J Cancer Res (Gann) 76:113–118

54. Aoki K, Ogawa H (1992) Familial cancer among cancer patients registered in the Aichi Cancer Registry. Heterogenity of aggregation of familial cancer. In: Weber W (ed) Familial cancer control. Springer, Berlin Heidelberg New York London Paris Tokyo, pp 119–122

55. Leon DA (1988) Socioeconomic factors and the primary prevention of cancer. In: Eylenbosch WJ, Depoorter AM, Larebeke NV (eds) Primary prevention of cancer. Raven, NY, pp 213–223

56. Takahashi E (1978) Ecologic human biology in Japan. Medical Information Services, Tokyo

57. Kudo Y, Shomoto M, Takeda S (1976) Trends in acceleration of growth from the viewpoint of maximum growth age (in Japanese). Jpn J Hygeine 31:378–385
58. Cootes RJ (1966) The making of the welfare state. Longman, London Translated into Japanese by M Hoshino (1977) Fubaisha, Tokyo
59. Ichibangase Y (1963) History of the development of social welfare in the United States (in Japanese). Koseikan, Tokyo

Evaluation of Mass Screening for Stomach Cancer*

Shigeru Hisamichi, Akira Fukao, and Yoshitaka Tsubono[1]

Key words. Gastric cancer—Mass screening—Evaluation—Case-control study

Introduction

According to the world cancer mortality statistics [1], the age-adjusted death rate for stomach cancer for males during 1984–1985 among the 40 listed countries was the highest in Costa Rica, followed in descending order by Japan, Chile, Poland, and Hungary. In females, the rate was again the highest in Costa Rica, followed in descending order by Japan, Guatemala, Chile, and Portugal.

In Japan, the deaths of males due to stomach cancer in 1960 accounted for more than one-half of all cancer deaths (51.6%). In females, the deaths due to stomach and uterine cancer amounted to 54.6% of all cancer deaths. Accordingly, the main target organs of cancer control activities in Japan were the stomach and the uterus. The main purposes of any cancer mass screening should be the early detection and prompt treatment to reduce the cancer mortality in a given population.

In 1988, although the age-adjusted death rate for stomach cancer has been decreasing in Japan, it still accounted for 24.6% and 21.6% of all cancer deaths in males and females, respectively. Thus, stomach cancer still remains the prime target for cancer control in Japan.

Under these circumstances, it is not only significant and important to review the history and current status of the mass screening program for stomach cancer, but also to evaluate this program from several aspects.

* Presented at the European School of Oncology (ESO), Course on "Gastric Cancer", Moscow, Russia, CIS, May 26–29, 1992
[1] Department of Public Health, Tohoku University School of Medicine, 2-1 Seiryo-cho, Sendai, 980 Japan

16

Table 1. History of cancer control activities in Japan.

1933	The Japanese Foundation for Cancer Research was established.
1958	The Japan Cancer Society was established.
	The first nationwide survey on the actual state of malignant neoplasm was conducted.
1960	Mass survey for stomach cancer by mobil X-ray units was inaugurated.
1961	Mass survey for cervix cancer was initiated.
1962	The National Cancer Center Research Institute was founded.
1965	The proposal for cancer control was approved by the Cancer Control Committee of Vice-ministers.
1983	The Cabinet Council for Cancer Control was organized and "Comprehensive 10-Year Strategy for Cancer Control" was established.
	The Health and Medical Services Law for the Aged was enacted.
1987	The Second 5-Year Plan for Cancer Screening was initiated.
1992	The Third 8-Year Plan (through the year 2000) for Cancer Control was initiated.

History of Cancer Control Activities in Japan

Table 1 outlines the history of cancer control activities in Japan. In 1960, mass screening for stomach cancer by mobile X-ray units was initiated in Miyagi Prefecture. Since then, a mass screening program for gastric cancer has been carried out on a nationwide level [2, 3]. In 1983, the Health and Medical Services Law for the Aged was enacted. Thereafter, mass screening programs for stomach and cervical cancer were conducted as part of the national policy, under the direction of the respective municipalities. In 1987, the Second 5-Year Plan of Cancer Screening was established, including mass screening programs for lung and breast cancer. In April, 1992, the Third 8-Year Plan for Cancer Control was instituted, including the screening for colon cancer by examination of fecal occult blood. Therefore, five types of mass screening programs designed to detect cancer of the stomach, cervix, lung, breast, and colon are presently available for local residents on a nationwide scale in Japan.

Screening Method for Gastric Cancer

There were two major diagnostic methods for stomach cancer, X-ray and gastro-camera examination. In the period around 1960, we considered the indirect X-ray examination as the best method for gastric mass screening in Japan for reasons of efficiency, effectiveness, accuracy, and being balanced in cost-benefit. The 5-year survival rate after surgery at that time remained at around a meager 20%. Therefore, we felt it mandatory to extend our efforts into the general population to perform examinations for early detection. Motor vehicles were designed with a built-in photofluorographic apparatus. According to the nationwide statistics of 1989 [4], 867 mobile X-ray units were in active duty.

Presently, the indirect X-ray examination is performed using a roll of film 100 mm in width, and 6 or 7 pictures (75.4%) are taken in various positions to

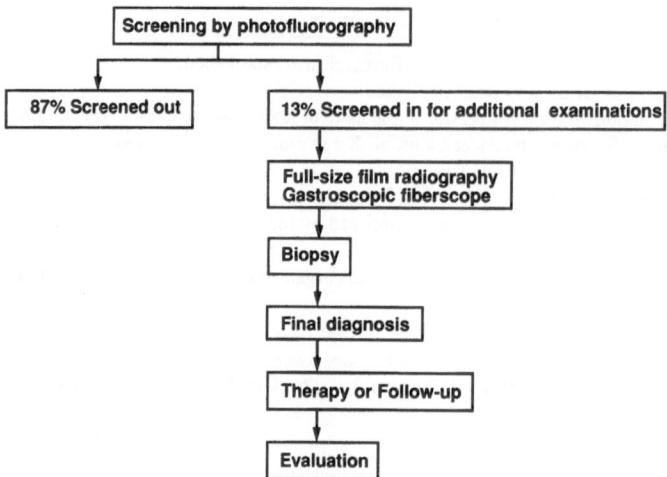

Fig. 1. System of mass screening for gastric cancer

cover all aspects of the stomach. These pictures include the barium-filling method, the mucosal study, and the double-contrast method which are important
for early detection of gastric cancer. This procedure, which minimizes economical
expenditures and X-ray hazards without sacrificing diagnostic ability, is recommended as one of the standard methods by the Japanese Society of Gastroenterological Mass Survey, and takes only 3 to 4 minutes to examine one person.

Figure 1 shows the screening system of mass survey for gastric cancer. Approximately 87% of the initial examinees are screened out, with the remaining 13%
being subjected to further examinations. The second-step studies include the
direct X-ray examination, fiberscopic examinations, and biopsy. Finally, we
evaluate the accuracy of the screening method, as well as the efficacy and
effectiveness of the screening program.

Results of Mass Screening for Gastric Cancer

According to the report from the Japanese Society of Gastroenterological Mass
Survey [4], the number of examinees in Japan has been increasing annually,
and approximately 5.2 million people over the age of 40 years, the high-risk age
group, were examined in 1988 (Fig. 2).

Table 2 shows the detection rate of stomach cancer and the proportion of early
stage cancer among the detected cases and among the resected cases in the mass
screening program. More than one-half (53.7%) of the stomach cancer cases
detected and 62.4% of the resected cases were in an early stage. These early stomach cancers are important, for they demonstrate quite a different clinical picture
and prognosis in comparison with the cases of gastric cancer ordinarily seen in the

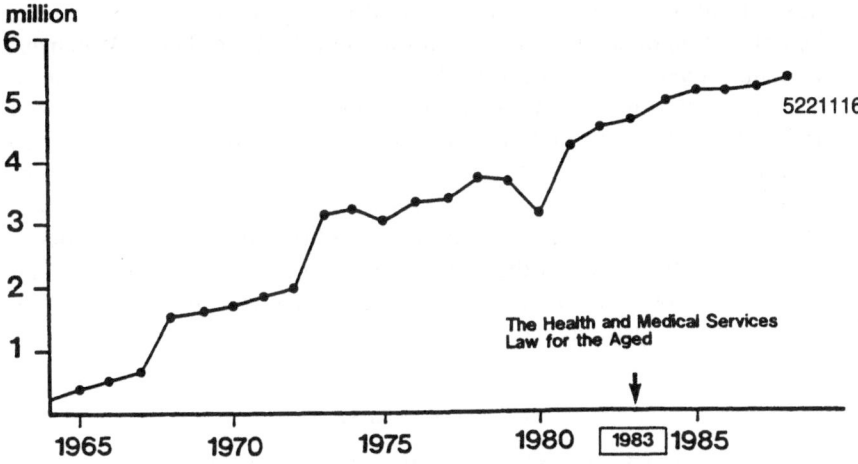

Fig. 2. Trend in numbers of subjects examined by mass screening program for gastric cancer (nationwide statistics)

Table 2. Results of mass screening for stomach cancer in Japan, 1988 (nationwide statistics).

Total screened (A)	5 221 116
Stomach cancer cases detected (B)	6 414
% of B/A	0.12
% Operated on	97.7
% With early cancer	
In detected cases	53.7
In resected cases	62.4

out-patient clinic. The survival rate of cases detected by mass survey is remarkably higher than that of cases detected in out-patient clinics [5].

Evaluation of Mass Screening for Stomach Cancer

Many studies have evaluated the effectiveness of mass screening for gastric cancer which were carried out in Japan. The objective of cancer screening is to achieve a reduction of mortality associated with the cancer in question through early detection and early treatment. The randomized controlled trial (RCT) is considered the best method for such an evaluative technique due to the lack of bias in the results [5–7].

Although the concept of RCT may be relatively simple, its practical execution is difficult. Specifically, in studies involving humans, randomization in the true sense is very difficult. Furthermore, since the same activity as that to be studied by the trial already exists, or is being practiced among the target group of the population, allocation of subjects into a control group is also difficult. Moreover, long-term commitments and vast financial resources are rquired to obtain meaningful results. Nevertheless, RCT by group randomization has been carried out for stomach cancer screening in Miyagi Prefecture, Japan, by our joint research group. Unfortunately, however, the results are still unavailable [8]. Accordingly, as the second-best alternatives, we carried out case-control studies, nonrandomized cohort studies, a kind of time-trend studies comparing the incidence with the mortality rate, studies of the relationship between the screening rate and the change of death rate. In this paper, we review three examples, case-control studies, time-trend analysis, and cost-effectiveness analysis.

Case-Control Studies

Oshima et al. [9] applied the case-control study to evaluate the effectiveness of mass screening for gastric cancer. From the matched analysis of the distribution of screening history in case-control combinations, the odds ratio of screened vs unscreened subjects dying from stomach cancer was calculated as 0.6 among males and 0.38 among females. These results suggest the effectiveness of the screening program in reducing stomach cancer mortality.

Fukao et al. [10] conducted a case-control study to evaluate the effectiveness of mass screening for gastric cancer and to determine the optimal interval between screenings. Cases and controls were selected as shown in Table 3. The study evaluated the relative protective effect of the diagnosis for advanced stomach cancer. Odds ratios of each respective interval group are shown in comparison with the group that had never been screened (Table 4). The odds ratio of the group that was screened 1 year before with a negative result was 0.4. This means that the chance of a person developing advanced cancer from a group screened every year is reduced to one-half. Accordingly, we recommend that the screening intervals for gastric cancer should not be greater than 3 years.

Time Trend Analysis

Figure 3 shows the trends of age-specific incidences and the mortality rates of stomach cancer in males and females of Miyagi Prefecture from 1960 to 1987 [8]. In this prefecture, since the population-based cancer registration was started in

Table 3. Case-control study on optimal interval of screening for stomach cancer. (From [10]).

Cases
  All advanced stomach cancer cases detected by mass screening in Miyagi Prefecture 1979–1983:
  241 males, 126 females
Controls
  Sex- and age- (±3 years) matched subjects were randomly selected from the examinees of the same
  precinct who were not diagnosed as having advanced stomach cancer: 367 controls

Table 4. Evaluation of mass screening for gastric cancer with case-control study design. (From [10]).

Decrease of advanced stomach cancer: Odds ratio for screened vs unscreened subjects of detected advanced stomach cancer (ss, s)	
Year(s) since last screening	Odds ratio
1	0.40[a]
2	0.60[b]
3	0.73[b]
4	0.71 ns
$\geqslant$5	1.0

[a] $P < 0.05$; [b] $P < 0.01$
ns, Not significant; ss, carcinoma infiltrating to the subserosa; s, carcinoma infiltrating to the serosa or beyond

1952 by the late Professor Segi of Tohoku University School of Medicine, it has continued uninterruptedly; therefore, we have data on both the incidence rate and the mortality rate of cancer covering a considerably long time period. The reliability of the cancer registration is considered to be high, as shown by a death certificate only (DCO) value of 9.5%, an incidence-death ratio of 1.8, and a histological identification per reported cases of 82% in 1986. For the evaluation of the reliability of a population-based cancer register, it is generally recommended that the percentage of registrations from DCO among all registered cancer patients should not be more than 30%. If the registration for DCO accounts for a large part of all registered cases, many cancer patients who do not die (within the period being evaluated) may be excluded from registration. The reliability of the registration (cancer *incidence*, not cancer *mortality*) would then be lower. The DCO percentage is considered to be a good index of the reliability of a cancer register. According to the Miyagi cancer register, the incidence rate of stomach cancer shows a decreasing trend in males, especially in recent years. Until around 1970, the mortality rate had decreased in parallel with the decreased incidence; however, since 1975, the decreasing trend has become more prominent, and a definite separation of the two curves can be seen, especially in the age group from 50 to 79 years, the main target age population for the screening. The same phenomenon can be seen in females and also in the study in Osaka by Oshima and Fujimoto [11]. Kuroishi et al. [12], who compared the trends in the death rates of stomach cancer between the model areas of mass screening of gastric cancer and their control areas, and Arisue et al. [13] reported similar results. Therefore, we consider this separation of the two curves to be attributable to the improvement of medical care and the widespread screening program that had been carried out during the last 25 years. However, it can not be denied that the

S. Hisamichi et al.

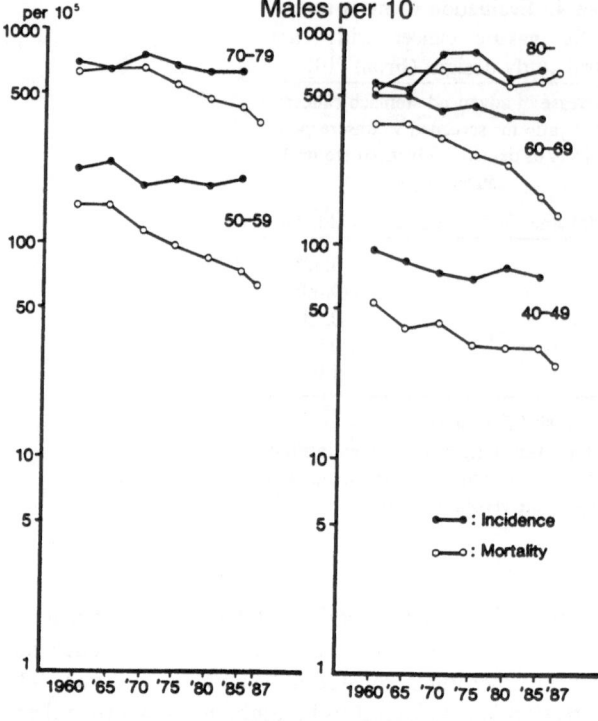

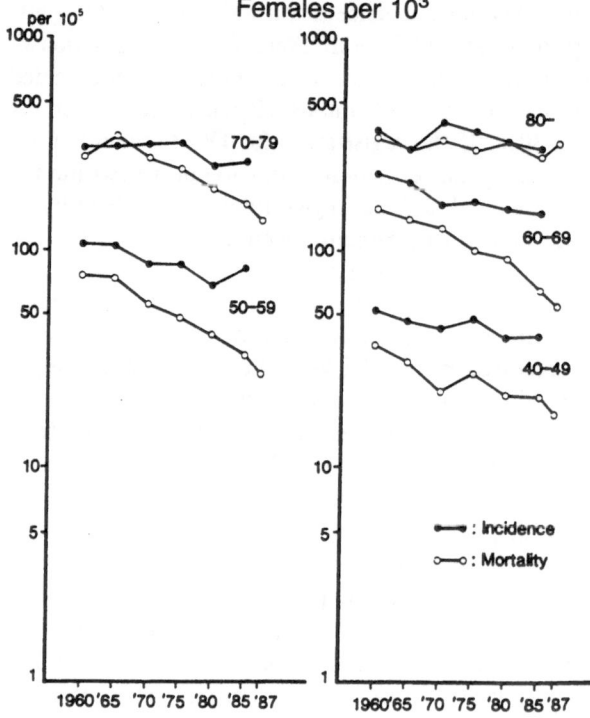

Fig. 3. Trends in age-specific incidence (in years) and mortality rates of stomach cancer (Miyagi Prefecture, Japan)

time-trend analysis is influenced by the advancements in medical technology as well as the system of data collection during the periods in question.

Mass Screening for Gastric Cancer in Venezuela

Venezuela is one of the countries with the highest mortality from stomach cancer in the world [14]. In 1981, stomach cancer ranked first among all cancer deaths in males (20.7%) and second in females (14.5%). The Andes Mountains area especially had a high mortality from stomach cancer. In the same year, a gastric cancer screening project was inaugurated in Tachira, in the western part of the Andes Mountains. In the following year, a joint venture was conducted by Venezuela and Japan with financial support from the Japan International Cooperation Agency (JICA). Mass screening for gastric cancer has been performed by the barium X-ray method used in Japan. Consequently, Oliver et al. [15] reported that of the 126 623 subjects examined, 44 562 underwent gastroscopic examinations and 14 589 received biopsy examinations. As a result, 133 early and 371 cases of advanced gastric cancer were diagnosed. The mortality of stomach cancer in Tachira has been decreasing while no changes have been seen in other neighboring areas.

Cost-Effectiveness Analysis

Various studies have evaluated the cost-effectiveness of mass screening program for gastric cancer in Japan [16–18]. Tsuji et al. [16] calculated the cost-effectiveness ratios of this mass screening by age and sex using simulation models, and concluded that it was negative among males older than the age of 65 years. Furthermore, the total cost of the screening program was less than that of not screening. It is suggested that the total cost for prevention and the deaths from gastric cancer in this age population were reduced by having implemented the screening program. Many other studies also demonstrated the extensive economic benefit, including the savings in medical expenditures, by mass screening for gastric cancer in Japan.

Discussion

The positive results of numerous studies evaluating the effectiveness of a mass screening program for stomach cancer, despite its being the second-best way without using randomized trials, strongly indicate that the widespread program in Japan is effective in reducing the mortality rate in the target population.

Strictly speaking, scientific pre-evaluations are necessary to conduct cancer screening on a mass scale for local residents. However, the mass screening program for stomach cancer in Japan can be considered to have thus far been carried out by a "do now, think later" design, or a way of, as we say in Japan, "thinking while walking".

The UICC Workshop on the evaluation of cancer screening, which was held in Cambridge, United Kingdom in 1990, concluded, "There are data from Japan that suggest stomach cancer screening can reduce mortality. Screening programs should continue in these regions with high stomach cancer incidence where they are already under way, but stomach cancer screening cannot be recommended in other countries as public health policy" [6].

In conclusion, the widespread program of mass screening for gastric cancer is considered to be effective in reducing the mortality rate of stomach cancer in the target age population. Furthermore, the decreasing trend of the mortality rates has accelerated during the last 15 years in Japan.

Acknowledgments. This work was supported in part by a Grant-in-Aid for Cancer Research (No. 4–22) from the Ministry of Health and Welfare of Japan.

References

1. Kurihara M, Aoki K, Hisamichi S (eds) (1989) Cancer mortality statistics in the world 1950–1985. University of Nagoya Press, Nagoya
2. Hisamichi S, Sugawara N (1984) Mass screening for gastric cancer by X-ray examination. Jpn J Clin Oncol 14:211–223
3. Hisamichi S, Sugawara N, Fukao A (1988) Effectiveness of gastric mass screening in Japan. Cancer Detect Prev 11:323–329
4. Hisamichi S, Doi H, Iwasaki M, Arisue T, Yamada T, Yoshikawa K, Kita S, Koga M, Ono Y, Hojyo K (1991) Nationwide statistics of mass screening for digestive organs in 1989 (in Japanese). J Gastroenterol Mass Survey 92:150–168
5. Hisamichi S (1989) Screening for gastric cancer. World J Surg 13:31–37
6. Miller AB, Chamberlain J, Day NE, Hakama M, Prorok PC (1990) Report on a workshop of the UICC project on evaluation of screening for cancer. Int J Cancer 46:761–769
7. U.S. Preventive Services Task Force (1989) Guide to clinical preventive services: An assessment of the effectiveness of 169 interventions. Williams and Wilkins, Baltimore
8. Hisamichi S, Fukao A, Sugawara N, Nishikouri M, Komatsu S, Tsuji I, Tsubono Y, Takano A (1991) Evaluation of mass screening programme for stomach cancer in Japan. In: Miller AB, Chamberlain J, Day NE, Hakama M, Prorok PC (eds) Cancer screening, UICC. Cambridge University Press, Cambridge, pp 357–370
9. Oshima A, Hirata N, Ubukata T, Umeda K, Fujimoto I (1986) Evaluation of a mass screening program for stomach cancer with a case-control study design. Int J Cancer 38:829–833
10. Fukao A, Hisamichi S, Sugawara N (1987) A case-control study on evaluating the effect of mass screening on decreasing advanced stomach cancer (in Japanese). J Gastroenterol Mass Survey 75:112–116
11. Oshima A, Fujimoto I (1979) Evaluation of mass screening program for cancer. In: Bailar JC (ed) Second symposium on epidemiology and cancer registries in the Pacific basin. NCI Monograph 53 NIH, Bethesda, pp 181–186

12. Kuroishi T, Hirose K, Nakagawa N, Tominaga S (1983) Comparison of trends in death rate of stomach cancer between the model areas of stomach cancer screening and their control areas (in Japanese). J Gastroenterol Mass Survey 58:45–52
13. Arisue T, Tamura K, Yoshida Y, Tebayashi A, Ikeda S, Otsuka S (1986) Comparisons of the changes in the mortality from stomach cancer between the model areas of mass screening for stomach cancer and the control areas (in Japanese). J Gastroenterol Mass Survey 73:26–32
14. Kurihara M, Aoki K, Tominaga S (1984) Cancer mortality statistics in the world. University of Nagoya Press, Nagoya
15. Oliver WE, Anderson L, Cano E, Peraza S, Sanchez V, Anderson O, Castro D, Alvarez N (1991) Screening of gastric cancer in the Venezuelan Andes. Report of the GI Cancer Center, San Cristobal, Venezuela
16. Tsuji I, Fukao A, Sugawara N, Shoji T, Kuwajima I, Hisamichi S (1991) Cost-effectiveness analysis of screening for gastric cancer in Japan. Tohoku J Exp Med 164:279–284
17. Hisamichi S, Nozaki K, Shirane A, Sugawara N, Ohshiba S (1977) Cost-effectiveness analysis of screening for gastric cancer (in Japanese). Igaku no Ayumi 98:81–85
18. Iinuma T, Tateno Y (1990) The future of gastric cancer screening from the viewpoint of cost-effectiveness (in Japanese). J Gastroenterol Mass Survey 88:164–166

Part 2
Experimental Carcinogenesis

Experimental Gastric Cancers

Takashi Sugimura[1]

Introduction

Gastric cancer is still one of the most abundant cancers in the world, with high incidences generally related to low socioeconomical status. The intestinal type of adenocarcinoma of the stomach is associated with intestinal metaplasia resulting from chronic gastritis and is observed more frequently in Asian, Eastern European and South American countries. Some gastric cancers are related to atrophy of the mucosa in the fundus portion with involvement of pernicious anemia.

In schirrus-type gastric cancers, the growth of stromal fibroblasts is possibly dominated by excretion of a growth factor for stromal cells from gastric cancer cells. Recently, an increase in adenocarcinomas has been noted in the cardiac region of the stomach located close to the oesophageal orifice, in individuals of high socioeconomic class in the United States. Gastric carcinogenesis is known to be a complicated multiple-step process and gastric cancers possess multiple genetic alterations. Factors determining carcinogenesis include genetic background, preceding pathological conditions, dietary habits and components, and the presence of Helicobactor pylori infections. Scientists have therefore concentrated attention on inducing gastric cancers in experimental animals to facilitate analysis of the involved mechanisms of carcinogenesis and to find effective approaches to treatment and prevention. Animals used include mice, rats, hamsters, and guinea pigs. Various carcinogenic agents were examined, including polycyclic aromatic hydrocarbons and 4-nitroquinoline 1-oxide. The administration route was by way of food, gastric intubation, or local submucosal injection. Even local transplantation of thread impregnated with polycyclic aromatic hydrocarbon was attempted. However, while some abnormal glandular proliferative lesions were noted, none of the attempts made were successful in inducing malignant adenocarcinomas in the glandular stomach of rodents before 1967. Instead, squamous cell carcinomas were very often produced in the

---

[1] National Cancer Center, 1-1 Tsukiji 5-Chome, Chuo-ku, Tokyo 104, Japan

28

forestomach of rodents or at the limiting ridge between the forestomach and glandular stomach. For a classical review, refer to Sugimura and Kawachi [1].

First Successful Induction of Adenocarcinomas in the Glandular Stomach of Rats by N-Methyl-N'-Nitro-N-Nitrosoguanidine

A Mutagen was Proven to Be Carcinogenic for the Glandular Stomach

N-Methyl-N'-nitro-N-nitrosoguanidine (MNNG) has been widely used as a potent and convenient microbial mutagen since the work of Mandell and Greenberg in 1960 [2]. Its carcinogenecity was reported in 1966, by Schoental in London [3] and Sugimura and his colleagues in Tokyo [4], demonstrating production of subcutaneous fibrosarcomas after subcutaneous injection as a solution in oil or water. When the experiments were extended and MNNG was administered to rats in their drinking water, the outcome was unexpected and exciting. Almost all Wistar strain rats which received continuous MNNG exposure (50–150 µg/ml drinking water) developed adenocarcinomas in the glandular stomach as shown in Fig. 1 [5]. The location was mainly in the pyloric region but the antrum and fundus portions were also affected. Histological findings demonstrated most of these gastric carcinomas were well-differentiated adenocarcinomas, some of them occasionally metastasizing to the liver. Signet-ring cell type carcinomas were also produced with metastasis found in the adjacent lymph nodes [5, 6]. This pattern of metastases is also characteristic in human beings. A single administration of MNNG also induced adenocarcinomas

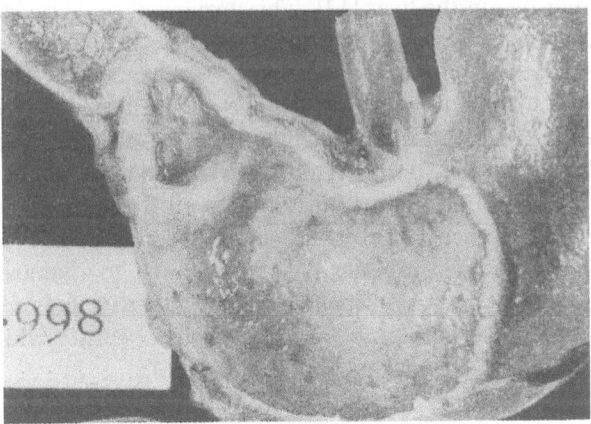

Fig. 1. Adenocarcinoma development in the glandular stomach of a rat given MNNG in its drinking water

in the glandular stomach of rats, but squamous cell carcinomas in the forestomach were more frequent [1].

Sequential Changes During Glandular Stomach Carcinogenesis Induced by MNNG

The time course of carcinogenesis was carefully investigated by Saito et al. by serially sacrificing rats receiving continuous MNNG [7]. A series of morphological changes was recognized. The first reaction was erosion of the mucosa in the glandular stomach and the induction of regeneration. Then, downward or upward adenomatous hyperplasias were observed with the presence of slight cellular and structural atypia. Longer administration of MNNG eventually resulted in the formation of malignant adenocarcinomas with more definite cellular and structural atypia and frequent mitoses. Sometimes pyloric stenosis and gastric dilation, resulting from gastric cancer formation, were observed. MNNG can also produce intestinal metaplasia in the glandular stomach of rats [8]. This is of interest given the widely accepted idea that intestinal metaplasia is related to the development of adenocarcinomas in the human stomach [9].

Possible Mechanisms of MNNG Carcinogenesis

MNNG has been used as a methylating agent in organic synthesis. A nascent intermediate produced from MNNG methylates the bases of DNA, mainly forming 7-methylguanine, with smaller amounts of 3-methyladenine, 1-methyladenine, 3-methylcytosine and O^6-methylguanine. O^6-Methylguanine may be the crucial adduct for production of mutations resulting in carcinogenesis [10, 11]. The glandular stomach contains much less O^6-methyltransferase activity, only one fiftieth of that in the liver [12]. This enzyme plays a crucial role in DNA repair by removing methyl moieties, with levels reflecting the sensitivity among various organs. Methylation of DNA bases is enhanced by the presence of sulfhydryl groups such as reduced glutathione and cysteine residues of proteins [11, 13] which are contained in large amounts in the glandular stomach. These facts may partly explain the specificity of MNNG carcinogenesis in the glandular stomach. MNNG can modify proteins in two different ways. One involves methylation and the other a nitroamidination reaction which occurs on the ε-amino group of lysine residues, converting it to homoarginine [13]. Modification of proteins may be responsible for cell damage induced by MNNG, followed by regenerative cell proliferation, which in turn could enhance the possibility to fix the DNA damage and cause mutations.

Variation in Susceptibility of Animal Strains to MNNG

Various Strains of Rats

There is considerable variation between rat strains; in particular, the Buffalo strain which was much more resistant to MNNG than Wistar-May-Furth animals, as reported by Bralow et al. [14]. Ohgaki carried out genetic analyses between sensitive ACI and resistant Buffalo strains and thereby proved the resistance to be a dominant trait [15]. The amount of O^6-methylguanine formed did not differ between the two strains and the concentrations of glutathione in the glandular stomach were the same. However, expansion of the width of the DNA synthesizing zone in the gastric mucous membrane which was cuased by MNNG was more marked in sensitive than in resistant animals. This difference in proliferative response could partly explain the sensitivity difference [15].

Mice and Hamsters

Many strains of mice are not susceptible to induction of gastric cancer by MNNG [1]. Golden hamsters do respond but develop fibrosarcomas from the submucosal layer of the stomach more frequently and more quickly than adenocarcinomas after continuous administration of MNNG [16]. N-Ethyl-N'-nitro-N-nitrosoguanidine (ENNG) on the other hand produces more adenocarcinomas in the glandular stomach of golden hamsters than MNNG [1].

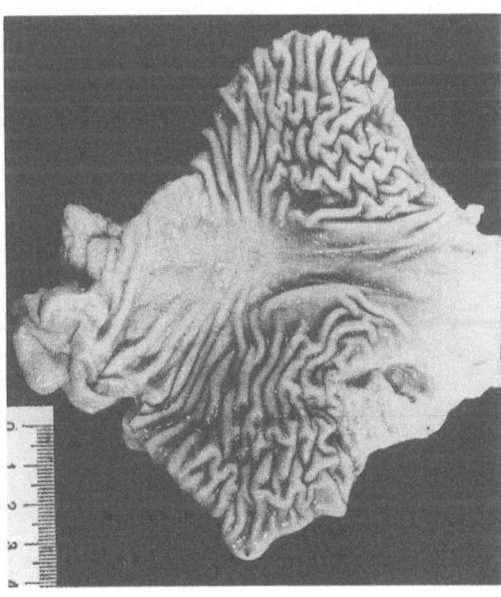

Fig. 2. Gastric cancer induced in a dog with MNNG

Dogs

Gastric carcinomas can be successfully induced in mongrel and Beagle dogs with continuous administration of MNNG (50–83 µg/ml) in their drinking water as shown in Fig. 2. The resultant well-differentiated adenocarcinomas are most frequently found in the fundus, but also in the antrum [17, 18]. However, many dogs concomitantly develop fibrosarcomas in the small intestine and therefore various improvements have been tried to enhance the specificity to produce only gastric carcinomas. For example, Kurihara et al. developed a better approach by soaking pellet diet in a solution of ENNG just before feeding the dogs [19]. The histological findings included well-differentiated carcinomas, poorly differentiated adenocarcinomas and signet-ring cell carcinomas, depending on the concentration of MNNG or ENNG, the duration, and the method of administration. It should be mentioned that in dogs, metastasis often occurs to the regional lymph nodes, and occasionally to the lungs and peritoneal cavity [20, 21].

Monkeys

When Macaca monkeys (rhesus and cynomolgus) were administered ENNG continuously at a concentration of 200 or 300 µg/ml in the dinking water for 11–26 months, periodic examination with radiography and fiber endoscopy revealed gastric carcinomas in the pyloric region after 11–38 months as shown in Fig. 3 [22]. Histologically they included poorly differentiated adenocarcinomas,

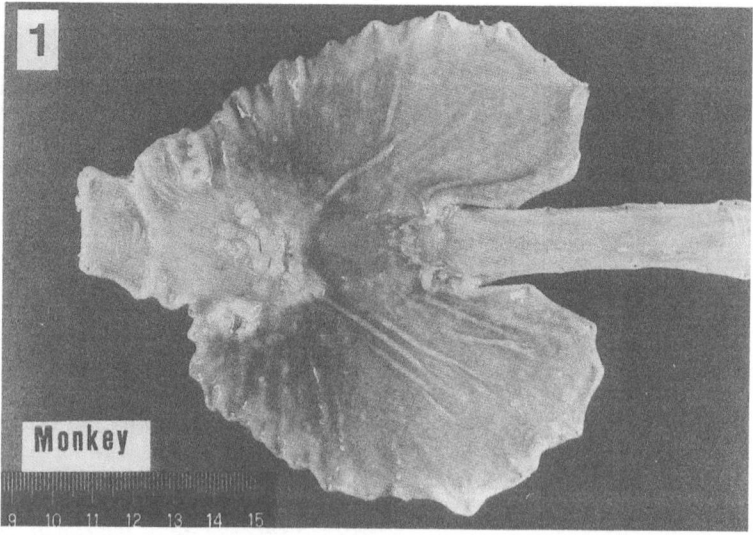

Fig. 3. Development of gastric carcinomas in the pyloric region of a monkey administered ENNG

signet-ring cell carcinomas, and moderate to well-differentiated adenocarcinomas, all similar to the respective human cancers.

One cynomolgus monkey given ENNG for 26 months and followed up for 108 months demonstrated an early carcinoma in the angulus of the stomach at the 31st month, but at autopsy, 71 months later this tumor had hardly progressed [23]. This experience indicates that monkeys may be more resistant to MNNG and ENNG than rats or dogs.

Modulation of the Carcinogenic Process

The carcinogenic process generally requires a long-time, during which multiple genetic alterations accumulate. However, the entire multiple step process is subject to modulation and can be either enhanced or suppressed. In this context, experimental production of stomach cancer has been widely used as a model for the human situation.

Enhancement of Gastric Carcinogenesis

Among various conditions under which gastric carcinogenesis was found to be promoted, the influence of sodium chloride is most relevant in the case of humans. Takahashi's group carried out extensive studies on the effects of sodium chloride on MNNG-induced carcinogenesis by simultaneous administration of sodium chloride in the feed along with the carcinogen MNNG in the drinking water solution which enhanced the carcinogenicity of MNNG [24]. This effect has been called the "co-initiating effect" [25]. The administration of excessive sodium chloride in feed after cessation of MNNG exposure also enhanced the development of adenomas and adenocarcinomas [26, 27]. Furthermore, administration of sodium chloride itself caused hemorrhagic lesions [28]. When excess sodium chloride is given to rats, malondialdehyde is formed in the mucosa of the glandular stomach and excreted in urine, indicating lipid peroxide formation in the tissue damaged by sodium chloride [29]. The results described above are in accordance with epidemiological findings suggesting the involvement of excessive intake of sodium chloride in areas where the incidence of stomach cancer is high as described in Chapter Epidemiology of Stomach Cancer of this volume.

In addition to sodium chloride, catechol, a substance occurring naturally in foods and beverages including onions and crude beet sugar was demonstrated to enhance gastric carcinogenesis induced by MNNG. Moreover, catechol itself alone produced adenocarcinomas in the glandular stomach of rats [30].

There are many other reports indicating substances or conditions which enhance MNNG or nitrosourea induced carcinogenesis. They include sodium taurocholate, bile and bile acid [31], gastrectomy and duodenal reflux [32], and iodoacetamide. Another factor of possible significance is chronic gastritis which often results in inflammation and intestinal metaplasia. In the course of these chronic changes more oxygen radicals and nitrogen oxide (NO) may be produced.

NO is released from L-arginine by nitric oxide synthase (NOS) which is increased by inflammation.

Suppression of MNNG-Induced Carcinogenesis

Suppression of carcinogenesis by MNNG has also been reported under several conditions or through substance administration, including exposure to estradiol [33]. However, only the effect of calcium is reviewed here, because it is the most relevant to the development of human gastric cancers.

A possible counter activity of calcium ions against gastric carcinogenesis was noted by Furihata et al. [34] who found the DNA synthesis induced by sodium chloride treatment to be reduced by administration of calcium chloride. Takahashi's group carried out experiments in which rats were given solutions of MNNG and sodium chloride and then water with or without calcium chloride at 1% or 0.2%. Inhibitory effects of calcium chloride administration during the post initiation phase of carcinogenesis in the glandular stomach were exerted in a dose-dependent manner [35]. Furthermore, calcium significantly reduced the formation of malondialdehyde in the mucosa of the glandular stomach and its excretion into the urine of rats [35]. The concentration of calcium ions which counterbalanced the effect of sodium chloride is close to that found in cow's milk [28]. The previous report of a lower frequency of gastric cancer among milk drinker's in Japan is therefore of interest [28].

Other Chemicals which Induce Glandular Stomach Cancers

An analogue of MNNG, ENNG, has also been used to induce stomach cancer [1]. Its potential is almost the same as that of MNNG whereas N-propyl-N'-nitro-N-nitrosoguanidine (PNNG) is weakly carcinogenic [36].

Working with nitroso compounds, Druckrey and his associates reported induction of cancers in the glandular stomach of rats by acetyl-N-methyl-N-nitrosourea [37]. N-Methyl-N-nitrosourea (MNU) has also been reported to induce adenocarcinomas in the glandular stomach of ACI/N strain rats but at a lower frequency [38]. A more recent report by Hirota et al. that MNU can produce, very specifically, adenocarcinomas in the glandular stomach of F344 male rats at very high frequency is clearly of interest. The best condition was to give a solution of 400 ppm MNU in the drinking water for 25 weeks and then sacrifice the animals 20 weeks after the cessation of carcinogen exposure. The authors called their method a "stop experiment" approach [39]. All these chemicals with nitroso groups are agents which can alkylate DNA bases.

Future Prospects

Through the efforts of many investigators, methods to develop gastric cancers specifically in the glandular stomach of rats, and in the stomach of dogs have been established. Sequential changes can be followed. Gastric cancers are the one of the most common human cancers and therefore investigations for their diagnosis, treatment, and of their molecular biology have been extensively carried out on human patients, as described in this volume (see Chapters 4, 5, and 6), yielding successful results. However, new challenges to treatment could be attempted on experimentally-induced gastric cancers in situ as reported previously [40]. Studies on genetic alterations, especially during carcinogenic processes, could be researched on animal models as follow-up studies. Modulation of carcinogenesis using animal models could be especially valuable for studies on prevention.

References

1. Sugimura T, Kawachi T (1973) Experimental stomach cancer. Methods in Cancer Res 7:245–308
2. Mandell JO, Greenberg J (1960) A new chemical mutagen for bacteria, 1-methyl-3-nitro-1-nitrosoguanidine. Biochem Biophys Res Commun 3:575–577
3. Schoental R (1966) Carcinogenic activity of N-methyl-N'-nitro-N-nitrosoguanidine. Nature 209:726–727
4. Sugimura T, Nagao M, Okada Y (1966) Carcinogenic action of N-methyl-N'-nitro-N-nitrosoguanidine. Nature 210:962–963
5. Sugimura T, Fujimura S (1967) Tumor production in glandular stomach of rat by N-methyl-N'-nitro-N-nitrosoguanidine. Nature 216:943–944
6. Sugimura T, Fujimura S, Baba T (1970) Tumor production in the glandular stomach and alimentary tract of the rat by N-methyl-N'-nitro-N-nitrosoguanidine. Cancer Res 30:455–465
7. Saito T, Inokuchi K, Takayama S, Sugimura T (1970) Sequential morphological changes in N-methyl-N'-nitro-N-nitrosoguanidine carcinogenesis in the glandular stomach of rats. J Natl Cancer Inst 44:769–783
8. Matsukura N, Kawachi T, Sasajima K, Sano T, Sugimura T, Hirota T (1978) Induction of intestinal metaplasia in the stomachs of rats by N-methyl-N'-nitro-N-nitrosoguanidine. J Natl Cancer Inst 61:141–144
9. Correa P, Cuello C, Duque, E (1970) Carcinoma and intestinal metaplasia of the stomach in Columbian migrants. J Natl Cancer Inst 44:297–306
10. McCalla DR (1968) Reaction of N-methyl-N'-nitro-N-nitrosoguanidine and N-methyl-N-nitroso-p-toluenesulfonamide with DNA in vitro. Biochim Biophys Acta 155:114–120
11. Lawley PD, Shah SA (1970) Methylation of deoxyribonucleic acid in cultured mammalian cells by N-methyl-N'-nitro-N-nitrosoguanidine. The influence of cellular thiol concentrations on the extent of methylation and the 6-oxygen of guanine as a site of methylation. Biochem J 116:693–707
12. Weisburger JH, Jones RC, Barnes WS, Pegg AE (1988) Mechanisms of differential strain sensitivity in gastric carcinogenesis. Jpn J Cancer Res 79:1304–1310
13. Sugimura T, Fujimura S, Nagao M, Yokoshima T, Hasegawa S (1968) Reaction of N-methyl-N'-nitro-N-nitrosoguanidine with protein. Biochim Biophys Acta 170:427–429

14. Bralow SP, Gruenstein M, Mevanze DR (1973) Host resistance to gastric adenocarcinomatosis in three strains of rats, ingesting N-methyl-N'-nitro-N-nitrosoguanidine. Oncology 27:168–180

15. Ohgaki H, Tomihari M, Sato S, Kleiheus P, Sugimura T (1988) Differential proliferative response of gastric mucosa during carcinogenesis induced by N-methyl-N'-nitro-N-nitrosoguanidine in susceptible ACI rats, resistant Buffalo rats, and their F_1 hybrid cross. Cancer Res 48:5275–5279

16. Fujimura S, Kogure K, Oboshi S, Sugimura T (1970) Production of tumors in the glandular stomach of hamsters by N-methyl-N'-nitro-N-nitrosoguanidine. Cancer Res 30:1444–1448

17. Sugimura T, Tanaka N, Kawachi T, Kogure K, Fujimura S, Shimosato Y (1971) Production of stomach cancer in dogs by N-methyl-N'-nitro-N-nitrosoguanidine. Gann 62:67

18. Shimosato Y, Tanaka N, Kogure K, Fujimura S, Kawachi T, Sugimura T (1971) Histopathology of tumors of canine alimentary tract produced by N-methyl-N'-nitro-N-nitrosoguanidine with particular reference to gastric carcinomas. J Natl Cancer Inst 47:1053–1070

19. Kurihara M, Shirakabe H, Murakami T, Yasui A, Izumi T, Sumida M, Igarashi A (1974) A new method for producing adenocarcinomas in the stomach of dogs with N-methyl-N'-nitro-N-nitrosoguanidine. Gann 65:163–177

20. Fujita M, Taguchi T, Takami M, Usugane M, Takahashi A (1975) Lung metastasis of canine gastric adenocarcinoma induced by N-methyl-N'-nitro-N-nitrosoguanidine. Gann 66:107–108

21. Sunagawa M, Takeshita K, Nakajima A, Ochi K, Kabu H, Endo M (1985) Duration of ENNG administration and its effect on histological differentiation of experimental gastric cancer. Br J Cancer 52:771–779

22. Ohgaki H, Hasegawa H, Kusama K, Morino K, Matsukura N, Sato S, Maruyama K, Sugimura T (1986) Induction of gastric carcinomas in nonhuman primates by N-ethyl-N'-nitro-N-nitrosoguanidine. J Natl Cancer Inst 77:179–186

23. Szentirmay Z, Ohgaki H, Maruyama K, Esumi H, Takayama S, Sugimura T (1990) Early gastric cancer induced by N-methyl-N'-nitro-N-nitrosoguanidine in a cynomolugus monkey six years after initial diagnosis of the lesion. Jpn J Cancer Res 81:6–9

24. Tatematsu M, Takahashi M, Fukushima S, Hananouchi M, Shirai T (1975) Effects in rats of sodium chloride on experimental gastric cancer induced by N-methyl-N'-nitro-N-nitrosoguanidine or 4-nitroquinoline 1-oxide. J Natl Cancer Inst 55:101–106

25. Takahashi M, Kokubo T, Furukawa F, Kurokawa Y, Tatematsu M, Hayashi Y (1982) Effect of high salt diet on rat gastric carcinogenesis induced by N-methyl-N'-nitro-N-nitrosoguanidine. Carcinogenesis 3:1419–1422

26. Ohgaki H, Kato T, Morino K, Matsukura N, Sato S, Takayama S, Sugimura T (1984) Study of the promoting effect of sodium chloride on gastric carcinogenesis by N-methyl-N'-nitro-N-nitrosoguanidine in inbred Wistar rats. Gann 75:1053–1057

27. Takahashi M, Okayama H, Furukawa F, Sato H, Hasegawa R, Shimoji N, Jang JJ, Hayashi Y (1988) Promoting effect of lower dose sodium chloride on rat gastric carcinogenesis. In: Proceedings of the Japanese Cancer Association, 47th Annual Meeting, Takyo, p 83

28. Sugimura T, Wakabayashi K (1990) Gastric carcinogenesis: Diet as a causative factor. Med Oncol Tumor Pharmacother 7:87–92

29. Takahashi M, Hasegawa T, Furukawa F, Okamiya H, Shinoda K, Imaida K, Toyoda K, Hayashi Y (1991) Enhanced lipid peroxidation in rat gastric mucosa caused by NaCl. Carcinogenesis 12:2201–2204

30. Hirose M, Kurata Y, Tsuda H, Fukushima S (1987) Catechol strongly enhances rat stomach carcinogenesis: A possible new environmental stomach carcinogen. Jpn J Cancer Res (Gann) 78:1144–1149

31. Kobori O, Shimizu T, Maeda M, Atomi Y, Watanabe J, Shoji M, Morioka Y (1984) Enhancing effect of bile and bile acid on stomach tumorigenesis induced by N-methyl-N'-nitro-N-nitrosoguanidine in Wistar rats. J Natl Cancer Inst 73:853–861

32. Salmon RJ, Merle S, Zafrani B, Decosse JJ, Sherlock P, Deschner EE (1985) Gastric carcinogenesis induced by N-methyl-N'-nitro-N-nitrosoguanidine: Role of gastrectomy and duodenal reflux. Jpn J Cancer Res (Gann) 76:167–172

33. Furukawa H, Iwanaga T, Koyama H, Taniguchi H (1982) Effect of sex hormones on carcinogenesis in the stomachs of rats. Cancer Res 42:5181–5182

34. Furihata C, Sudo K, Matsushima T (1989) Calcium chloride inhibits stimulation of replicative DNA synthesis by sodium chloride in the pyloric mucosa of rat stomach. Carcinogenesis 10:2135–2137

35. Nishikawa A, Furukawa F, Mitsui M, Enami T, Kawanishi T, Hasegawa T, Takahashi M (1992) Inhibitory effect of calcium chloride on gastric carcinogenesis in rats after treatment with N-methyl-N'-nitro-N-nitrosoguanidine and sodium chloride. Carcinogenesis 13:1155–1158

36. Wang X, Williams GM (1987) Comparison of stomach cancer induced in rats by N-methyl-N'-nitro-N-nitrosoguanidine or N-propyl-N'-nitro-N-nitrosoguanidine. Cancer Lett 34:173–185

37. Druckrey H, Ivankovic S, Preussmann R (1970) Selektiv Erzeugung von Carcinomen des Drüsenmagens bei Ratten durch Orale Gabe von N-Methyl-N-nitroso-N'-acetylharnstoff (AcMNH). Z Krebsforsch 74:22–33

38. Maekawa A, Matsuoka C, Onodera H, Tanigawa H, Furuta K, Ogiu T, Mitsumori K, Hayashi Y (1985) Organ-specific carcinogenicity of N-methyl-N'-nitro-N-nitrosourea in F344 and ACI/N rats. J Cancer Res Clin Oncol 109:178–182

39. Hirota N, Aonuma T, Yamada S, Kawai T, Saito K, Yokoyama T (1987) Selective induction of glandular stomach carcinoma in F344 rats by N-methyl-N-nitrosourea. Jpn J Cancer Res (Gann) 78:634–638

40. Ebihara K, Ekimoto H, Itchoda Y, Abe F, Inoue H, Aoyagi S, Yamashita T, Koyu A, Takahashi K, Yoshioka O, Matsuda A (1978) Studies on antitumor activities and pulmonary toxicity of pepleomycin sulfate (NK631) (in Japanese). Jpn J Antibiot 31:872–885

Part 3
Pathology

Histological Typing and Grading of Gastric Carcinomas

Paul Hermanek[1] *and Christian Wittekind*[2]

Key words. Classification, histological—Grading—Histology—Inflammation, peritumorous—Laurén classification—Ming classification—Pluriform structure—Typing, histological—WHO classification

Introduction

The aim of a tumor classification is to arrange tumors into specifically defined groups and subgroups. The tumors comprising one group are not usually replicas of each other, but resemble one another more closely than they resemble those in other groups. Such a system is convenient, but has inherent limitations which must be clearly recognized. The pathologist must be aware of the difficulties in the classification of tumors, including gastric carcinomas. Individual tumors exhibit a wide range of structures and behavior, so that subdivisions within groups are largely arbitrary.

The classifications discussed in this chapter are based on microscopic tumor characteristics, such as histological patterns and cytological criteria. From clinical and oncological points of view, a tumor classification is useful when groups and subgroups of tumors show a different biological behavior and thus carry a different prognosis. We consider to what extent the various classifications fulfill these criteria.

Grading of tumors of the individual histological groups and subgroups is undertaken with the premise that the grade of differentation might correlate with biological aggressiveness and prognosis. A grading system considers the degree of cytological and histological similarity of the tumor to the tissue of origin, as well as its nuclear abnormalities and mitotic activity.

[1] Department of Surgery, The University of Erlangen, Maximiliansplatz, D91054 Erlangen, Germany
[2] Institute of Pathology, The University of Erlangen, Department of Pathology in the Department of Surgery, Maximiliansplatz, D91054 Erlangen, Germany

The Accepted Systems of Histological Typing

Historically, there are numerous systems for histological typing of gastric carcinoma, most of which will not be dealt with here. The complexity of the systems might explain why some pathologists—particularly from North America—doubt the value of any histological classification. In 1977, the WHO [1] introduced a relatively simple and reproducible classification, which will herein be referred to as conventional or traditional typing. However, conventional WHO typing does not carry much prognostic or therapeutic significance. Therefore, in the second edition of the WHO International Histological Classification [2] two other classifications have been included, i.e., that of Laurén [3], predominantly used in Middle and Northern Europe, and that of Ming [4].

Traditional Typing

Most carcinomas of the stomach are adenocarcinomas which are defined as malignant tumors of glandular epithelium composed of tubulary, acinar, or papillary structures. The tumors may resemble either intestinal or gastric epithelium. While variable numbers of Paneth's or endocrine cells may be present, the presence of these specialized elements does not alter the classification.

Papillary Adenocarcinomas

These lesions are composed of either pointed or blunt finger-like epithelial processes with fibrovascular cores. The tumor cells are cylindrical or cuboidal and usually maintain a polarized surface orientation. The papillary subtype may show focally tubular differentiation (papillotubular).

Tubular Adenocarcinomas

These tumors are composed predominantly of branching tubules embedded in or surrounded by fibrous stroma (Fig. 1). The diameters of the tubules show some variation and occasionally cystic dilation can be found. The tumor cells are cylindrical or cuboidal, but may be flattened by the accumulation of luminal mucin or cell debris. Adenocarcinoma with both acinar (glandular) and solid structures as well as adenocarcinoma with lymphoid stroma are, by definition, included in this category.

Mucinous Adenocarcinomas

These are defined as tumors in which a substantial amount of extracellular mucin (more than 50% of the tumor) is retained within it. This type sometimes has been designated as mucoid, colloid, and muconodular adenocarcinoma.

The mucin can be observed macroscopically with a glassy or slippery cut surface. Several growth patterns can be seen: (a) glands lined by a columnar mucous-secreting epithelium with interstitial mucin (so-called well-differentiated type), and (b) chains of irregular nests of cells surrounded by mucous (so-called poorly

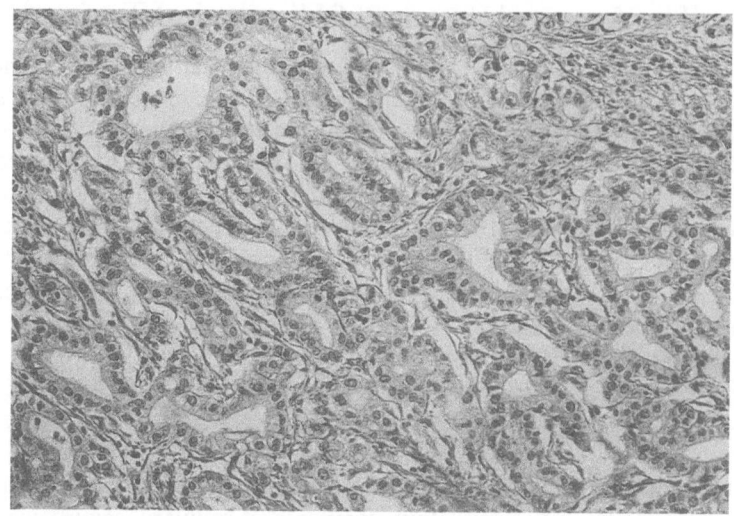

Fig. 1. Well differentiated tubular adenocarcinoma (H & E, ×160)

differentiated type). Some tumors show both growth patterns. Not infrequently, signet-ring cells may be present. However, more than 50% of a tumor should consist of signet-ring cells before classifying it as signet-ring cell carcinoma.

Signet-Ring Cell Carcinoma

This is an adenocarcinoma in which more than 50% of the tumor is made up of isolated or small groups of malignant cells containing intracytoplasmic mucin. The tumor is sometimes referred to as mucocellular carcinoma. Although signet-ring cells do not form tubules, they have a glandular capacity and, thus, there is often a glandular component, particularly in the deep mucosa of intramucosal signet-ring cell carcinoma. This is why it is appropriate to classify signet-ring cell tumors as adenocarcinomas.

Classically, the intracytoplasmic mucin presses the nucleus against the periphery of the cell into a banana-like form, thus causing the signet-ring cell appearance. However, the amount of intracytoplasmic mucin varies from cell to cell, thus the four types of tumor cells: (a) cells with an intracytoplasmic cyst filled with acid mucin (Fig. 2), (b) cells distended with secretory granules of neutral or acid mucin, (c) cells with eosinophilic cytoplasmic granules containing neutral mucin, and (d) cells without mucin, occurring in the deep layers of the gastric wall. All these cells may occur independently or in combination within any one tumor. Signet-ring cells tend to infiltrate diffusely and may be associated with considerable stromal fibrosis (they were occasionally called scirrhous carcinomas in the past). The malignant nature of the condition may be obscured by the extensive fibrosis suggesting an ulcerative scar. Stains for mucin or an immunohistochemical demonstration of cytokeratin should clarify the diagnosis. In

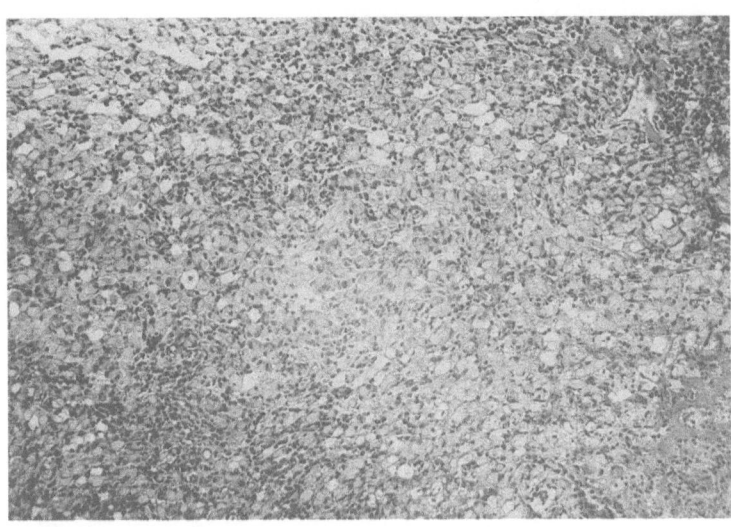

Fig. 2. Poorly differentiated signet-ring cell carcinoma with diffuse stromal invasion (H & E, ×80)

some cases, such as carcinomas involving the entire stomach, a phenomenon radiographically described as linitis plastica occurs.

Adenosquamous Carcinomas

These are tumors in which both adenocarcinomatous and squamous carcinomatous components are present. Not included are adenocarcinomas with small foci of squamous metaplasia: these should be classified as adenocarcinomas, with the squamous element referred to in the description.

Squamous Cell Carcinomas

These malignant tumors are composed of cells resembling those of squamous epithelium. In the majority of cases reported as gastric squamous cell carcinomas, a thorough histological examination will reveal small foci of adenocarcinoma. Most squamous cell carcinomas of the cardia are the result of spread of an esophageal cancer.

Small Cell Carcinomas

These are uncommon malignant tumors similar in histology, histochemistry, ultrastructure, and clinical behavior to small cell carcinoma of the lung. These tumors have solid or sheet-like structures with occasional acinar patterns and vascular stroma. Many of the tumor cells contain argyrophil granules or dense core granules. These granules may be positive for serotonin, somatostatin, gastrin, and other neuroendocrine markers. Positive cells are unevenly distributed.

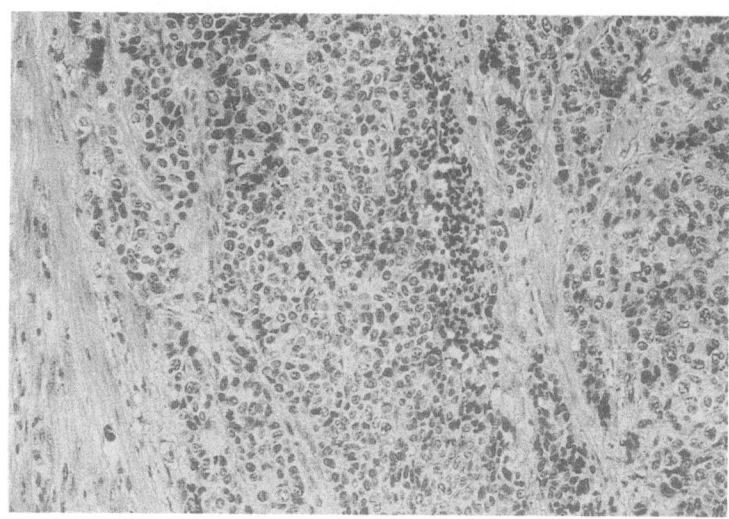

Fig. 3. Undifferentiated carcinoma with diffuse stromal invasion (H & E, ×160)

This tumor type has been called endocrine cell or neuroendocrine carcinoma. The tumor usually contains adenocarcinomatous components, particularly in the mucosa, and has been called adeno-endocrine cell carcinoma (see Endocrine Cell Tumor of the Stomach by Ito and Tahara, this Volume).

Undifferentiated Carcinomas

These are malignant epithelial tumors that have no glandular structures or other features to indicate definite differentiation (Fig. 3). Undifferentiated carcinomas should be distinguished from poorly differentiated adenocarcinomas, small cell carcinomas, lymphoma, and leukemic infiltrates by the use of mucin stains and immunohistochemical methods.

Histological typing and grading as recommend by the Japanese Research Society for Gastric Cancer 1981 [5] are very similar to the traditional WHO classification (see Classification of Gastric Carcinoma by Nagayo, this Volume).

Other Carcinomas

Additional types include choriocarcinoma [6], embryonal carcinoma (endodermal sinus tumor) [7], parietal cell carcinoma [8], and hepatoid carcinoma [9, 10]. The very uncommon mixed carcinoid-adenocarcinoma is classified as an endocrine tumor (see Endocrine Cell Tumor of the Stomach by Ito and Tahara, this Volume).

Laurén Classification

In addition to the traditional classification presented above, the Laurén classification has recently come into the foreground, because it has proven useful for epidemiological purposes [11] and clinical planning of therapy. The spread of the intestinal and diffuse types are different in the neighboring macroscopically normal-appearing stomach wall, and thus require different surgical approaches with respect to margins of clearance [12–14].

The Laurén classification is a further development and simplification of the ideas of Mulligan and Rember [15]. These authors differentiated between intestinal cell, pylorocardiac gland, and mucous cell carcinoma, the latter corresponding to the diffuse type of Laurén. The pylorocardiac carcinoma is included in Laurén's intestinal type.

The *intestinal type* is characterized by a predominance of glandular epithelium with cells similar to intestinal columnar cells. Focally, there may be brush borders, goblet cells secreting mucins, or clear cell differentiation. Cellular cohesion is good, and the tumor is usually sharply demarcated by a pushing margin.

The *diffuse type* is composed of scattered individual cells or small clusters of cells with wide and diffuse infiltration of the gastric wall. The cells are poorly cohesive and show a poorly demarcated margin. Many of the cells contain mucus and can show the typical signet-ring cell appearance, but nonmucus-producing cells occur as well. Some glandular arrangement may be seen in the superficial part of the tumors.

The Ming Classification

Ming's classification divides gastric carcinomas into two types, expanding and infiltrating. Thus, it exclusively considers the behavior of the tumor margin. The expanding type, with its pushing growth margin, is relatively well demarcated, whereas the infiltrating type shows a diffusely spreading pattern at the infiltrative margin. This classification can be performed only in the resection specimen, not in the biopsy specimen.

The Problem of Pluriform Gastric Carcinomas

Any classification of gastric carcinoma is complicated by the fact that more than 50% of tumors are pluriform, i.e., show considerable diversity in different parts. In an unpublished study of 100 unselected cases, only 22 cases had uniform histological structure, 78% had two or more histological components according to the traditional classification (44% had two, 29% had three, 3% had four, and 2% had five components). Therefore, any classification has to provide recommendations for categorizing these tumors with pluriform histology.

Traditional Typing

Classification should be based on the predominant type, with the minor component(s) referred to in the description.

The Laurén Classification

For *clinical purposes*, tumors with structures of both intestinal and diffuse types should be classified as diffuse type, independent of the relative proportions. The pathologist's report to the clinicians must always follow this rule.

In *epidemiological and histogenetic studies*, the Laurén classification should be followed according to the predominant structures [11]. Whereas the great majority of gastric carcinomas can be subdivided into intestinal and diffuse types, a minority cannot be thus classified. These include tumors with about equal proportions of intestinal and diffuse characteristics, and others that are undifferentiated and have a solid compact growth pattern. These are placed into an indeterminate category. Squamous cell carcinoma and adenosquamous carcinoma are categorized separately.

The Ming Classification

In this clinically oriented typing system, tumors with infiltrating margins are classified as infiltrating, independent of any additional component with expanding margins.

Correlation Between the Various Classifications

The intestinal-type carcinoma generally corresponds to tubular, papillary, or mucinous adenocarcinoma, mostly well or moderately, but possibly poorly differentiated. Diffuse-type carcinomas are signet-ring cell carcinomas, poorly differentiated adenocarcinomas or undifferentiated carcinomas. Ming's expanding type corresponds roughly to Laurén's intestinal type, and the infiltrative to the diffuse type.

Incidence of the Various Histological Types

About 45%–50% of gastric carcinomas are tubular adenocarcinomas, about 20% (15%–25%) are signet-ring cell carcinomas, and less than 5% are undifferentiated carcinoma. Papillary and mucinous adenocarcinoma are each observed in 5%–10%. The other types occur only in about 1%. These data relate to the total of carcinomas as observed in the two German multicenter studies [16, 17]. In relation to resection specimens only, the proportion of signet-ring cell and undifferentiated carcinoma is reduced. In the Erlanger Cancer Center (ECC), out of 1134 resected carcinomas, 553 (48.8%) were the intestinal type and 581 (51.2%) the diffuse type according to Laurén (Fig. 4). The Ming classification of 1120 resected carcinomas resulted in 481 (42.9%) being typed as expansive and 639 (57.1%) as infiltrative carcinomas.

Grading of Gastric Carcinomas

According to the WHO International Histological Classification [2], adenocarcinomas may be graded predominantly by consideration of the degree of architectural and cytological similarity to the presumed tissue of origin.

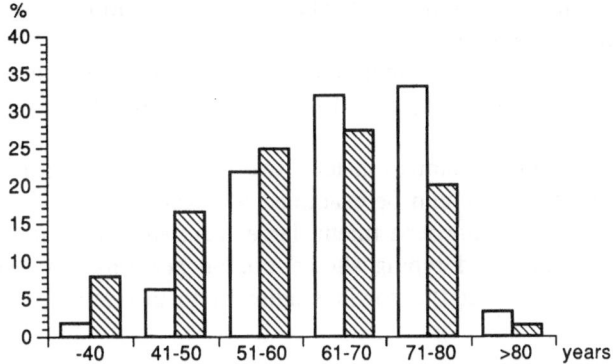

Fig. 4. Distribution of intestinal- (*open columns*; n = 553, median 68 years of age) and diffuse- (*hatched columns*; n = 581, median 61 years of age) type carcinomas in different age groups

1. *Well differentiated (G1):* adenocarcinomas with a regular glandular structure that often resembles metaplastic intestinal epithelium
2. *Moderately differentiated (G2):* adenocarcinomas intermediate between well differentiated and poorly differentiated
3. *Poorly differentiated (G3):* adenocarcinomas composed either of highly irregular glands that are recognized with difficulty or consist of single cells or cells in small or large solid cell clusters with mucus-secreting cells or abortive glandular structures

Signet-ring cell carcinoma is by definition considered as being poorly differentiated (G3). Adenosquamous and squamous cell carcinomas may be graded as in other sites. Small cell and undifferentiated carcinomas are considered as being G4 (undifferentiated). Well and moderately differentiated tumors can be grouped together as low grade, and poorly and undifferentiated as high grade.

While Laurén's intestinal type carcinoma may correspond to G1–G2, but rarely to G3, the diffuse type is assigned a high grade (G3, G4). Similarly to the occurrence of different histological types, one may observe different grades in a gastric carcinoma. In that case, the highest grade should determine the final categorization.

In 1107 graded resected gastric carcinomas registered in the ECC during 1978 −1989, 12% (133) were G1, 17% (188) G2, 45% (498) G3, and 26% (288) G4.

Prerequisites for Typing and Grading

An optimal result of the histopathological examination of a biopsy can only be achieved if the pathologist has all the information regarding the patient's clinical data and the findings of the endoscopic examination. The biopsied material should be fixed quickly in 4% buffered formalin or special fixation media for special immunohistochemical studies.

With respect to treatment planning, Laurén's classification should be used in reporting forceps and snare biopsies. If this is not possible, the biopsy should be repeated.

In a radical resection specimen, at least two blocks each from the center and the margin of the tumor should be examined to precisely quantify the extent of different components. In our department, large area (whole-mount giant) sections are preferred. Grading and typing should not be performed at the advancing margins of the tumor or at the portions adjacent to ulcerative or inflammatory processes.

Reproducibility of Typing and Grading

In 1984, 14 pathologists participating in the German multicenter TNM study [16] examined 17 large area sections of stomach carcinomas. Agreement of typing with the accepted diagnosis of the reference pathology was 88% (210/238) for the traditional and 89% (212/238) for the Laurén classification; however, it was only 63% (150/238) for grading (P. Hermanek and P. Schmitz-Moormann, unpublished data).

In 1990, 100 cases from the new German multicenter study on stomach cancer [17] were independently classified by two examiners. With the traditional classification, agreement was obtained in 78/100 cases. Each of the 22 cases with a discordant classification showed more than one histological type. In using the Laurén classification, only 2/98 cases were discrepant (in two cases the Laurén classification was not applicable). In using the grading system with four different grades, there was agreement in 76/100 cases. In a grading system with the categories of low-grade and high-grade, agreement reached 88% (C. Wittekind, unpublished data).

The common pluriform histology explains differences between histological typing in biopsies and resection specimens. In particular, in about 10%–15% of biopsy diagnoses of intestinal carcinoma, the resection specimen shows tumor structures of a diffuse type carcinoma in some deeper areas, i.e., the carcinoma has to be classified as being a diffuse type.

Correlation of the Laurén Classification to Clinical Features and Pathological Staging

The sex ratio (male/female) in the intestinal type is 2.31 (386/167) and 1.49 (343/238) in the diffuse type ($P < 0.001$) (ECC data 1978–1989, resected patients only). The intestinal and diffuse types of carcinoma differ in age distribution (Fig. 4): patients with the intestinal type are older than those with the diffuse type ($P < 0.01$), with the difference in the median age being 7 years.

There are also significant differences (Table 1) in tumor site (in the cardia and fundus there is predominance of the intestinal type, while there are more over-

Table 1. Data of Erlangen Cancer Center (ECC) 1978–1989. Only patients with resection of the carcinoma.

	Intestinal (n = 553)	Diffuse (n = 581)	Differences (P)
Tumor site			
Cardia	135 (24.4)	65 (11.2)	
Fundus	83 (15.0)	68 (11.7)	
Corpus	82 (14.8)	88 (15.1)	0.001
Antrum and pylorus	154 (27.8)	139 (23.9)	
Overlapping	99 (17.9)	221 (38.0)	
Macroscopic type			
Early	137 (24.8)	79 (13.6)	
Borrmann I	64 (11.6)	25 (4.3)	
II	172 (31.1)	92 (15.8)	0.001
III	139 (25.1)	178 (30.6)	
IV	35 (6.3)	204 (35.1)	
Unclassified	6 (1.1)	3 (0.5)	
Residual tumor classification (UICC)			
No residual tumor (R0)	473 (85.5)	422 (72.6)	0.001
pT Classification			
pT1 Mucosa	63 (11.4)	34 (5.9)	
Submucosa	63 (11.4)	36 (6.2)	
pT2 Muscularis propria	58 (10.5)	35 (6.0)	
Subserosa	215 (38.9)	148 (25.5)	0.001
pT3	118 (21.3)	257 (44.2)	
pT4	36 (6.5)	71 (12.2)	
pN Classification			
pN0	235 (42.5)	136 (23.4)	
pN1	125 (22.6)	126 (21.7)	
pN2	183 (33.1)	316 (54.4)	0.001
pNX	10 (1.8)	3 (0.5)	
(p) M Classification			
(p) M1	101 (18.3)	165 (28.4)	0.001
Stage grouping (UICC 1987)			
Ia	110 (19.9)	54 (9.3)	
Ib	106 (19.2)	55 (9.5)	
II	92 (16.6)	86 (14.8)	
IIIa	83 (15.0)	91 (15.7)	0.001
IIIb	45 (8.1)	107 (18.4)	
IV	108 (19.5)	186 (32.0)	
Unclassified	9 (1.6)	2 (0.3)	

Numbers in parentheses represent percent of total UICC, Union Internationale Contre Le Cancrum

lapping lesions in the diffuse type) and Borrmann type (in types I and II there is more intestinal and in types III and IV diffuse carcinoma is predominant). Curative resections are more frequently possible in intestinal carcinoma. The diffuse type carcinoma is generally more advanced in pTNM and stage grouping.

Table 2. Further conventional histological features of questionable independent prognostic significance.

Feature	Results of multivariate analysis of prognosis	
	Significant	Non-significant
Peritumorous inflammatory reaction	[23, 24]	[25–27]
Desmoplasia	[26]	[23–25, 27]
Tumor necrosis		[28]
Venous invasion	[26, 29]	[25, 28, 30]
Lymphatic invasion	[29]	[26, 28, 30, 31]
Perineural invasion		[28]

Other Histological Features Used for Classification

There are some histological features which can be assessed by conventional histology and which are not included in the accepted classifications listed above, but are frequently mentioned in pathology reports (Table 2). No independent prognostic significance of these features could be proven by multivariate analyses, and the respective results are either controversial or negative.

The favorable influence of peritumorous inflammation observed by some authors is in confirmation with the reported less aggressive behavior of carcinomas "with lymphoid stroma" [18]. In this pattern, mainly poorly differentiated tubular adenocarcinomas are diffusely infiltrated by lymphocytes and plasma cells, with occasional lymph follicles.

In 1987, Haraguchi et al. [19] distinguished between the funnel, column, and mountain types of stomach carcinoma using morphovolumetry. These types are defined according to the relationship between the volume of tumor in the mucosa (exophytic) and the deeper gastric wall. This classification correlates with stage and histological type, but has no independent prognostic significance.

Several authors have analyzed the cytologic differentiation using electron microscopy, mucin histochemistry, and immunohistology [20–22]. Various groupings have been proposed, but difficulties arise as a result of the common multidirectional differentiation as well as from the inhomogeneity of structure of carcinomas when employing conventional histology. Furthermore, no independent prognostic significance of these sophisticated classification attempts has thus far been proven.

References

1. Oota K, Sobin LH (1977) Histological typing of gastric and oesophageal tumours. WHO International Histological Classification of Tumours. WHO, Geneva
2. Watanabe H, Jass JR, Sobin LH (1990) Histological typing of oesophageal and gastric tumours, 2nd edn. WHO International Histological Classification of Tumours. Springer, Berlin Heidelberg New York London Paris Tokyo Hong Kong

3. Laurén P (1965) The two histologic main types of gastric carcinoma: Diffuse and so-called intestinal-type carcinoma. Acta Pathol Microbiol Scand 64:31–49
4. Ming S-Ch (1977) Gastric carcinoma. A pathobiological classification. Cancer 39:2475 –2485
5. Japanese Research Society for Gastric Cancer (1981) The general rules for the gastric cancer study in surgery and pathology. Jpn J Surg 11:127–145
6. Krulewski T, Cohen LB (1988) Choriocarcinoma of the stomach. Pathogenesis and clinical characteristics. Am J Gastroenterol 83:1172–1175
7. Motoyama T, Saito K, Iwafuchi M (1985) Endodermal sinus tumor of the stomach. Acta Pathol Jpn 39:497–502
8. Capella C, Frigerio B, Cornaggia M, Solcia E, Pinzon-Trujillo Y, Chejfec G (1984) Gastric parietal cell carcinoma—a newly recognized entity: Light microscopic and ultrastructural features. Histopathology 8:813–824
9. Ishikura H, Kirimoto K, Shamoto M, Miyamoto Y, Yamagiwa H, Ito T, Aizawa M (1986) Hepatoid adenocarcinoma of the stomach: An analysis of 7 cases. Cancer 58:119–126
10. Rothacker D, Müller W, Borchard F (1991) Hepatoide Differenzierung im Magen-karzinom. Verh Dtsch Ges Pathol 75:390
11. Munoz N, Correa P, Cuello C, Duque E (1968) Histologic types of gastric carcinoma in high- and low-risk areas. Int J Cancer 3:809–818
12. Gall FP (1986) Histologie- und stadiengerechte Therapie beim Magenkarzinom. In: Gall FP, Hermanek P, Hornig D (eds) Magenkarzinom. Epidemiologie, Pathologie, Therapie, Nachsorge. Zuckschwerdt, München
13. Hermanek P (1986) Prognostic factors in stomach cancer surgery. Eur J Surg Oncol 12:241–246
14. Hornig D, Hermanek P, Gall FP (1987) The significance of the extent of proximal margin of clearance in gastric cancer surgery. Scand J Gastroenterol 22 [Suppl] 133:69–71
15. Mulligan RM, Rember RR (1954) Histogenesis and biologic behavior of gastric carcinoma. Arch Pathol Lab Med 58:1–25
16. Rohde H, Gebbensleben B, Bauer P, Stützer H, Zieschang J (1989) Has there been any improvement in the staging of gastric cancer? Findings from the German Gastric Cancer TNM Study Group. Cancer 64:2465–2481
17. Siewert JR, Böttcher K, Roder JD, Busch R, Hermanek P, Meyer HJ and the German Gastric Carcinoma Study Group (1993) Prognostic relevance of systematic lymph node dissection: Results of the German Gastric Carcinoma Study. Br J Surg 80 (in press)
18. Watanabe H, Enjoji M, Imai T (1976) Gastric carcinoma with lymphoid stroma: Its morphologic characteristics and prognostic correlations. Cancer 38:232–243
19. Haraguchi M, Okamura T, Sugimachi K (1987) Accurate prognostic value of mor-phovolumetric analysis of advanced carcinoma of the stomach. Surg Gynecol Obstet 164:335–339
20. Tahara E, Ito H, Nakagami K, Shimamoto F, Yamamoto M, Sumii K (1982) Scirrhous argyrophil cell carcinoma of the stomach with multiple production of polypeptide hormones, amine, CEA, lysozyme and HCG. Cancer 49:1904–1915
21. Fiocca R, Villani L, Tenti P, Solcia E, Cornaggia M, Frigerio B, Capella C (1987) Characterization of four main cell types in gastric cancer: Foveolar, mucopeptic, intestinal columnar and goblet cells. Pathol Res Pract 182:308–325
22. Borchard F (1990) Classification of gastric carcinoma. Hepatogastroenterology 37: 223–232

23. Davessar K, Pezzullo JC, Kessimian N, Hale JH, Jauregui HO (1990) Gastric ade-
    nocarcinoma: Prognostic significance of several pathologic parameters and histologic
    classifications. Hum Pathol 21:325–332
24. Schmitz-Moormann P, Hermanek P, Himmelmann CW (1992) Morphological pre-
    dictors of survival in early and advanced gastric carcinoma. J Cancer Res Clin Oncol
    118:296–302
25. Maruyama K (1987) The most important prognostic factors for gastric cancer pa-
    tients. A study using univariate and multivariate analyses. Scand J Gastroenterol 22
    [Suppl] 133:63–68
26. Ribeiro MM, Seoxas M, Sobrinho-Simoes M (1988) Prognosis in gastric carcinoma.
    The preeminence of staging and futility of histological classification. Dig Dis Pathol
    1:51–68
27. Schmitz-Moormann P, Pohl C, Büttich C, Himmelmann CW (1987) Prediction of
    prognosis in patients with gastric cancer by quantitative morphology and multivariate
    analysis. Scand J Gastroenterol 22 [Suppl] 133:58–62
28. Bedikian AY, Chen TT, Khankhanian N, Heilbrun LK, McBride CM, McMurtrey,
    MJ, Bodey, GP (1984) The natural history of gastric cancer and prognostic factors
    influencing survival. J Clin Oncol 2:305–310
29. Gabbert HE, Meier S, Gerharz CD, Hommel G (1991) Incidence and prognostic
    significance of vascular invasion in 529 gastric cancer patients. Int J Cancer 49:203
    –207
30. Meier S, Gerharz CD, Ramp U, Hommel G, Gabbert HE (1991) Bedeutung der
    Tumorzelldissoziation für die Prognose von Magenkarzinompatienten. Verh Dtsch
    Ges Pathol 75:344
31. Baba H, Korenaga D, Okamura T, Saito A, Sugimachi K (1989) Prognostic factors in
    gastric cancer with serosal invasion. Univariate and multivariate analysis. Arch Surg
    124:1061–1064

Classification of Gastric Carcinoma

Takeyo Nagayo[1]

Key words. Gastric cancer—Classification—Gross appearance—Histological type
—Histogenesis—Early stage—Advanced stage

Introduction

The gross appearance of gastric cancer, which can be observed clinically by X-ray and endoscopic examination and can be detected more clearly by postoperative macroscopic examination of surgically resected stomachs, varies quite widely from case to case, not only in terms of its nature of growth but also in its developmental stage.

For the purpose of macroscopic classification, therefore, it is necessary to first put various features of the cancer into early and advanced stages, and classify each stage of the cancer into several types, according to its commonly shared macroscopic characteristics. Because of the ever-increasing number of cases which seems to fall between early and advanced stages, much attention and discussion have recently been elicited in Japan on how to both delineate and treat these cases.

In general, morphological manifestations of gastric cancer become more prominent in parallel to its grade of intramural growth. Therefore, the gross appearance of the cancer in an obviously advanced stage will mainly be described according to their common biological characteristics, with brief reference to the courses of the development from early to advanced stages.

---

[1] Aichi Cancer Center, Kanokoden 1-1, Chikusa-ku, Nagoya, 464 Japan

Gross Appearance

Advanced gastric cancer can be classified by its common macroscopic characteristics into the following four main types as proposed by Borrmann [1] in 1926. This is rather a classic system, but it has been used by many investigators as the standard for the macroscopic classification of advanced gastric cancer [2–6], owing to its usefulness for both clinical and research purposes. However, in light of the problems mentioned earlier, it was proposed that the macroscopic classification of gastric cancer of all stages and types should be redesigned into a more systematic one, and this was the object of recent discussion by the Committee of the Japanese Research Society for Gastric Cancer. The discussions produced the agreement of the Committee members to omit Borrmann's name from the nomenclature of macroscopic classification of advanced gastric cancer, and express it simply as follows, even though the basic standard of the criteria remains unchanged:

1. Type I: polypoid protrusion
2. Type II: circumscribed excavation
3. Type III: induration with ulceration
4. Type IV: diffuse thickening

The factors for the classification are based principally on the presence or absence of a (a) well-defined boundary, (b) protrusion, (c) excavation or ulceration, (d) ill-defined induration, and (e) deformity. The usefulness of the classification is dependent not only on its adequacy for clinical purposes, especially as a guide for the methods of postoperative treatments and for the assessment of prognosis, but also on its utility in epidemiological, statistical, and research investigations.

Type I: Polypoid Protusion

This type of advanced gastric cancer is characterized macroscopically by a large (usually more than 3 cm in diameter), elevated, polypoid, or fungating protrusion toward the lumen of the stomach, with a well-defined boundary.

Unlike the earlier stages of this type, the shape of the protrusion is more or less irregular, and its surface is uneven, nodular, lobulated or bumpy; it frequently assumes an appearance similar to that of cauliflower and, in almost all cases, it is sessiled with a more or less broad base. Deep ulceration at the surface of the polypoid tumor is scarcely visible, even though erosion or superficial ulceration is not uncommon. The protruded mass is usually not hard but rather tends to be soft, fragile, and dark red in color due to the presence of venous congestion and hemorrhage (Fig. 1).

The site of the lesion is varied, but it is found more often (71.2%) in the antrum or angulus than in the corpus or fundus. In most cases, the lesion is unifocal and more often is seen in a relatively older population (the average age among 81 patients was 59.0 years) [6]. Borrmann designated this type of advanced gastric

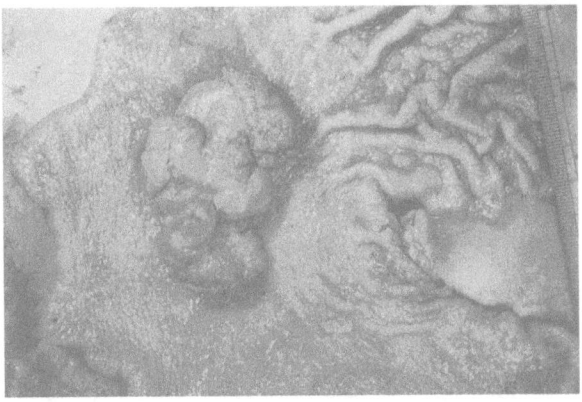

Fig. 1. Type I: polypoid protrusion

cancer as type I. The frequency of this type among all the cases resected surgically is around 2.0% and the sex ratio (m/f) is 2.4.

From the viewpoint of histogenesis, this type of carcinoma commences in two different ways, one being malignant transformation of gastric polyp, most of which is not hyperplastic but adenomatous in nature, and the other being focal upward growth of the mucosal cancer from its very beginning. The frequency is far greater in the latter type.

Type II: Circumscribed Excavation

Circumscribed advanced gastric cancer with excavation also has a clear boundary with the surrounding mucosa but it is characteristically large, (usually more than 2 cm in diameter), round, and deeply excavated in the central part of the cancerous lesion, giving it a crater-like appearance. The base of the crater is uneven, hemorrhagic, and often covered by grayish-white exudates with necrotic mass. It is also characteristic of this type that the deep, round, or oval-shaped crater is always surrounded by elevated mucosa which forms a rampart-like marginal wall. This type differs in appearance from the ulcerated and indurated types, which will be described below, in that the convergence of the mucosal folds toward the center of the excavation is seldom seen, and the marginal wall forms a well-defined boundary with the surrounding mucosa (Fig. 2).

This type of lesion is seen most frequently in the mucosa of the antrum (55.3%), especially in older subjects (the average age of the patients was 56.3 years) [6], and is accompanied quite often by widespread and severe grades of intestinal metaplasia, which can be detected by a dye-scattering method with the aid of an endoscope. This type of advanced gastric cancer was predominant in incidence (58.7%) up to the latter half of the 1970s in Japan, but its frequency has gradually declined in recent years and, at present, it was delegated into a minor group.

T. Nagayo

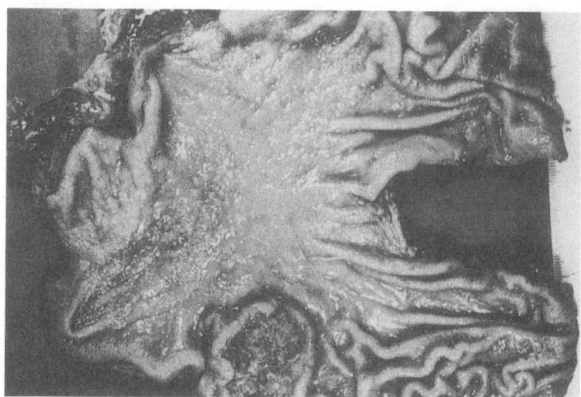

Fig. 2. Type II: circumscribed evacuation

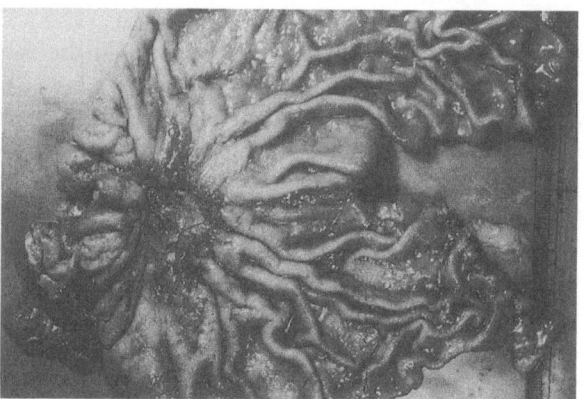

Fig. 3. Type III: induration with ulceration

Another typical feature of this type is that it is seen more often in the anterior or posterior wall of the antrum. Its sex ratio (m/f) is 2.6.

The earliest change of this type is a focal, shallow and well-defined mucosal depression less than 1 cm in diameter. Marginal elevation of the mucosa can only be noticed when the depression becomes larger and deeper.

Type III: Induration with Ulceration

Unlike the previous two types, the boundary of the indurative cancerous growth is more or less ill-defined, while a relatively shallow ulcer is present in the central part of the indurated lesion (Fig. 3).

The ulceration, which is easily detectable by routine X-ray and endoscopic examinations, is irregular in shape, varied in size, but usually not very deep. The mucosa around the ulcer is more or less elevated, but forms no clear marginal wall because of the infiltrative nature of the growth process of this cancer. Convergence of the mucosal folds toward the center of the ulcerated lesion is frequently seen, but the degree of convergence is not so intense as in the cases of chronic peptic nulcer.

Together with the his tological findings, this type of gastric cancer has a nature intermediate between types II and IV, which will be described later. The frequency of this type among all gastric cancers resected surgically is close to that of type II (24.1%). The relative frequency has been increasing during the last few years. The average age of these patients is the lowest (51.3 years) among all the types of advanced gastric cancer [6]. The sex ratio (m/f) is lower than for the previous two types, but males predominate in number.

Ulceration of the cancerous lesion is secondary in nature in almost all cases. When malignant transformation of the chronic peptic ulcer occurs in the mucosa around the ulcer, and the malignant change progresses into an advanced stage, it may take the form of this type. Advanced gastric cancer showing such change of an ulcer-cancer sequence did exist in the past, but is seldom encountered in recent years due to the drastic decrease of cases of chronic peptic ulcer.

Type IV: Diffuse Thickening

No well-defined focal lesion in the stomach is recognizable whatsoever in this type, and the main change occurring in the stomach is diffuse thickening and hardening of the gastric wall. This type is often called scirrhous cancer.

Even though the surface of the mucosa is relatively flat and atrophic, a detailed macroscopic examination of the resected stomach may reveal a shallow ulcer or erosion of the mucosa in more or less indurated lesions, which signify the site of origin in this pattern of advanced gastric cancer. Most of the affected area is seen in the mucosa of the antrum or angulus. When the scirrhous changes occur in the area of the prepylorus or of the antrum, stenosis of the pylorus due to the constriction of the pyloric ring inevitably occurs in the advanced stage, and dilatation of the proximal part of the stomach may result (Fig. 4). Earliest feature of

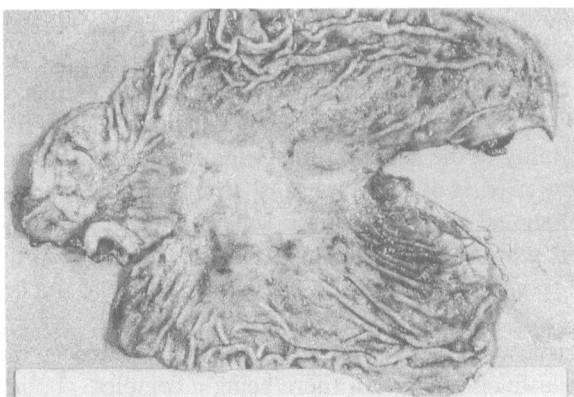

Fig. 4. Type IV: diffuse thickening in the absence of any well-defined focal lesion

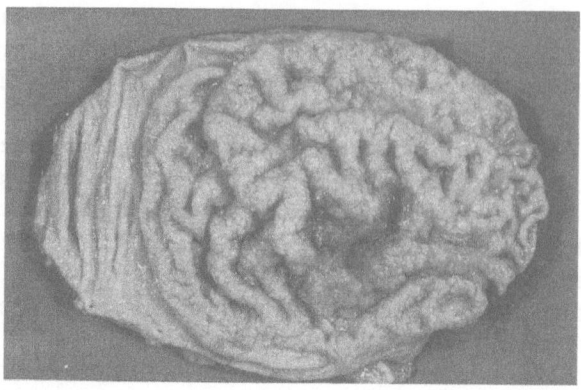

Fig. 5. Linitis plastica, an extreme type IV lesion

this type of advanced cancer is various size and various shape of mucosal erosion with zig-zagged margin.

Linitis plastica, which is characterized by diffuse thickening and hardening of almost the entire gastric wall without any noticeable focal lesion, is an extreme example of this type of advanced gastric cancer. This type is also characterized by the presence of extensive hypertrophy of the mucosal folds in the area of the corpus or fundus. At first glance, it resembles the giant rugae of Ménétrier's disease, but the giant fold in this type is the result of secondary or reactive hyperplasia of the mucosa to the widespread fibrosis evoked by cancer cell infiltration underneath the layer of the mucosa, especially the submucosa (Fig. 5).

As mentioned previously, this specific type of advanced gastric cancer commences as a small cancerous erosion in the fold-rich anterior or posterior mucosa of the corpus and, unlike the cases of mucosal erosion in the antrum or angulus, the erosion does not produce extensions over the surface but the cancer cells are prone to infiltrate into the submucosa and then stimulate prominent extensive lateral growth.

It is noteworthy that this scirrhous type of gastric cancer is relatively frequent in younger age groups and in middle-aged females (average age in our series [6] was 52.7 years), even though the type as a whole belongs to a minor group (15.1%). Some cases of this type, however, escaped being included in the statistics because of the nonresectability of the stomach due to the continuous infiltrative growth of the cancer into lower parts of the esophagus. From the recent advances of cancer chemotherapy, it should also be mentioned that quite a few cases of the scirrous type of advanced gastric cancer are quite sensitive to some sort of anti-cancer drugs including cysplatine, and remarkable improvement of the lesions has been achieved.

The characteristic tendencies of the age and sex incidences in this type are partly explained histologically, with there being a complete absence of intestinal metaplasia in the affected mucosa. The male/female sex ratio is nearly 1.0.

Morphological classification itself almost always involves some intrinsic problems, and this is also true for gastric cancer. There are some cases of advanced gastric cancer in which the gross appearance seems to be in-between the types described above, while in the others, the macroscopic changes are more complicated than those of the typical ones, probably due to fusion of double or multiple cancers or heterogeneity of the original cancer itself. Thus, it is inevitable that the same case is classified as being another type by different examiners. Morever, there are some features of advanced gastric cancer which can not be classified into any of the types described above because of their uncommon or unusual characteristics. Such cases of advanced gastric cancer should better be put into the category of "peculiar or unclassified type".

Histological Appearance

In contrast to colorectal cancer, which almost always produces relatively uniform histological picture of highly differentiated tubular adenocarcinoma, gastric cancer takes several histological forms, even in its early stage, and this variability in its histology increases in accordance with the advancement of intramural growth of the cancerous tissues.

The wide variety of histological classifications of gastric cancer, as devised by different investigators using several methods, is due primarily to the histological structure of the normal gastric mucosa itself. The mucosa covering the various parts of the stomach is histologically composed of rather different glandular components, even though the basic structure of the mucosa is uniform. Moreover, the biologically disparate differentiation potentials of the stem cells—a source of malignant transformation of the mucosal epithelia—by age and disease conditions may be an another reason for the nature of the histological manifestations of such cancer.

It should be noted that in some cases of advanced gastric cancer, the original histological features are frequently modified by secondary alterations of the intramural tissue environment, such as circulatory disturbances, fibrosis due to ulceration or scar formation, and others, and that this variability of the histological picture can sometimes be accelerated by the intrinsic heterogeneity of the tumorforming cancer cells.

As a result of this diversity, the histological features of advanced gastric cancer have been classified by a number of investigators into different types [7–14]. From my experience and studies, it seems most reasonable and practical to classify it into the following three prototypes, on the basis of the grade of glandular formation of the cancerous tissues [6]:

1. Well-differentiated tubular adenocarcinoma (tub. 1)
2. Moderately differentiated tubular adenocarcinoma (tub. 2)
3. Poorly differentiated adenocarcinoma (por)

Regardless of the histological types, when the connective tissue stroma in the cancerous tissue is either extremely sparse or extremely abundant, the above classifications are supplemented by the adjectives medullary or scirrhous (e.g., well-differentiated medullary would be "tub. 1, med.", and poorly differentiated scirrhous carcinoma would appear as "por. scir.").

Well-Differentiated Adenocarcinoma

This type of cancer is characterized by a high grade of glandular formation. The lesions obviously show features of being glandular, tubular, tubulo-papillary, or cystic-papillary adenocarcinomas and are mostly composed of columnar epithelia with a brush border, sometimes containing goblet and Paneth's cells. Their oval-shaped or elongated nuclei show several grades of atypia, ranging from normal-looking arrangements to a more or less pleomorphic and irregular distribution (Fig. 6).

The stroma of the cancerous tissue is generally sparse but is rich in capillaries, especially when there is polypoid protrusion, and focal degeneration or necrosis of the cancerous tissue is quite often seen in the central part of a medullary malignancy. In most cases, mucus production is entirely lost in this type but, on the contrary, it is quite abundant in the other ones, leading to the diagnosis of mucinous, mucoid or muconodular carcinoma.

Adenocarcinoma with this histological picture tends to grow expansively in the stomach, as indicated by tight connections of the cancerous epithelia, while invasion of the cancer cells into the lymphatic system and metastasis into the regional lymph nodes are quite frequently seen in its advanced stages by enlargement of the nodes. Furthermore, direct invasion of the cancer cells into intra- and

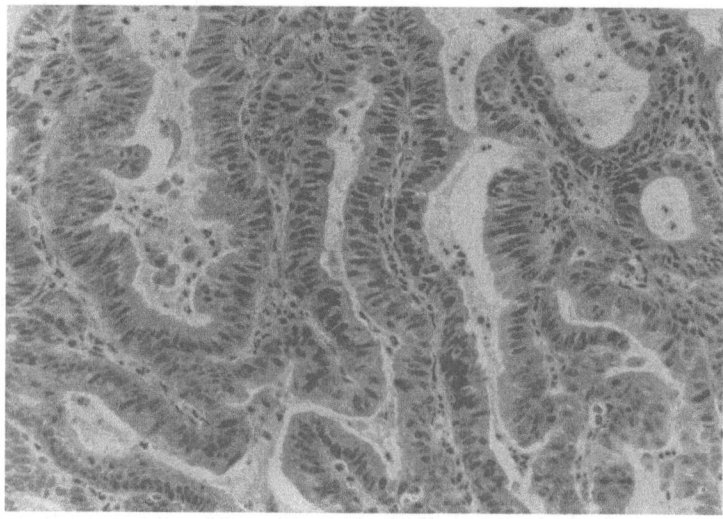

Fig. 6. Well-differentiated adenocarcinoma

extramural venules, causing liver metastasis by means of the portal vein, is also quite common in an advanced stage.

Thus, the histological and biological nature of this type of cancer is similar in several respects to that of colorectal cancer, and for these reasons, together with the histological, histochemical, and electron-microscope findings, Laurén and Jaervi named this type of gastric cancer the "intestinal type" [15–17].

Moderately Differentiated Adenocarcinoma

Even though the diagnosis of adenocarcinoma is made from its gland-forming structure, nests of the cancerous tissue are relatively small or sparse, and the cancerous epithelia forming the glands are mostly cuboidal or sometimes flat and lacking in a brush border, goblet cells, and Paneth's cells. Thus, unlike the cases of the previous type, the characteristic of intestinal metaplasia of the cancerous epithelia is not apparent in this type (Fig. 7).

Most of the cancerous lesion shows an alveolar structure with several glandular patterns (cribriform, acinar, solid, reticular, etc) similar in nature to those of lobular carcinoma of the breast. It is by no means uncommon to see cancerous tissues composed of this type of cancer coexisting with well- or poorly differentiated adenocarcinoma in a single focus. Furthermore, both types often show transitional features. The amount of the stroma is moderate in most cases, but fibrous changes of the affected mucosa are not very rare. The border of the cancerous lesion and the surrounding tissue is more or less ragged, but is neither expanding nor diffusely infiltrating.

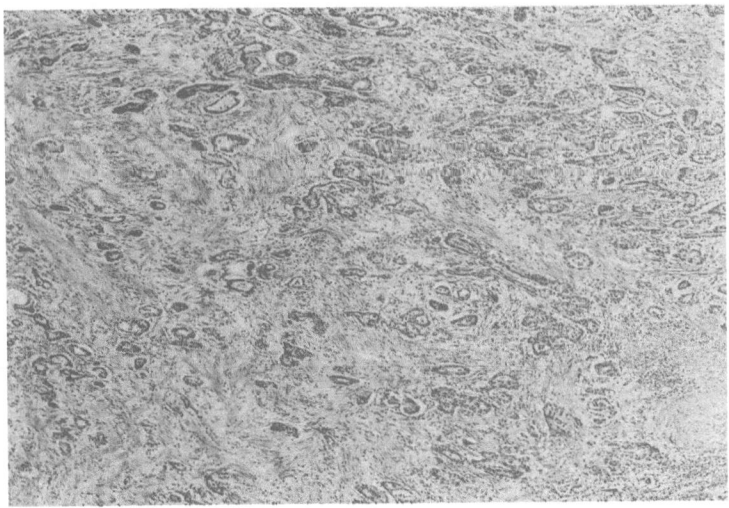

Fig. 7. Moderately differentiated adenocarcinoma

From the findings described above, this type of histology corresponds neither to the "intestinal type" nor to the "diffuse type" as defined by the Laurèn-Jaervi classification. In my opinion, it rather called "gastric type" adenocarcinoma originating from the non-metaplastic proper gastric mucosa.

Poorly Differentiated Adenocarcinoma

In this type, the formation of glands of the cancerous tissues is very poor and they often take the form of minute, solid clusters of anastomosing, reticular, or trabecular arrangements and are composed of nonmucin-producing small, immature cells. The infiltrative growth pattern of the detached cancer cells from the main focus to the surrounding tissues, which is often accompanied by fibrous reaction of the stroma, makes the affected gastric walls indurative and the boundary of the lesion more or less ill-defined. It is by no means rare that the diagnosis of adenocarcinoma is made only by the presence of a faint and sparse glandular arrangement in some parts of the cancerous lesion (Fig. 8).

Unlike that in cases of well- and moderately differentiated adenocarcinoma, mutual cohesion of the tumor-forming cancer cells is weak and tends to be detached from the clusters and the cells thus liberated from the main mass, which freely and diffusely invade actively into the surrounding tissues and provoke fibrous proliferation of the connective tissue by specific "cell-mesenchyme interaction". This growth behavior results in diffuse and desmoplastic changes of the gastric wall without any focal change even at the advanced stages. Because of these macroscopical and microscopical characteristics, this type of malignancy is often clinically called scirrhous cancer.

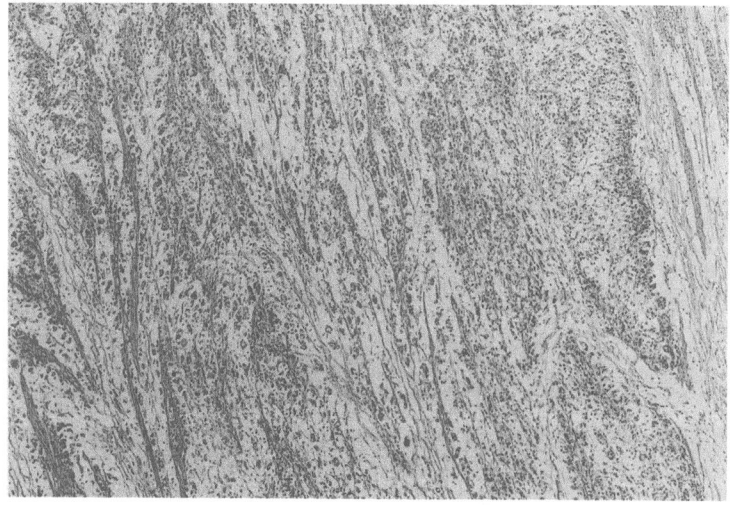

Fig. 8. Poorly differentiated adenocarcinoma

Permeation of the cancer cells into the lymphatic system, especially of the submucosa, is not uncommon and may cause the state of lymphangitis carcinomatosa. However, penetration of the cancer cells directly into capillaries or small venules is hardly ever seen in routine histological examinations. Infiltrative growth of the cancer cells beyond the serosa into the neighboring tissues results in dissemination of the cancer cells onto the surface of the peritoneum and/or omentum, leading to peritonitis carcinomatosa with concomitant ascites. This type of cancer corresponds exactly to the gastric cancer of the "diffuse type" histology as defined in Laurén-Jaervi's classification.

There is another type of carcinoma which is histologically classified into poorly differentiated adenocarcinoma because of its scanty glandular formation. This type of cancer, however, tends to take the form of a solid mass or have a focus with an alveolar arrangement and a relatively well-defined boundary. Many of them have medullary stroma and/or are characterized by intense reactive formation of the lymph follicles in and around the cancerous tissues.

When infiltrative cell growth of the cancer is limited to the mucosa or has only slightly invaded into the upper layer of the submucosa—the state of which is detectable macroscopically by cancerous erosion—the cancer cells infiltrating within the mucosa frequently show abundant mucin in their cytoplasm and these are called "signet-ring cells". However, when infiltrative cell growth of these cancers are further advanced beyond the submucosa into the deeper layers, and fibrous proliferation of the gastric walls does occur, signet-ring cells become scarcely visible in the fibrotic and indurative cancerous lesion. Thus, in an advanced stage, they essentially break up into minor components.

The Relationship Between Gross Appearance and Histological Features

It is reasonable to say that various histological changes of gastric cancer form the basis of gross types of the developing cancer. In other words, the appearance of cancer as seen by the naked eye allows us to infer their cytological, histological, and biological natures.

In general, in any kind of advanced gastric cancer showing a well-defined boundary with the surrounding mucosa, such as the large polypoid, fungating, or bulging tumors in type I, and the large, roung, and deep excavation surrounded by prominent marginal elevation such as those classified into type II, the histological picture almost always shows well-differentiated adenocacinoma characterized by expansive growth because of the tight connection of the tumor-forming cancerous epithelia. Alternatively, in the carcinomas characteristically having an ill-defined boundary with (type III) or without (type IV) prominent ulcerations in the indurated lesion, poorly differentiated adenocarcinoma predominates in both number and frequency.

The correlation between macroscopical and histological findings of advanced gastric cancer is highest (90.7%) in the type I cases followed by type II (74.2%)

Table 1. Relationship between macroscopic and histological types.

Macroscopic type	Histological type (grade of differentiation)			No. of cases
	Well	Moderate	Poor	
Borrmann's classification				
Type I	90.7	9.3	0	54
Type II	74.4	20.3	5.3	2024
Type III	20.4	32.9	46.7	828
Type IV	5.5	22.0	72.5	473
Type O	37.7	39.4	22.9	188
Total				3567

Table 2. Crude correlation between macroscopic and histologic types of advanced gastric carcinoma.

Macroscopy (Borrmann type)	Histology (type)
I:	Intestinal
II:	Intestinal
III:	Diffuse
IV:	Diffuse

and then by type IV (72.5%). Most of the first two types show the histology of well-differentiated adenocarcinoma with features similar to those of colorectal cancers, while no such close a correlation between macro- and microscopic types was observable in type III cases (46.5%) (Table 1).

When the criteria of the histological classification proposed by Laurèn and Jaervi are applied to this problem, characteristics of the above-mentioned correlation of gross appearances of advanced gastric cancers with their histological features can be summarized as shown in Table 2.

References

1. Borrmann R (1926) Makroskopishe Formen des vorgeschritteten Magenkrebses. In: Henke F, Lubarsch O (eds) Handbuch der speziellen pathologischen Anatomie und Histologie, vol 4/1. Springer, Berlin
2. Kuru M, Sano R (1967) Histopathological study of gastric carcinoma in the Japanese. UICC Monoger Ser 10
3. Kajitani T (1976) Surgical treatments for gastric cancer. Their contribution to improvement in the five-year survival rate. Asian Med J 19:915–935
4. Hermanek P (1982) Surgical pathology. The TNM system. Langenbecks Arch Chir 358:57–63

5. Morson BC, Dawson IMP (1972) Macroscopical features and topography. Gastrointestinal pathology. Blackwell. Oxford
6. Nagayo T (1986) Histogenesis and precursors of human gastric cancer. Research and practice. 3 Background data to the study of advanced gastric cancer. Springer, Berlin, pp 17–39
7. Evans RW (1956) Histological appearance of tumours. Livingstone, Edinburgh, pp 426–452
8. Takizawa N (1972) Histopathological classification of gastric carcinoma for standard reporting system used in Japan. Acta Pathol Jpn 22:11–18
9. Ota K, Tanaka N (1952) Histological types of gastric carcinomas and their topographical incidence. Gann 43:367–370
10. Imai T (1968) Some comments on the geographical-pathologic aspects of gastric carcinogenesis. Gann Monogr 3:123–127
11. Willis RA (1953) Carcinoma of the stomach. Pathology of tumours. Butterworth, London, pp 391–411
12. Broders AG (1941) The microscopic grading of cancer. Surg Clin North Am 21:947–962
13. Ming SC (1977) Gastric carcinoma. A pathological classification. Cancer 39:2475–2485
14. Stout AP (1953) Tumors of the stomach. Atlas of tumor pathology, section 6. AFIP, Washington
15. Jaervi Q, Laurén P (1952) On the pathogenesis of gastric cancer. Acta UICC 8:393–394
16. Laurén P (1965) The two main histological types of gastric carcinoma, diffuse and so-called intestinal type carcinoma. An attempt at a histo-clinical classification. Acta Pathol Microbiol Immunol Scand [A] 64:31–49
17. Jaervi O, Nevalainen T, Ekfors T, Kulatunga A (1974) The classification and histogenesis of gastric cancer. Excerpta Med Int Congr Series 6:228–234

Pathology of Early Gastric Cancer

Teruyuki Hirota[1], Si-Chun Ming[2], and Masayuki Itabashi[3]

Introduction

Gastric cancer is one of the main causes of cancer death in the world, though its incidence rates vary greatly from country to country. Because Japan shows one of the highest rates of gastric cancer in the world [1, 2], and because the disease causes the highest mortality in Japan in both sexes, great efforts have been made to promote early diagnosis and treatment, especially mass screening by double contrast radiography.

As a result, many early gastric cancers have been detected, and the overall cure rate has been greatly improved. Clinicopathological study of gastric cancer at the early stage helps to elucidate its pathogenesis and precursors [3, 4].

During the thirty years from 1962 to December 1991, 6439 patients with gastric cancer were treated surgically at the National Cancer Center Hospital in Tokyo. Early gastric cancer was found in 2400 patients (37.3%) (Fig. 1); advanced gastric cancer was found in the remaining 62.7%. The data presented in this chapter were based on the study with these cases at the National Cancer Center, where the authors worked from 1966 to 1992 (1966–1992 for Hirota, 1976–1992 for Itabashi).

Concept and Definitions

The concept of early gastric cancer was defined by the Japanese Society For Gastric Cancer Study in 1963 [5–7]. According to the Society, early gastric cancer is a primary carcinoma of the stomach which invades either the mucosa or

[1] Pathology Division, Tokyo Medical College Hospital. 6-7-1 Nishishinjuku, Shinjuku-ku, Tokyo, 160 Japan
[2] Department of Pathology, School of Medicine, Temple University. 3400 North Broad Street, Philadelphia, PA 19140, USA
[3] Clinical Pathology Division, Ibaraki Prefectural Central Hospital. 6528 Koibuchi, Tomobe-machi, Nishiibaraki-gun, Ibaraki, 309-17 Japan

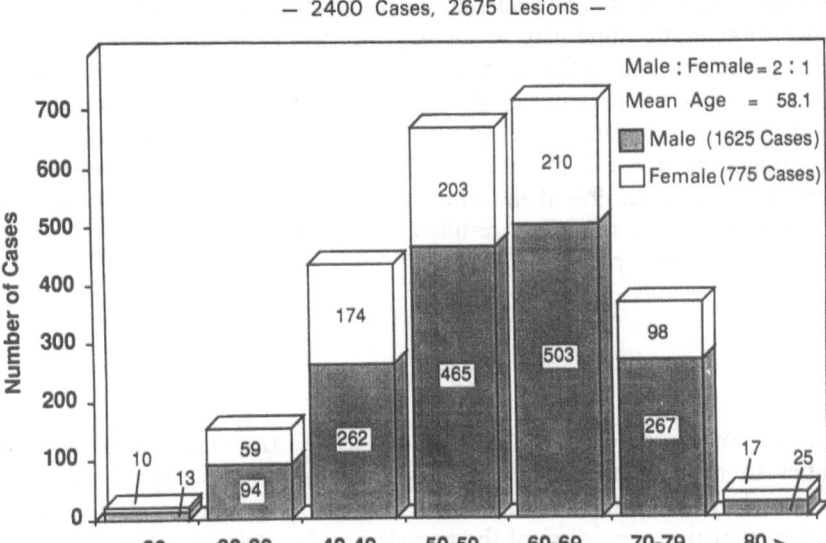

Fig. 1. Age and sex distribution of early gastric cancer cases (National Cancer Center Hospital, Tokyo, Japan, May, 1962–Dec, 1991)

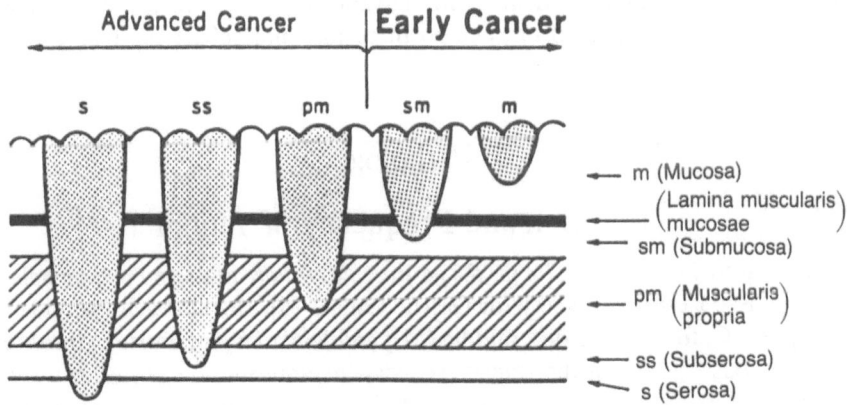

Fig. 2. Definition of early and advanced gastric cancers according to the level of cancerous invasion in the gastric wall (from [33], with permission)

the submucosal layer (Fig. 2), regardless of the presence or absence of lymph node metastasis.

Discussions as to whether carcinomas with positive lymph node metastasis should be excluded from "early" gastric cancer were subsequently carried out.

Although there is an intimate relationship between nodal status and prognosis, it is very difficult for internists to identify the nodal metastases preoperatively. Based on the opinions of internists participating in the diagnosis, a decision was made not to take the presence of metastasis into consideration. The word "early" here indicates the possibility of complete surgical resection and does not imply a time dimension. Even if metastases are found, those with positive metastases represent less than ca. 9% of the whole series of early gastric cancers. Adequate regional lymphadenectomy has resulted in a 5-year survival rate of over 95% which is an excellent prognosis [8, 9].

Age and Sex

Figure 1 shows a wide age distribution of early gastric cancer patients in their twenties to their eighties, with the highest peak in the sixties, and with a male:female ratio of approximately 2:1. This ratio is nearly constant in world mortality statistics, regardless of the prevalence of gastric cancer in each country [2]. A slight increase in patients over 60 years of age has been noted since the early 1970s [10]. According to mass surveillance health data, there is a female predominance until the fourth decade. Men predominate in the forties and fifties, and a peak is reached in the sixties for both men and women. Among surgical cases, little male:female difference was noted in the small number of patients in their eighties. Among patients with advanced age, however, a considerable number were not operated on; and so these may not reflect the true prevalence rate.

Pathology

Location and Frequency of Tumor

According to *The general rules for the gastric cancer study in surgery and pathology* by the Japanese Research Society for Gastric Cancer [5], the stomach is divided into the upper (C, for cardia side), middle (M), and lower (A, for antrum) thirds along the long axis [5]. Along the transverse axis, the anterior and posterior walls, the greater and lesser curvatures, and the whole circumference are distinguished.

Data from the National Cancer Center Hospital in Tokyo showed the highest (55.5%) rate of occurrence of early gastric cancer in the M region, followed by the A and C regions (Fig. 3). This tendency was greater in the group which had ulcers within the cancer. In the whole series of patients subjected to surgery for gastric cancer in the Japan Registry, including advanced cases, occurrences of cancer in the pyloric portion or A region was the highest (44.6%), followed by the M region (39.3%) and the C region (16.1%). Instead of presenting the true regional incidence, these data probably reflect multiple factors, including the rate of detection and feasibility of surgical resection.

Fig. 3. Location of early gastric cancer (National Cancer Center Hospital, Tokyo, Japan, May, 1962–Dec, 1991) *A*, distal third; *M*, middle third; *C*, proximal third, *Ant*, anterior wall; *Less*, lesser curvature; *Post*, posterior wall; *Great*, greater curvature

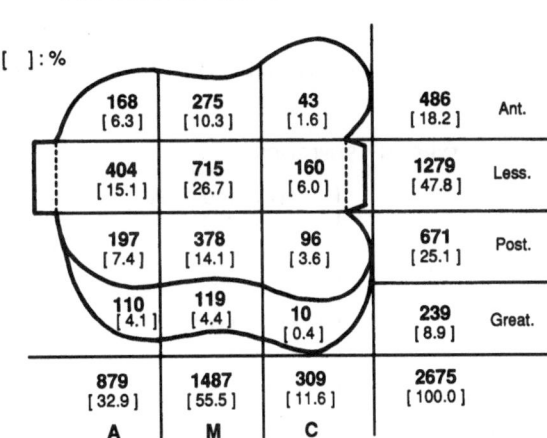

Early gastric cancer occurs most frequently on the lesser curvature (47.8%), followed by the posterior wall (25.1%), anterior wall (18.2%), and greater curvature (8.9%) (Fig. 3). A considerable difference is found in comparison with advanced cancers, probably because of the difference in the rate of detection.

Macroscopic Features and Classification

Japanese macroscopic classification, especially for advanced gastric cancer, is mainly based on Borrmann's classification of gastric carcinoma according to its gross morphologic features [11]. He classified the tumors into four types: type 1 for polypoid tumors, type 2 for fungating tumors, type 3 for ulcerated tumors, and type 4 for diffusely infiltrating tumors. Early gastric cancer was not included in the above classification but has been classified as type 0 in recent years [5].

The macroscopic classification of early gastric cancer is shown in Fig. 4 and includes type I (protruding type), type II (superficial type), and type III (excavated type).

A type I tumor is a tall, nodular or polypoid lesion that often shows an irregular surface with crevices between the papillary projections (Fig. 5).

Type II lesions are further subdivided into three types. Type IIa lesions (superficial and slightly elevated type) consist of a slight elevation of the lesion approximately twice or greater the thickness of the mucosa upto 5 mm (Fig. 6A–B). Type IIb lesions (superficial and flat type) are approximatly level with the surrounding mucosa, and type IIc lesions (superficial and slightly depressed type), have a shallow depression.

Type IIc cancer is the most frequent and most important lesion in clinical diagnosis (Table 1). In this type, the erosive surface of the carcinoma is slightly depressed from the surrounding mucosa. It varies in size (Figs. 7, 8). Nagayo subdivided type IIc lesions into two types: IIc', well-demarcated and less than

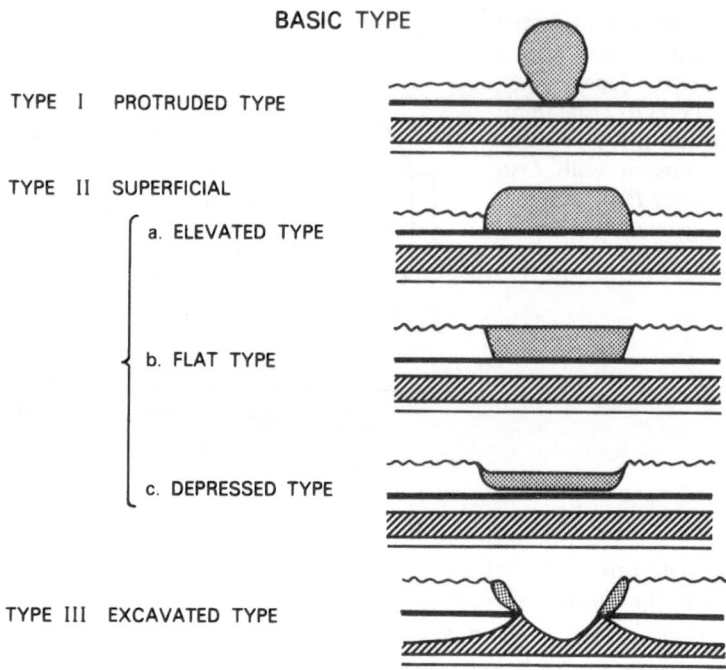

Fig. 4. Macroscopic classification of basic types of early gastric cancer

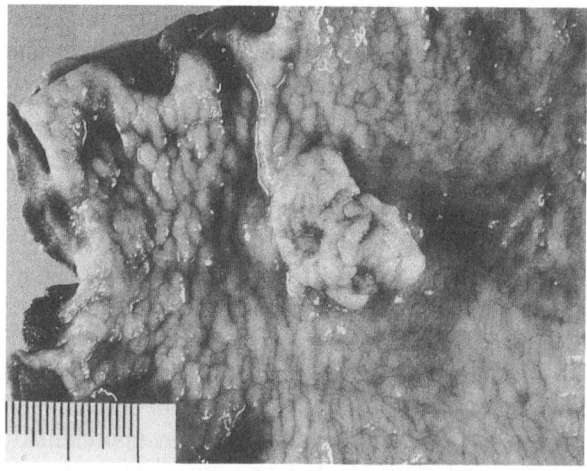

Fig. 5. Type I (protrude type) early gastric carcinoma (from [33], with permission). Scale indicates cm

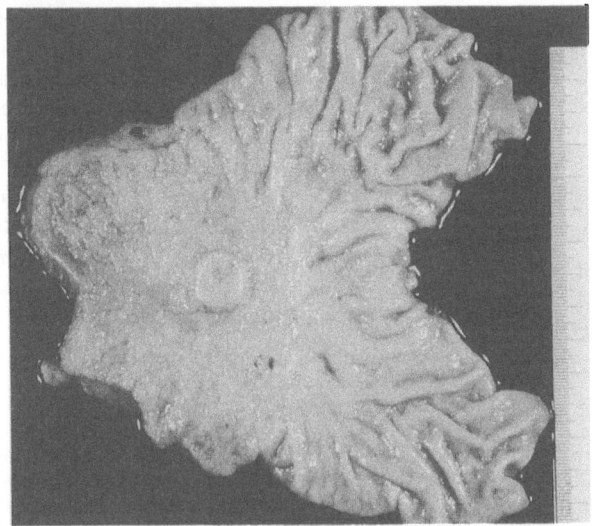

Fig. 6a,b. Type II (superficial and slightly elevated type) early gastric carcinoma. **a** Gross appearance; **b** Scanning view of the microscopic morphology. H&E

Table 1. Macroscopic types of early gastric cancer

Macroscopic type	Lesions	%	
I	160	6.0	
IIa	227	8.4	23.0 [A]
IIa + IIc	232	8.6	
IIb	80	3.0	3.0 [B]
IIc	1659	62.1	
IIc + III	174	6.5	
IIc + IIa	72	2.7	74.0 [C]
III	15	0.6	
III + IIc	56	2.1	
Total	2675	100.0	100.0

2400 cases; 2675 lesions
National Cancer Center Hospital, Tokyo. May 1962–
Dec. 1991

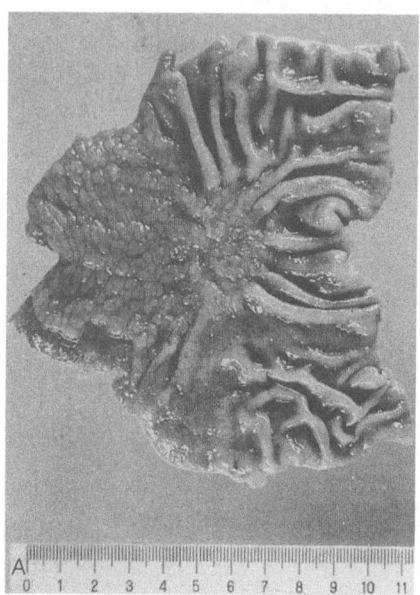

Fig. 7a–c. Type IIc (superficial and slightly depressed type) early gastric carcinoma (from [33], with permission). **a** Gross appearance (scale indicates cm); **b** Scanning view of the microscopic morphology. Both open ulcer (*white arrow*) and scar tissue (*black arrow*) are present in the lesion (H&E). The *line* marks the extent of the carcinoma. **c** Higher magnification of the tumor showing poorly differentiated adenocarcinoma (H&E)

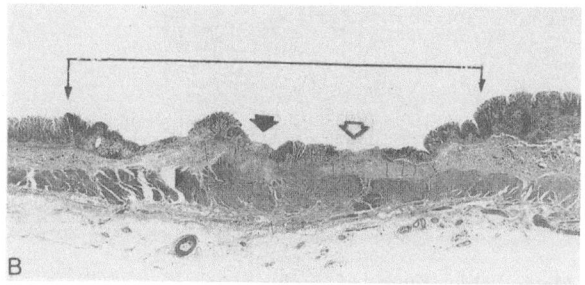

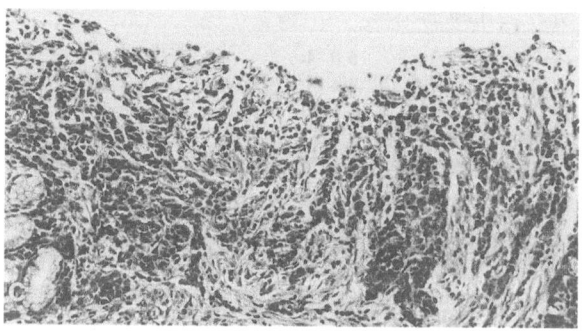

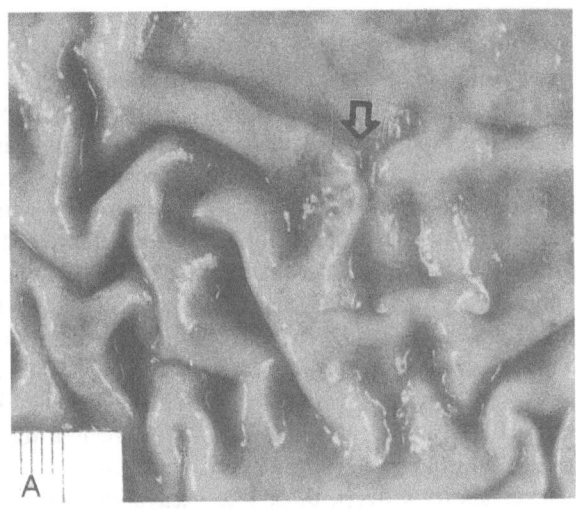

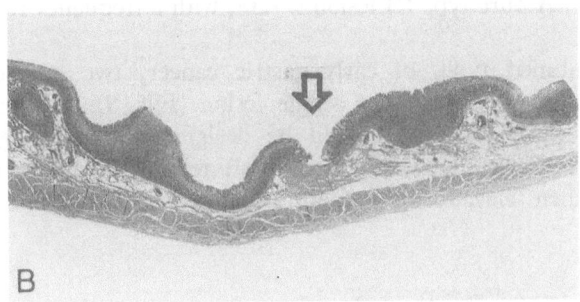

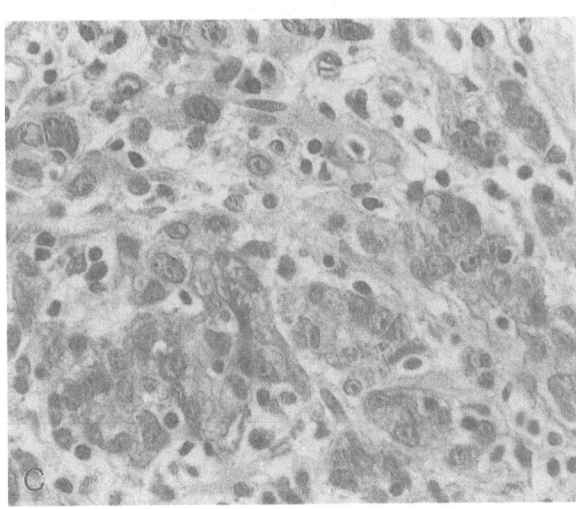

Fig. 8a–c. Minute type IIc early gastric carcinoma (from [33], with permission) **a** Gross appearance (scale indicates cm); **b** Scanning view of microscopic morphology. *Arrow* point to the depressed cancer (H&E). **c** High magnification of the tumor showing poorly differentiated carcinoma cells. H&E

3 cm in diameter, and IIc″ poorly demarcated and larger than 3 cm in diameter. The larger one has also been called superficial spreading type [12]. The term "superficial spreading type" was originally proposed by Stout in 1942 [13].

The tips of the mucosal folds converging toward the center of type IIc lesions show characteristic pen-tip-like narrowing, i.e., narrowing with indentation and an abrupt borders (Fig. 7A). The border of the depressed lesion from the surrounding normal mucosa shows a characteristic irregular margin called "moth-eaten appearance" (Fig. 7A). The depressed surface of the type IIc lesion is characterized as follows: (1) unlike the surrounding normal mucosa, it is flattened and occasionally accompanied by granular changes of various sizes (Fig. 7), (2) within the depressed area, an ulcer scar or an open ulcer may be present, which may be shallow (Fig. 7) or deep (Fig. 11), (3) there is a disappearance of the glistening surface, and (4) there are changes in color tone.

Type III cancer shows a deep, ulcer-like excavation surrounded by a narrow rim of carcinomatous tissue along the ulcer border. The lesion may resemble a benign ulcer. A pure type III lesion is rare, with a frequency rate of less than 1% (Table 1).

In a combined types of early gastric cancer, two or more of the basic macroscopic types coexist in a single lesion (Fig. 9). Discussions are still in progress as to which type should be designated first. In general, the type occupying the larger area is written first, regardless of the histogenesis. For example, when elevation and depression coexist, opinions may be divided

COMBINED TYPE

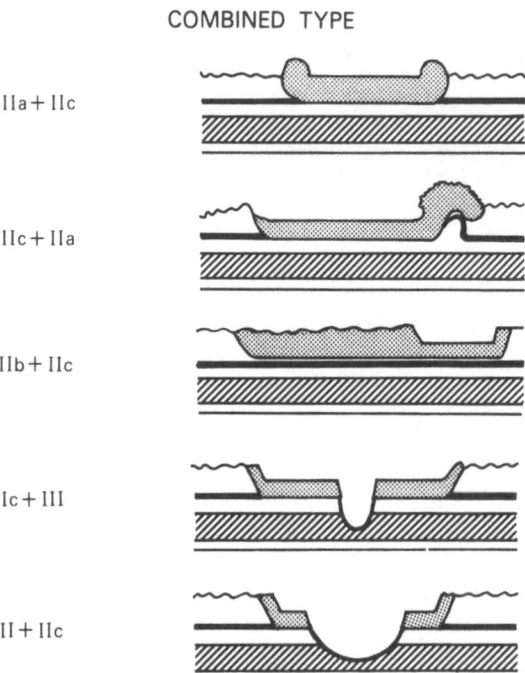

IIa + IIc

IIc + IIa

IIb + IIc

IIc + III

III + IIc

Fig. 9. Macroscopic classification of combined types of early gastric cancer

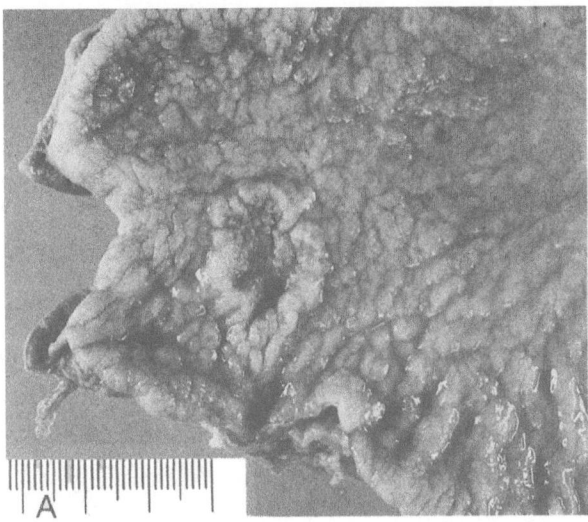

Fig. 10. IIa + IIc (combined type) early gastric cancer (from [33], with permission). Gross appearance (scale indicates cm)

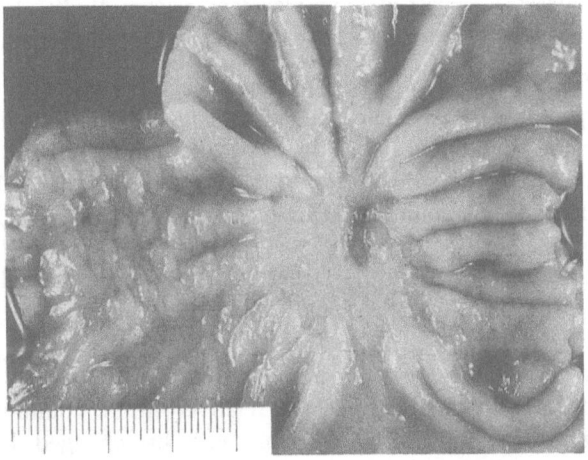

Fig. 11. IIc + III (combined type) early gastric cancer (from [33], with permission) Gross appearance (scale indicates cm)

between calling it type IIa + IIc or type IIc + IIa (Fig. 10), but according to our statistical data, these designations make little difference as to the rate of lymph node metastasis or prognosis. When ulceration beyond the muscularis mucosa is found within a type IIc lesion and the type IIc lesion is more conspicuous than the type III lesion, the combined lesion is called type IIc + III (Fig. 11). As

Table 2. Chronological trend in macroscopic types of early gastric cancer

Macroscopic type	I (1962–1963)	II (1964–1968)	III (1969–1973)	IV (1974–1978)	V (1979–1983)	Total
I	9 (18)	37 (15.2)	30 (8.1)	30 (8.3)	13 (3.3)	119 (8.4)
IIa	2 (4)	18 (7.4)	43 (11.6)	40 (11.1)	41 (10.3)	144 (10.1)
IIa + IIc	5 (10)	18 (7.4)	38 (10.3)	29 (8.1)	32 (8.1)	122 (8.6)
IIb	0 (0)	5 (2.0)	13 (3.5)	9 (2.5)	12 (3.0)	39 (2.7)
IIc	18 (36)	97 (40.0)	198 (53.7)	213 (59.2)	267 (66.3)	793 (55.6)
IIc + III	8 (16)	38 (15.7)	29 (7.9)	23 (6.4)	18 (4.5)	116 (8.2)
IIc + IIa	0 (0)	2 (0.8)	5 (1.4)	11 (3.0)	14 (3.5)	32 (2.3)
III + IIc	6 (12)	24 (9.9)	9 (2.4)	5 (1.4)	4 (1.0)	48 (3.4)
III	2 (4)	4 (1.6)	4 (1.1)	0 (0)	0 (0)	10 (0.7)
Total	50 (100)	243 (100)	369 (100)	360 (100)	401 (100)	1423 (100)

1300 cases; 1423 lesions

described previously, attempts were made to avoid terminology associated with preexisting concepts for the definition, classification, and designation of gastric cancer, and abstract expressions were employed instead.

The gross types can be combined into three groups according to the dominating features: A, protruded or elevated lesions; B, flat lesions; and C, depressed or excavated lesions. Their frequencies are listed in Table 1.

Prevalence and Chronological Changes of Macroscopic Types. The prevalence of macroscopic types of early gastric cancer varies somewhat among institutions. In the Japanese national statistics, type IIc was seen most frequently (33.8%), followed by type IIc + III (23.4%), type I (9.7%), and type IIa + IIc (6.5%). In our data, type IIc also was found most frequently (62.1%) (Table 2). Of the 1252 cases studied by Nagayo [3], type IIc″ was the most frequent (41.9%), followed by type III (22.6%), IIc′ (19.3%), IIa (8.1%), I (6.2%), and IIb (1.9%). In contrast, among cases studies by Johansen [14], 13.3% of the tumors were type IIb.

The polypoid lesions are generally more common in the elderly, whereas the large depressed and ulcerated lesions are relatively more common in younger patients [3]. The distribution of macroscopic types has changed during the past 25 years. The elevated type is decreasing in frequency but the depressed type, initially accounting for 68.0% of cases increased recently to 75.3%. The relatively shallow type IIc lesion has become more frequent, while the type III lesion has virtually disappeared since 1974 [10].

Size

In the early 1960s, 86% of early gastric cancers were larger than 2 cm. Smaller lesions have increasingly been diagnosed in recent years (Fig. 12), reflecting the progress in diagnostic methods. The diagnosis of small cancers (less than 10 mm

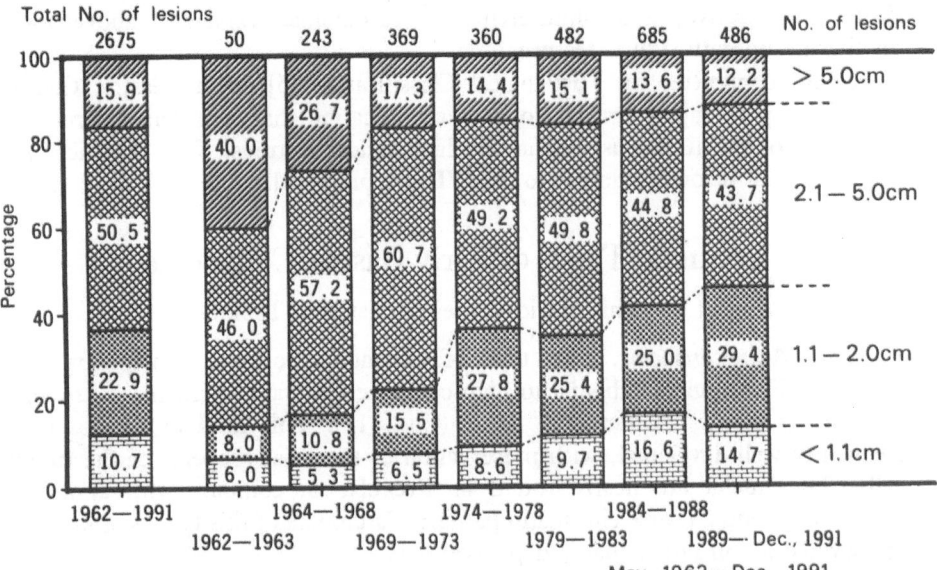

Fig. 12. Chronological trend in percentage of early gastric cancer by size at the National Cancer Center Hospital, Tokyo, Japan

in size) and particularly of the minute cancers (less than 5 mm in size) is important, not only in its potential for a complete cure but also in its contribution to the understanding of premalignant lesions [15]. Type IIb cancer consists of 58.3% of tumors less than 5 mm in diameter and 0% of tumors larger than 5 mm [16], which indicates that as the tumor grows larger, the originally flat lesion becomes either protruding or depressed.

Histologic Features and Classification

The classification proposed by Lauren [17] and the World Health Organization (WHO) [18] are often used. In the former, gastric carcinomas of the ordinary type are classified into two types; intestinal and diffuse. In the latter, the traditional histologic classifications are used. Gastric carcinomas have also been classified, according to growth patterns, into expanding and infiltrative types [19]. In Japan, Nakamura [20] often classifies gastric carcinomas into differentiated and undifferentiated types. The differentiated type of adenocarcinomas in this classification includes papillary adenocarcinoma and well-differentiated to moderately differentiated tubular adenocarcinomas. The undifferentiated type shows little or no glandular formation but include such differentiated tumors as signet-ring cell carcinoma and mucinous adenocarcinoma, as well as poorly differentiated adenocarcinoma and undifferentiated solid tumors (Tab. 3). The intestinal, expanding, and differentiated carcinomas often show a great deal of similarity, while the diffuse, infiltrative, and undifferentiated carcinomas explained above form another group with similar features.

The Subcommittee for Histological Classification [5] of the Gastric Cancer Study Group in Japan has developed a classification that considers the relative frequency of the tumor as well as the histological features. This classification, listed in detail below, is similar to the WHO typing [18].

Common Types of Early Gastric Carcinoma

The frequencies of these histological types are listed in Table 3.

Papillary Adenocarcinoma. This type of carcinoma consists of papillary and villous proliferation of cuboidal to high-cylindrical-shaped carcinoma cells along the narrow bands of interstitial tissue (Figs. 13). This kind of carcinoma is frequently well-developed, with preservation of the axial property of the tumor cells. The nuclei are nearly round or irregular in contour, with abundant nucleoplasm and a coarse chromatin pattern. Carcinoma of this type is often from an elevated lesion rather than a depressed one.

Tubular Adenocarcinoma. In this type, glandular formation is distinct. Depending on the degree of glandular lumen formation, this type is further divided into well-differentiated and moderately differentiated subtypes. The former type is defined as an adenocarcinoma with a distinct glandular structure without complex arborization, despite mild variations in size and irregularity in the glandular-structures (Fig. 14). Carcinoma cells are frequently high-cylindrical to cuboidal and arranged in a single layer. The nuclei are arranged evenly along the base of the cells, with occasional pseudostratification. The nuclei are irregular in shape, with thickening of the nuclear margin, abundant karyoplasm, and a coarse chromatin pattern.

Table 3. Histologic types of early gastric cancer

Histological type	Lesions	%	
Papillary adenocarcinoma	172	6.4	60.7 [D]
Tubular adenocarcinoma	1453	54.3	
Poorly diff. adenocarcinoma	355	13.3	39.3 [U]
Signet-ring cell carcinoma	676	25.3	
Mucinous adenocarcinoma	19	0.7	
Total	2675	100.0	

[D], Differentiated type; [U], Undifferentiated type
2400 cases; 2675 lesions
National Cancer Center Hospital, Tokyo. May, 1962–Dec, 1991

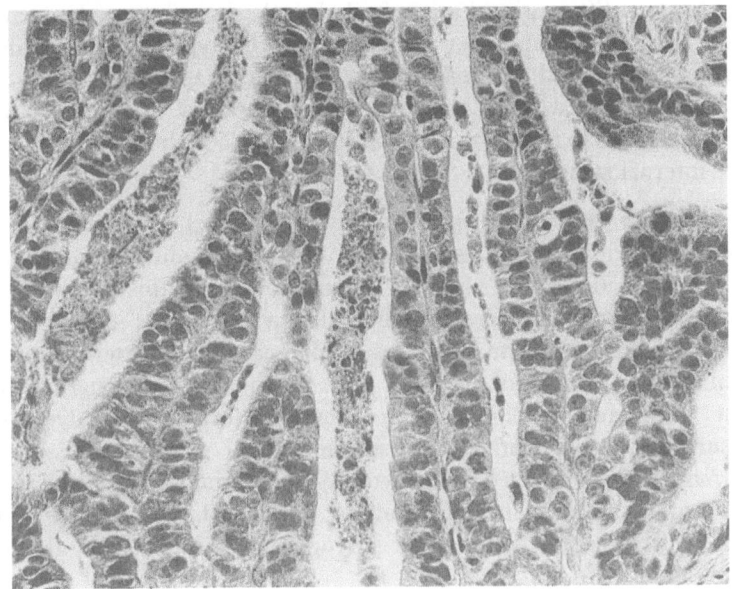

Fig. 13. Papillary adenocarcinoma (from [33], with permission). H&E, ×200

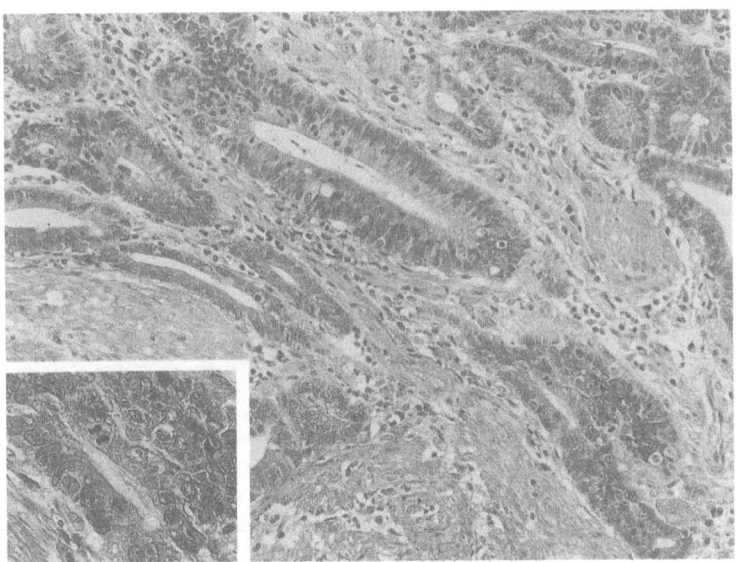

Fig. 14. Well-differentiated tubular carcinoma. H&E, ×200

In the moderately differentiated type of tubular adenocarcinoma, the glandular structures are irregular, complex, or incomplete. In this type of adenocarcinoma, in addition to the expected marked structural atypia, the axial property of the tumor cell is irregular, with frequent pseudostratification. The nuclei of the tumor cells appear nearly round or irregular in shape, with abundant karyoplasm and a coarse internal structure.

Poorly Differentiated Adenocarcinoma. In this histological type, few, if any, distinct glandular formations are seen. Acinar or microglandular structures may be seen only in a small number of areas. Carcinoma cells of this type may show different growth patterns, such as diffusely infiltrative growth of individual cells, like free cells, which often form scirrhous carcinoma. Other patterns consist of solid medullary structures of various sizes with an occasional cord-like arrangement. Individual carcinoma cells may also form small, alveolus-like structures surrounded by relatively coarse intercellular connective tissue (Fig. 15). Mucus may be demonstrated in the cytoplasm of tumor cells, but the amount of mucus is usually sparse. The nuclei of the tumor cells vary in size and are nearly round or irregular, with abundant karyoplasm. Numerous mitotic figures are commonly found.

Signet-Ring Cell Carcinoma. Within the cytoplasm of the tumor cells, a large amount of mucus is present. The nuclei are irregular, crescent-shaped, and pushed to one side (Fig. 16). The name of this carcinoma refers to the shape,

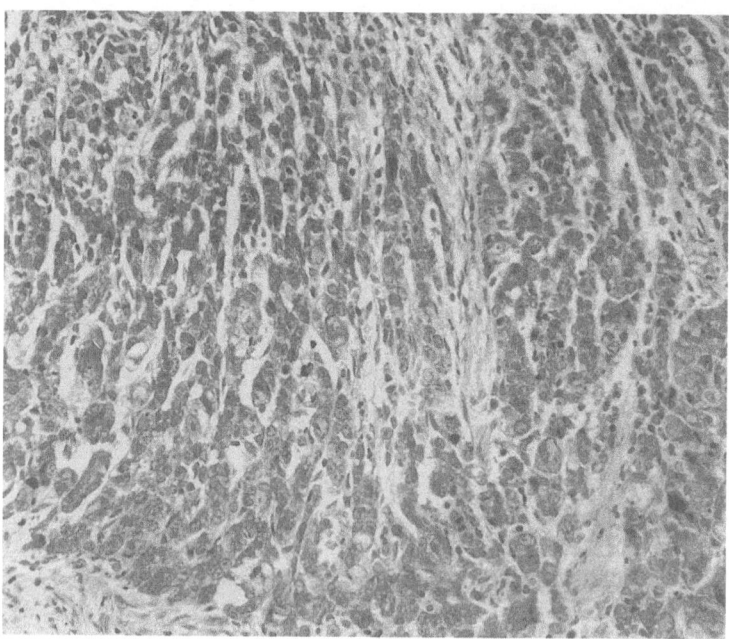

Fig. 15. Poorly differentiated adenocarcinoma (from [33], with permission). H&E, ×200

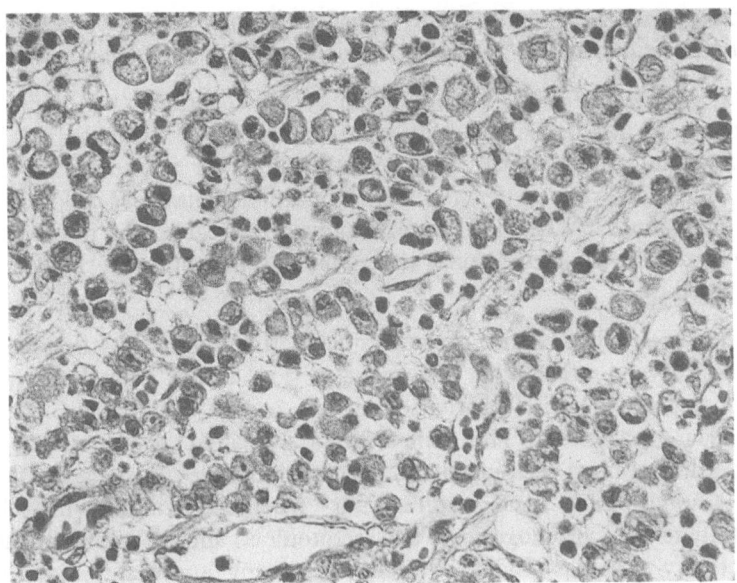

Fig. 16. Signet-ring cell carcinoma (from [33], with permission). H&E, ×200

which resembles a ring with a signet. A small alveolar or cord-like arrangement is noted, occasionally with a solid appearance. In many cases, individual cells proliferate in an isolated fashion, with a strong tendency toward diffuse infiltration. In the WHO classification [18], this type is further classified into goblet-cell, classical, and eosinophilic cytoplasm types.

Mucinous Adenocarcinoma. In this type, the carcinoma cells float within mucus pools, exhibiting nodular patterns of various sizes, or line the internal wall of the interstitium surrounding the mucus pools. Some of the carcinoma cells show a signet-ring-like appearance, and others appear cylindrical, with a tubular or papillary arrangement. This type of carcinoma may thus be a variant of either signet-ring cell carcinoma or glandular adenocarcinoma with abundant mucus secretion. It should be understood that all adenocarcinomas of the stomach secrete mucin, but the amount varies. To qualify for the term of mucinous carcinoma, the total amount of mucin must exceed 50% or more of the total tumor volume.

Special Types of Early Gastric Carcinoma

Adenosquamous Carcinoma. Within a single lesion, a mixed picture of adenocarcinoma and squamous cell carcinoma is seen in approximately equal proportions, or with one element occupying at least one third of the lesion. When a very small area of squamous metaplasia is found within the lesion of adenocarcinoma, the lesion is not classified in this category, and only the description of metaplasia is added to the main diagnosis of adenocarcinoma.

Squamous Cell Carcinoma. The carcinoma cells overlap in a multi-layered structure as in the squamous cell epithelium, with a tendency to lamellar arrangement toward the open surface of the tumor or in the center of tumor patches. There are varying degrees of keratinization. Squamous cell carcinoma is rare in the stomach. When it is seen in the cardiac region, the possibility of its being an extension of an esophageal carcinoma into the cardia must be considered and excluded.

Carcinoid Tumor. The main growth site of the tumor is frequently the submucosal layer, rather than the mucosa. The tumor cells have relatively abundant cytoplasm, with nearly round and evenly small nuclei filled with homogeneous karyoplasm. This tumor shows alveolar, cord-like ribbon-like, or lace-like structures and occasionally the formation of rosettes or glandular lumen. Positive argyrophilic and argentaffin reactions, immunohistochemical demonstrations of chromogranine and serotonine, and the demonstration of neurosecretory granules under electron microscopy are useful in differential diagnosis [21].

Undifferentiated Carcinoma. This kind of tumor lacks any specific picture of differentiation, structurally or functionally. It is therefore not possible to establish the origin from the point of view of histogenesis. It should be noted that the undifferentiated carcinoma in this classification is not the same as the undifferentiated type in the Japanese classification mentioned at the beginning of this section. The latter includes the poorly differentiated as well as some of the differentiated carcinomas described in this section. Undifferentiated carcinoma is rarely seen in association with lymphoid stroma.

Other Types. Choriocarcinoma or malignant chorioepithelioma with syncytio- and cytotrophoblastic cells in varying numbers may occur in the stomach [22]. This type of carcinoma is frequently accompanied by foci of ordinary histological types of carcinoma. An early small-cell carcinoma has been reported [23]. Finally, advanced carcinomas may simulate the early lesions.

Frequency of Histological Types

Among early gastric cancers diagnosed at the National Cancer Center Hospital in Tokyo (Table 3), the differentiated type of glandular adenocarcinoma (D) makes up 60.7%, while poorly differentiated and undifferentiated carcinoma (U) accounts for 39.3% of the total. In gastric cancer as a whole, including advanced gastric cancer, poorly differentiated and signet-ring cell carcinomas account for the majority of cancers (56.3%), and papillary and tubular adenocarcinomas account for 43.7%. Signet-ring cell carcinoma accounts for 25.3% of early gastric cancer, but only 22.7% of advanced gastric cancer. Conversely, the frequency of poorly differentiated adenocarcinoma was 13.3% in early cancer and much higher

(29.5%) in advanced cancer. Mucinous adenocarcinoma is rare and is located mainly in the submucosal or deeper layers, so that it accounts for only 0.7% of early gastric cancer; its frequency in advanced gastric cancer is 5.2%.

Ulceration in Early Gastric Cancer

Frequency of Ulceration. Secondary ulcer formation seems to occur frequently within the early gastric carcinoma. Ulceration was seen in about 65.4% of the whole group of early gastric cancer and in 80% of patients below the age of 65. Ulceration was less frequent in elderly patients (69.2%). The frequency of ulceration and/or ulcer scar had decreased from 93.5% in 1962 to 71.9% in 1983 [10]. According to the classification of Murakami [24], which expresses four levels of ulceration depth from Ul-I to Ul-IV, ulcers in early cancer appear most commonly at the level of Ul-II (involving the submucosa). Formation of an ulcer scar is the main cause of the convergence of muocsal folds toward the carcinomatous lesion.

Relation of Ulceration to Submucosal Invasion. At the National Cancer Center Hospital, a large number of early gastric carcinomas with submucosal invasion were found in the group with ulceration (360 of 529 cases, 68.1%) [25], but the prevalence rate of submucosal invasion was not much different for the tumors without ulceration (416 cases) and those with ulceration (786 cases), 40.6% and 45.8%, respectively. The prevalence rate of submucosal infiltration reversed in carcinomas larger than 3 cm. The presence of an ulcer therefore appears to contribute to the development of submucosal invasion in type IIc carcinomas measuring less than 3 cm, whereas in carcinomas larger than 3 cm, pronounced submucosal invasion was found in the absence of ulceration.

Multiple Occurrence of Early Gastric Cancer

Multiple carcinoma was found in about 8.3% of 500 early gastric cancer cases at the National Cancer Center Hospital [26]. In 77% of these, two lesions coexisted in the stomach. Coexistence of three lesions was found in 20% and more than four lesions in 3%. In patients over 65 years of age, the rate of multiple tumors was 13%, i.e., twice that of the group under 65 years of age. The back-ground gastric mucosa giving rise to multiple gastric carcinomas frequently revealed extensive distribution of intestinal metaplasia in the stomach. Among 77 specimens studied by Johansen [14], 8 had two or three early cancers, 6 had one advanced of them and one early cancer, and 1 had one advanced and two early cancers.

Metastasis to Lymph Nodes

It is reported that even early gastric cancer showed lymph node metastases at frequencies ranging from 0%–17% in intramucosal carcinomas, and 13%–30% in submucosal carcinomas in Japan [27]. The corresponding ranges in Europe were

1.5%–7% and 4%–12.3%, respectively. At the National Cancer Center Hospital, lymph node metastasis were seen in 2.1% of cases with tumors limited to the mucosa and in 13.9% of cases with submucosal invasion. The respective percentages in another report based on the data from multiple Japanese institutions were 4% and 19% [28]. The rate of lymph node metastasis was related to the size of the primary tumor: 4% in tumors less than 1 cm in diameter and 18% in tumor larger than 4 cm. The metastasis from mucosal cancer was limited to primary regional nodes, but the submucosal cancers may spread to secondary or tertiary nodes [29]. The frequency of metastases to lymph nodes also varied, depending on the presence or absence of ulceration in the carcinoma. Among cases with tumors limited to the mucosa, metastases were found in 0% of cases without ulceration and in 2%–3% of cases with ulceration. Conversely, in cases with submucosal invasion, lymph node metastases were found in 23.3% of those with ulceration.

Histogenesis

Histologic examination of early gastric cancer, particularly the minute lesions, allows the opportunity to evaluate the back-ground mucosa from which the early cancerous lesion arises. Such studies revealed that the glandular differentiated carcinoma was associated with intestinal metaplasias, whereas the nonglandular carcinoma arose from the nonmetaplastic gastric mucosa [30]. By serial-step sections, Hattori noted that carcinoma, metaplasia, and dysplasia all began at the neck region of the glands, where regeneration of the epithelium normally occurred, and concluded that these cellular abnormalities were coincidental lesions [31]. Similar cellular origin from the gland neck was demonstrated for the signet-ring cell carcinoma by Grundmann [32].

Precancerous Lesions and Conditions. The precancerous state of clinical conditions with a high expectancy of cancer development should be distinguished from a precancerous lesion, defined as a pathological entity showing distinct histopathological abnormalities and a significantly high frequency of malignant transformation. Our review of 1900 early gastric cancer cases revealed the frequency of elevated or depressed lesions or conditions in which carcinoma arised or coexisted [33]. Among the elevated lesions, adenoma was the most important (high-risk) lesion [34], followed by hyperplastic polyp and verrucous gastritis. Among the depressed lesion or almost flat lesion, atrophic (metaplastic) gastritis showed the highest frequency of association with early carcinoma. Chronic gastric ulcer, regarded as an important precancerous lesion in the past [35], showed an association with carcinoma in only 0.68% among the total early gastric cancer cases, when Hauser's criteria [36] of ulcer-carcinoma was applied. Our study as well as many other studies indicate that chronic atrophic gastritis—especially of the type accompanied by intestinal metaplasia—is the most important precancerous lesion [37]. Our data also showed that the intestinal metaplasia accompanying the cancerous lesion was often of the incomplete type [37]. The gastric remnant following partial resection and the stomach of patients with pernicious anemia is also thought to represent precancerous states.

Recurrence of Cancer after Surgery and Prognosis

Follow up data of early gastric cancer showed a 5-year postoperative recurrence rate of about 3% in cases of intramucosal carcinoma and of 8%–9% in cases of submucosal carcinoma [33].

The 10-year postoperative recurrence rate was as high as 8%–14% in intramucosal carcinoma cases, and 10%–22% in submucosal carcinoma cases. Recurrence in the relatively early period after the operation generally occurs in cases of submucosal carcinoma, while late recurrence is common in intramucosal carcinoma cases. Papillary and tubular differentiated-type adenocarcinomas frequently show hepatic metastases, whereas other types of carcinoma more often show local recurrence.

The postoperative survival rate in patients with early gastric cancer was calculated by means of the actuarial survival rate method. The 5-year survival rate was reported to be 95.5%, and the 10-year survival rate, 95.0%. When cases with intramucsal carcinoma and submucosal carcinoma were distinguished, almost 99.1% of patients with intramucosal carcinoma survived at the 10- and 20-year points, whereas 91.2% and 90.2% of patients with submucosal carcinoma survived at the 10- and 20-year points, respectively [38]. Prognosis is also influenced by other pathological factors. Data obtained so far, especially with multifactorial analysis, indicate the influence of lymph node metastases. The histologic type of the tumor has little importance in prognosis.

References

1. Segi M, Tominaga S, Aoki K, Fujimoto I (1990) World cancer mortality. In Segi M (ed) Cancer mortality and morbidity statistics, Japan and the world. Gann Monogr on Cancer Res, Japan Scientific Societies, Tokyo, 26:121–251
2. Aoki K, Kurihara M, Hayakawa N, Suzuki S (1992) Death rates for malignant neoplasms for selected sites by sex and five-year age groups in 33 countries, 1953–'57 to 1983–'87. UICC, International Union Against Cancer, Aichi Cancer Center, Nagoya, Japan, pp 103–135
3. Nagayo T (1986) Histogenesis and precursors of human gastric cancer. Springer, Berlin
4. Hirota T, Okada T, Itabashi M (1984) Significance of chronic gastritis as a precancerous condition of the stomach. In: Ming SC (ed) Precursors of Gastric Cancer. Praeger, New York pp 131–138
5. Japanese Research Society for Gastric Cancer (1981) The general rules for the gastric cancer study in surgery and pathology. Jpn J Surg 11:127–145
6. Kuru M (1967) Atlas of early carcinoma of the stomach. Nakayama-Shoten, Tokyo

7. Murakami T (1971) Pathological diagnosis. Definition and gross classification of early gastric cancer. Gann Monogr Cancer Res 11:53–55
8. Kajitani T, Miwa K (1979) Treatment results of stomach carcinoma in Japan, 1963–1966. In WHO-CC Monograph No. 2, WHO-CC for diagnosis and treatment of stomach cancer, National Cancer Center, Japan, pp 77–83
9. Green PHR, O'Toole KM, Slonim D (1988) Increasing incidence and excellent survival of patients with early gastric cancer: Experience in a United States medical center. Am J Med 65:658–661
10. Hirota T, Itabashi M, Daibo M (1984) Chronological changes in the morphological features of early gastric cancer, especially recent changes in macroscopic findings. Jpn J Clin Oncol 14:181–199
11. Borrmann R (1926) Geschwüre des Magens und Duodenums. In Henke F, Lubarsch O (eds) Handbuch der Speziellen Pathologischen Anatomie und Histologie, vol 4. Springer, Berlin, p 865
12. Nagayo T (1966) Mode of origin of gastric mucosal cancer with special reference to that of "superficial spreading type". Gann Monogr Cancer Res 3:113–121
13. Stout AP (1942) Superficial spreading type of carcinoma of the stomach. Arch Surg 44:651–657
14. Johansen A (1981) Early gastric cancer. Bispebjerg Hospital, Copenhagen, Denmark
15. Hirota T, Itabashi M, Suzuki K, Yoshida S (1980) Clinical study of minute and small early gastric cancer. Histogenesis of gastric cancer. Pathol Annu 15:1–19
16. Kurihara M, Miyasaka K, Shirakabe H (1981) Diagnosis of small early gastric cancer by x-ray, endoscopy and biopsy. Cancer Detect Prev 4:377–383
17. Lauren P (1965) The two histological main types of gastric carcinoma. Diffuse and so-called intestinal type carcinoma. An attempt at histochemical classification. Acta Path Microbiol Scand 64:31–49
18. Watanabe H, Jass JR, Sobin LH (1989) Histological typing of esophageal and gastric tumours. World Health Organization international histological classification of tumours (2nd ed). Springer, Berlin, vol 18, pp 20–26
19. Ming S-C (1977) Gastric carcinoma: A pathological classification. Cancer 39:2475–2485
20. Nakamura K (1983) Histogenesis of the gastric cancer and its clinical application. Tsukuba International Center, Ibaraki, Japan
21. Solcia E, Capella C, Fiocca R (1992) Disorders of the endocrine system. In Ming SC, Goldman H (eds) Pathology of the gastrointestinal tract. Saunders, Philadelphia, pp 240–263
22. Ozaki H, Ito I, Sano R, Hirota T (1971) A case of choriocarcinoma of the stomach. Jpn J Clin Oncol 1:83–94
23. Fukuda T, Onishi Y, Nishimaki T (1988) Early gastric cancer of the small cell type. Am J Gastroenterol 83:1176–1179
24. Murakami T (1960) Histogenesis of gastric cancer (in Japanese). Gan Chiryo No Shinpo 2:1–11
25. Hirota T, Yamamichi N, Itabashi M (1982) Clinicopathological study of the early gastric cancer with submucosal invasion. Relationship between macroscopic and microscopic findings (in Japanese). Stomach Intestine 17:497–508
26. Kikuchi S, Hirota T, Itabashi M (1984) Clinicopathological characteristics of 104 cases of multiple early gastric cancer including 11 cases which had malignancy in other organs (in Japanese). Prog Dig Endosc 24:121–125, 6
27. Bogomoletz WV (1984) Early gastric cancer. Am J Surg Pathol 8:381–391

28. Hukutomi H, Sakita T (1984) Analysis of early gastric cancer cases collected from major hospitals and institutes in Japan. Jpn J Clin Oncol 14:169–179
29. Murakami T (1979) Early cancer of the stomach. World J Surg 3:685–692
30. Nakamura K, Sugano H (1983) Microcarcinoma of the stomach measuring less than 5 mm in the largest diameter and its histogenesis. Prog Clin Biol Res 132D:107–116
31. Hattori T (1986) Development of adenocarcinoma in the stomach. Cancer 57:1528–1534
32. Grundmann E (1975) Histologic types and possible initial stages in early gastric carcinoma. Beits Pathol Bd 154:256–280
33. Hirota T, Ming SC (1992) Early gastric cancer. In Ming SC, Goldman H (eds) Pathology of the gastrointestinal tract. Saunders, Philadelphia, pp 570–583
34. Hirota T, Okada T, Itabashi M, Kitaoka H (1984) Histogenesis of human gastric cancer with special reference to the significance of adenoma as a precancerous lesion. In Ming SC (ed) Precursors of gastric cancer. Praeger, New York, pp 233–252
35. Ming SC (1984) Relationship between gastric carcinoma and chronic gastric ulcer. In Ming SC (ed) Precursors of gastric cancer. Praeger, New York, pp 265–272
36. Hauser G (1926) "Ulcus-Karzinom". In Henke F, Lubarsch O (eds) Hand-buch der speziellen Pathologischen Anatomie und Histologie, vol 4. Springer, Berlin p 1
37. Hirota T, Takizawa C, Itabashi M (1987) Minute carcinoma of the stomach. Its definition, pathomorphologic characteristics and lesions of background mucosa (in Japanese). Pathol Clin Med 5 (suppl):115–124
38. Maruyama K (1987) The most important prognostic factor for the gastric cancer patient. Scand J Gastroenterol 22 [suppl 133]:63–68

Growth Patterns of Gastric Cancer

Kiyoshi Inokuchi[1] and Keizo Sugimachi[2]

Key words. Growth patterns of cancer—Pen type—Super type—DNA distribution patterns—Early gastric cancer—Superficial gastric cancer—Mass screening

Summary. Early gastric cancer cases were analyzed in terms of growth patterns of the superficially speading (Super) type and the penetrating growth (Pen) type, the latter further subdivided into the Pen A-type which grows expansively and the Pen B type which has infiltration. This classification was then extended to include advanced cancer, and the natural history of gastric cancer was studied. While the Super type showed good prognosis after surgery, then Pen A type had a poorer prognosis except when confined to the mucosa. The prognosis of the Pen B type, which was good for cases in early stages, became poor once the lesion invaded the serosa. Such growth patterns were further studied in terms of cytophotometric DNA analysis. It was found that most Super-type cases have low ploidy, while most of the Pen A type have high ploidy and the Pen B type, which had retained low ploidy in the submucosal stage, developed high ploidy when the invasion reached the serosa. Such analyses led us to postulate that early cancer of the Super type progresses to the funnel-shaped advanced cancer with relatively good prognosis, while the Pen A type grows into box-shaped lesions corresponding to Laurén's intestinal type, while the Pen B type became the mountain-shaped ones of the diffuse type. Based on data from annual check-ups, it was estimated that initially occurring low and high ploidy cancer may be approximately equally distributed. Thus, it is important to bear in mind that diagnostic advances may actually favor the detection of slow growing, low-malignant lesions, overlooking rapidly growing highly malignant lesions in their early stage before detection, thereby allowing them to progress to an advanced stage.

---

[1] Emeritus Professor of Kyushu University, Terazuka 1-3-47, Minami-ku, Fukuoka, 815 Japan
[2] Professor of the 2nd Department of Surgery, Kyushu University School of Medicine, Maedahi 3-1, Higashi-ku, Fukuoka, 812 Japan

88

Introduction

With recent progress in techniques to diagnose cancers making it possible to detect minute lesions, and because mass surveys or periodic examinations for gastric cancer have become widely employed, the ratio of early gastric cancer among overall operated cases has reached more than 60% in most Japanese institutions with well-organized gastroenterology teams. Such a trend is undoubtedly a triumph of modern medicine, since such patients can expect a long survival rate after surgery. Nevertheless, it is also a current fact that from 20% to 30% of gastric cancer patients detected even in periodical examinations are already at an advanced stage. Recently, a "polarization phenomenon" become evident in gastric cancer patients; that is, either "early" or "advanced" cancers have become predominant in associated with a decrease in those in intermediate stages. Despite the high rate of early detection, gastric cancer still remains a leading cause of death in Japan. This strongly suggests that the disease involves considerably diverse growth patterns, reflected by very slow or rapid growth, and that more of the former are being detected while some of the latter are being overlooked. It may be the case that advances in diagnostic techniques are indeed prone to favor the detection of the less malignant cancers rather than the more malignant ones. We proposed the concept of growth patterns of gastric cancer involving the Super and Pen growth types in 1966 [1] and subsequently reported clinicopathological data related to this concept in terms of cytophotometric DNA analysis [2–4].

The present paper is a review of clinical gastric cancer from the viewpoint of its growth patterns and with special reference to the pitfalls of early detection.

Initial Experiences of Slow and Rapid Recurrence of Early Gastric Cancer

In the late 1950s and early 1960s when the concept of early cancer was not yet resolved, we treated several interesting cases of early gastric cancer with extremely slow or rapid recurrence [1]. Figure 1 demonstrates cases with late recurrence. They all consisted of mucosal cancers with a wide extension of several square centimeters and in which the cancer cells had remained at the oral gastric stump devised at the time of the first operation. An effective repeat resection was done 4–9 years after the first operation. This aroused the suspicion that superficial mucosal cancer might be characterized by extremely slow growth. Yet, we later treated five other patients with submucosal gastric cancers with early recurrence (Fig. 2), all of whom had an elevated lesion with a papillary adenocarcinoma located at the antrum. Liver recurrence occurred relatively soon after surgery. These findings suggested that there are two types of recurrencies in early gastric cancer, early and late ones, and this gave rise to a keen interest in the study of growth patterns of gastric cancer.

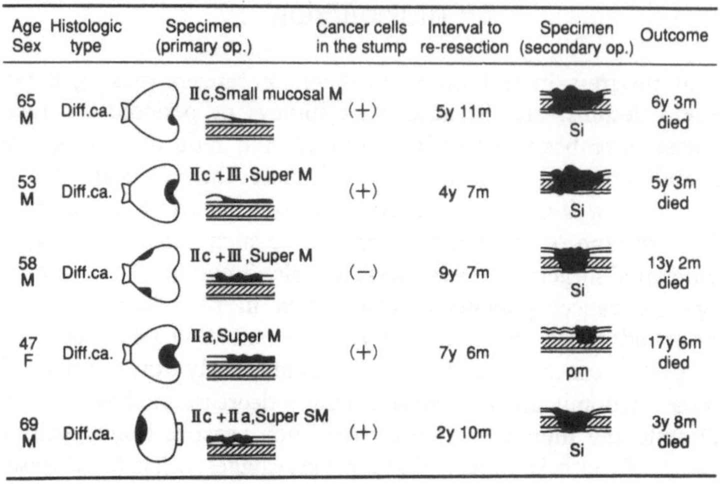

Age Sex	Histologic type	Specimen (primary op.)	Cancer cells in the stump	Interval to re-resection	Specimen (secondary op.)	Outcome
65 M	Diff.ca.	IIc,Small mucosal M	(+)	5y 11m	Si	6y 3m died
53 M	Diff.ca.	IIc + III ,Super M	(+)	4y 7m	Si	5y 3m died
58 M	Diff.ca.	IIc + III ,Super M	(−)	9y 7m	Si	13y 2m died
47 F	Diff.ca.	IIa,Super M	(+)	7y 6m	pm	17y 6m died
69 M	Diff.ca.	IIc + IIa,Super SM	(+)	2y 10m	Si	3y 8m died

Fig. 1. Late recurrence of early gastric cancer. *Diff.ca*, Differentiated cancer; *M*, mucosal; *SM*, submucosal; *y*, year; *m*, month

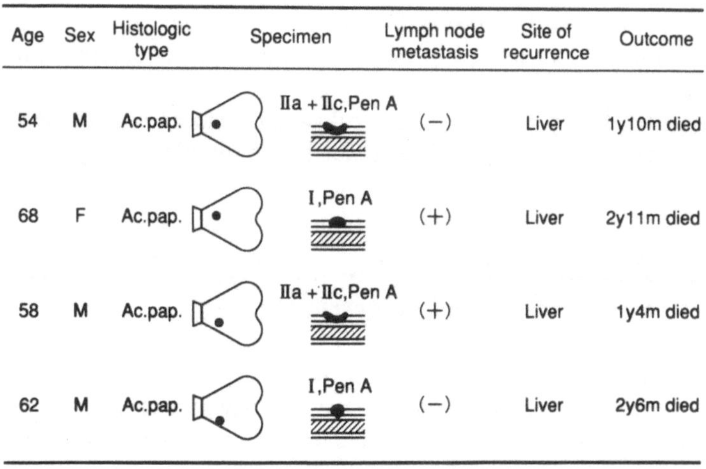

Age	Sex	Histologic type	Specimen	Lymph node metastasis	Site of recurrence	Outcome
54	M	Ac.pap.	IIa + IIc,Pen A	(−)	Liver	1y10m died
68	F	Ac.pap.	I,Pen A	(+)	Liver	2y11m died
58	M	Ac.pap.	IIa + IIc,Pen A	(+)	Liver	1y4m died
62	M	Ac.pap.	I,Pen A	(−)	Liver	2y6m died

Fig. 2. Early recurrence of early gastric cancer. *Ac.pap.*, papillary adenoearcinoma

Our Classification of Growth Patterns

Two types of growth patterns of early gastric cancer were classified according to the histologic appearance of the cut surface of the primary tumor as illustrated in Fig. 3 [2, 3]. The superficially spreading type (Super type) was designated to lesions with a diameter of over 4.0 cm and which were either confined to the

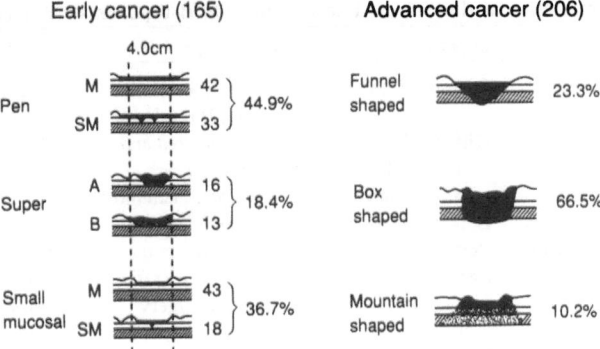

Fig. 3. Growth patterns of early and advanced cancers. Abbreviations as in Fig. 1

mucosa (Super M type) or were only partly invading the submucosa (Super SM type). A lesion less than 4.0 cm in diameter which invaded the submucosa in a penetrating fashion was designated as the Pen type, which was further subdivided into Pen A and Pen B subtypes according to the mode of cancerous invasion to the submucosa. The Pen A subtype showed complete destruction of the muscularis mucosae, and the Pen B subtype grew infiltratively downwards with network-like replacement of the muscularis mucosae.

An intramucosal carcinoma and the one limited to only slight submucosal invasion with a diameter of less than 4.0 cm were designated as being of a small mucosal type which could not classified as either Super or Pen. This mode of classification of growth patterns extended to advanced cancers as well. The abbreviations Super-PM, Super-S; Pen-PM, and Pen-S were used to describe the extent of invasion to the uppermost the proper muscle (PM) and serosa (S).

Features of Growth Patterns in Early Gastric Cancer

According to our previous study in 1985 [5], in which 167 cases of early gastric cancer treated from 1951 to 1972 in the Second Department of Surgery of Kyushu University Hospital were analyzed, we summarized the features of the growth patterns as follows:

1. Incidence: the Super type was found in 44.9%, the Pen type in 18.4%, and the small mucosal type in 36.7% among early cancers. On the other hand, the funnel shape was found in 23.3%, the box shape in 66.5%, and the mountain shape in 10.2% among advanced cancers.
2. Gross appearance: depressed lesions (IIc, IIc + III) dominated in the Super type (82.7%), while elevated lesions (IIa + IIc) were more numerous in the Pen A type (87.5%).
3. Histologic type: well-differentiated carcinoma with papillotubular structures was common in the Pen A type (81.3%), but poorly differentiated carcinoma

Table 1. Characteristics of the Super, Pen A, and Pen B types in early gastric cancer.

Features	Super type	Pen A type	Pen B type
Gross type	Depressed lesion	Elevated lesion (IIa, IIa + IIc)	Depressed lesion (IIc, IIc + IIa)
Histologic type	Differentiated and poorly differentiated	Differentiated and particularly papillary carcinoma	Poorly differentiated carcinoma
Lymphogenous metastasis	Low incidence	High incidence	Low incidence
Hematogenous metastasis	Very rare	Rather frequent	Rare
Recurrence	Remnant stomach long after initial surgery	To liver soon after initial surgery	Peritoneal when the lesion invades the serosa
Prognosis	Favorable	Poor	Not unfavorable, but poor when the invasion reaches the serosa
Progression	Slow	Rapid	Rapid

was most common in the Pen B type (61.5%). The Super type was almost equally divided between the well (58.7%) and the poorly (41.3%) differentiated forms. The small mucosal type was primarily composed of differentiated carcinoma (72.1%).

4. Vascular invasion and lymph node metastasis: a much higher rate of lymphatic invasion was seen in the Pen type, with an incidence of 43.8% in the Pen A and 30.8% in the Pen B type. The Super type showed an 18.7% rate of lymphatic invasion and one of 4.9% in the small type. Lymph node metastasis was highest in Pen A (25.0%), as opposed to 7.7% in Pen B and 10.7% in the Super type. Venous invasion was noted only in the Pen A group (25%).

5. Accompanying peptic ulcer: the Super type was found to be accompanying peptic ulcers in 62.5% of cases as opposed to 10% in the Pen A type and 24% in the Pen B type. The small mucosal type was accompanied by peptic ulcer at a rate of 50%.

Table 1 summarizes the above growth pattern features.

Prognosis

Late recurrence in the remnant stomach was common in the Super type cases, while early recurrence in the liver was often seen in cases of the Pen A type. The small mucosal, Super, and Pen B types had an excellent outcome, the 10-year survival rate being about 90%. In contrast, the 5-year survival rate of Pen A submucosal cancer was considerably poorer, being only 64.8%. As to the prognosis of advanced cancer with the respective growth types, the 5-year survival rate was over 75% in funnel-shaped cancer (Super-PM and -S). In the advanced

Table 2. Five-year survival rates of gastric cancer patients in terms of various growth patterns.

Depth of invasion	Super	Pen A	Pen B
Mucosal	100%·		
Submucosal	95.7%	64.8%	100%
Proper muscle	84.6%	53.3%	84.6%
Serosal	75.0%	35.7%	47.8%

Table 3. Duration of ulcer symptoms in each gastric cancer growth pattern.

Growth pattern	Ulcer history	No. of cases	Duration of symptoms (months)								
			0–3	3–6	6–12	12–24	24–36	36–48	48–60	60–72	72–
Super	(−)	16	6	7	1	2					
	(+)	19	1		4	4	2	1	3	3	1
Pen A	(−)	10	10								
	(+)	0									
Pen B	(−)	4	3	1							
	(+)	2		1					1		
Small	(−)	28	12	11	4	1					
mucosal	(+)	24	1	1	5	7	3	3	1	3	

Pen A type, the survival time was shorter in cases of deep invasion of the lesion, being 53.3% in Pen A-PM and 35.5% in Pen A-S. In the advanced Pen B type, the survival rate was favorable when the lesion was confined to the proper muscle (84.6%); however serosal invasion resulted in the much poorer rate of 47.8% (Table 2).

Speed of Growth in Super and Pen Type Cancers

In terms of the speed of growth of Super and Pen type cancers, after an investigation of duration of symptoms and follow-up of endoscopic examinations, Okabe [6] reached the conclusion that two forms of gastric cancer exist: one is rapid growing, presenting an elevated appearance (IIc + IIc), and the other is a slow growing one displaying a depressed lesion (IIc, IIc + III). His speculations lent support to our ideas of Pen and Super growth patterns.

Kusaba's systematic study on gastric cancer in terms of duration of symptoms and treatment history for ulcer provided interesting insights on the speed of tumor growth [7]. The symptoms lasted 60 months or more in the Super type, whereas in the Pen A type there was no patient with history of ulcer, and the clinical symptoms averaged only 3 months in duration (Table 3). The Pen B type showed similar statistics to those of the Pen A type. These findings strongly suggest that the speed of growth is slow in the Super type and rapid in the Pen type. The statistics for small mucosal cancers resembled those of the Super type. This may be explained by the unstated premise that the prototype of Super and Pen is included in small mucosal cancer. Kusaba also suggested that absence or shorter duration of GI symptoms with a minimal history of ulcer treatment, or, alternatively, longer duration of symptoms with a history of ulcer treatment are good indicators of the Super or Pen type of cancer [7].

Cytophotometric DNA Analysis of Early Carcinoma

Paraffin sections 10 micron, μ in latin, 10^{-6} m (meter) in thickness were made from the portions adjacent to H and E-stained sections. Feulgen-stained specimens were examined to obtain the cell nuclear DNA content. The DNA histogram patterns were graded into types I, II, III, and IV, according to the degree of DNA histogram ploidy. Types I and II and Types III and IV were designated as low ploidy and high ploidy, respectively.

The DNA distribution types in terms of growth pattern of early and advanced cancer are summarized in Fig. 4. Most cases of the Super type are in low ploidy. This propensity was similar in the small mucosal and Pen B types. On the other hand, more than 80% of the Pen A type showed types III or IV, i.e., high ploidy. Differences in DNA distribution patterns between the Pen A and Super and between the Pen A and Pen B were significant. All the normal gastric mucosa

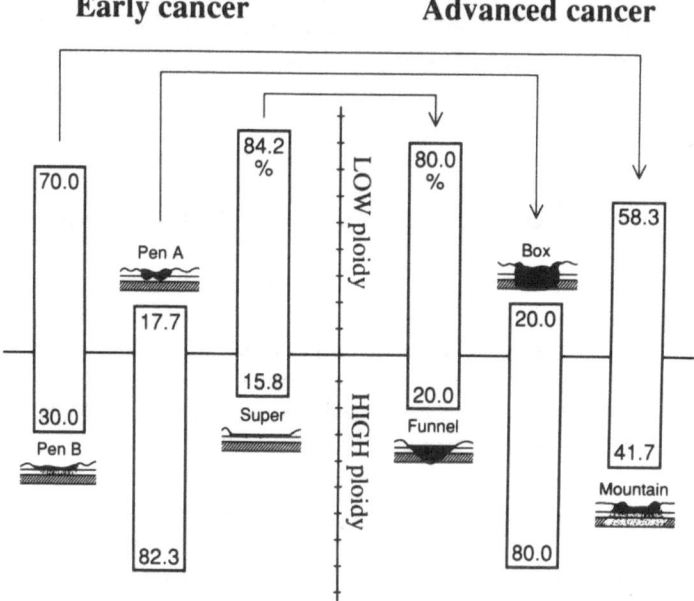

Fig. 4. Correlation of early and advanced cancer in relation to DNA ploidy patterns (expressed in percent)

showed type I. It should be noted that the DNA patterns provide a good reflection of the malignancy of the Pen A type.

As to the advanced cancer, funnel-shaped advanced cancer displayed a low ploidy DNA pattern similar to that of the Super type early cancer. The majority of the box- and mountain-shaped advanced cancers displayed high ploidy DNA patterns. The data on both sides of the center line of Fig. 4 seem to depict a mirror image of each other, reflecting the correlation between early and advanced gastric cancer in terms of DNA ploidy.

DNA Distrubution Patterns in Terms of Depth Invasion and Histologic Type

Figure 5 indicates the DNA ploidy according to various depths of invasion in terms of the degree of differentiation. The low and high ploidy patterns were generally equally distributed in every layer among the differentiated cancers, whereas the behavior was entirely different in poorly differentiated cancers, i.e., the low DNA ploidy which included all patients with mucosal cancer developed into high ploidy as the invasion advanced into the serosa, at which point cases with high ploidy cancer comprised about 60% of the total. Haraguchi et al. also noted the heterogeneity of DNA ploidy in undifferentiated gastric cancer [8]. These different features in relation to DNA ploidy may explain the prognostic characteristics of Pen B gastric cancer according to which the favorable outcome of early cancer becomes poor once the lesion invades the serosa.

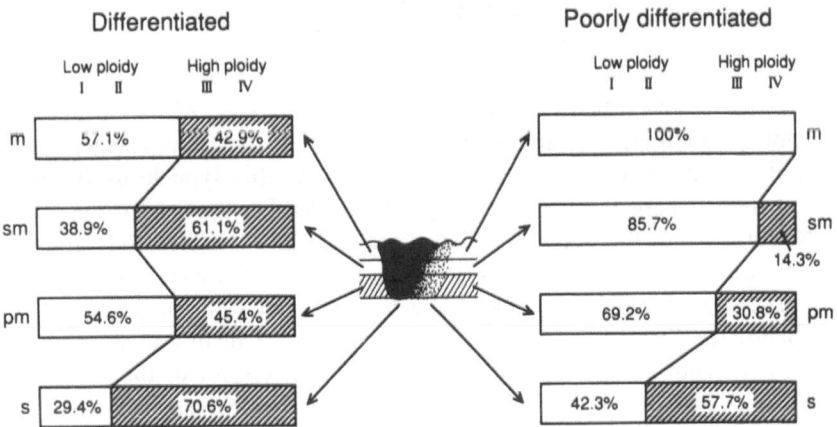

Fig. 5. DNA distribution patterns in terms of depth invasion and histologic types. *m*, Mucosal; *sm*, submucosal; *pm*, proper muscle, *s*, serosal

Consistency of DNA Ploidy in Primary and Recurrent Lesions

To determine the relationship between early and advanced cancer, it is essential to know whether DNA patterns remain consistent as the cancer grows. Korenaga et al. studied the consistency of DNA ploidy between primary and recurrent gastric cancer of 11 patients who had undergone a second resection of the lesion due to recurrence in the remnant stomach [9]. The same distribution patterns in the primary and recurrent lesions were seen in ten of them, while in the other patient with a type III primary lesion, a type II carcinoma was found at the time of recurrence. The DNA cytophotometric profile of cancer cells may thus be said to be a valid cell marker of a given tumor, and is thought to be applicable for determining the natural history of gastric cancer.

Postulated Correlation Between Early and Advanced Cancer

From the clinicopathological features of the Super and Pen growth types and from the corresponding similarity of DNA low and high ploidy patterns, it is probable that early cancer of the Super type progresses to funnel-shaped advanced cancer, which is often designated as "IIc-like advanced or non-Borrmann type cancer". As for the Pen types, it may be probable that early cancer of the Pen A type will advance to box-shaped lesions corresponding to the intestinal type in Laurén's classification, while that of the Pen B type will develop into the mountain-shaped lesion corresponding to the diffuse Laurén type. Figure 4 illustrates the probable relationship between early and advanced gastric cancer.

Why is the Pen Type Detected Less Frequently in Early Stages?

It seems paradoxical that the Pen type of cancer is less frequently detected at an early stage, despite the fact that this type leads to most cases of advanced cancers. The same question arises as to why the malignancy of the Super category is more detectable at an early stage, despite the fact that this type leads to the less frequent funnel-shaped cancer. These questions could be resolved if the different speeds of growth of the Super and Pen types were taken into consideration. The Pen type grows rapidly and develops into an advanced cancer with in a short time, hence the chance of detection may be decreased at an early stage. On the other hand, the Super type may be detected more frequently at an early stage because it remains there for a longer time. The discrepancy of the rate between the actual occurrence and of detection may be large in cases of cancer with rapid growth patterns, but relatively smaller in cases of slow-growing cancer. In addition, since the Super type is often accompanied by a peptic ulcer, this may cause a detection bias in those patients with the Super type who visit hospitals

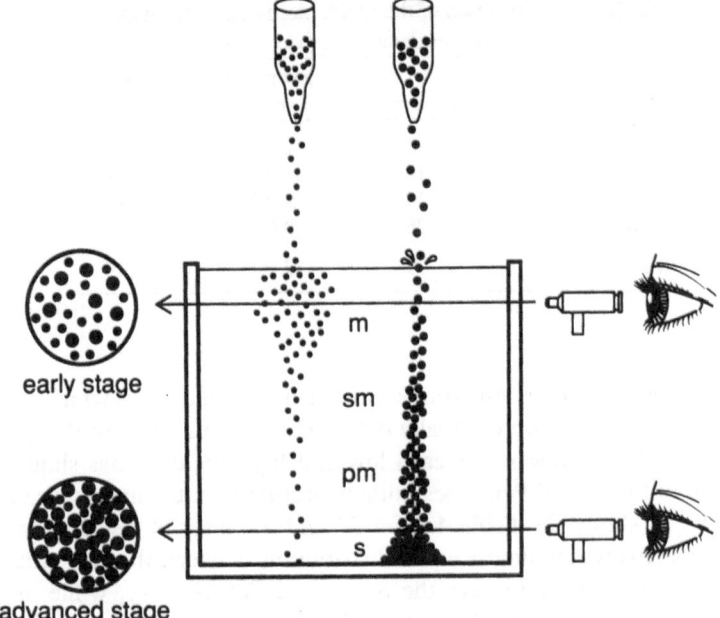

Fig. 6. Natural history of gastric cancer in relation to growth patterns. Abbreviations as in Fig. 5

more often than do those with cancer of the Pen type who tend to have fewer peptic ulcers.

Figure 6 is an explanatory illustration of this mechanism, in which two kinds of particles of small and large sizes are simultaneously placed into water and the sedimentation status is observed from the outside of the container at various depths. According to Stokes' sedimentation law, small particles sink slowly, while large ones sink rapidly. Then, the phenomenon will have resulted in small particles being initially located more in the upper part of the water while the large particles would be nearer the bottom of the water. The small and large particles are clearly analogous to the slow and rapid growth types of cancer, Super and Pen, respectively.

Approximately Estimated True Occurrence Rate of Super and Pen Growth Types in the Development of Human Gastric Cancers

It is obviously important to estimate the rate of Super and Pen type cancers at the initial stage of occurrence of the disease. Table 4 indicates the DNA ploidy patterns in terms of depth of invasion of the gastric cancer which was detected in

Table 4. Distribution of the DNA ploidy patterns in gastric cancers which were not detected a year previously.

Depth of invasion	No. of cases	Low ploidy (% of total)	High ploidy (% of total)
Mucosal	13	8 (62)	5 (38)
Submucosal	18	11 (61)	7 (39)
Proper muscle	15	9 (60)	6 (40)
Serosal	26	9 (35)	17 (65)
Total	72	37 (51)	35 (49)

successive annual examination groups. Provided that all cancers which had initially appeared in the mucosa were actually detected in any one layer of the gastric wall, the total number of cancers for each low and high ploidy series should indicate the amount of Super and Pen types initially occurring in the mucosa, respectively. The results as shown in Table 4 were 37 and 35 cases of low and high ploidy cancer, respectively, an almost equal distribution between the two groups. Since low ploidy early cancers involve the Super and Pen B types, while high ploidy cancer consists mostly of the Pen A type, it is assumed that the rate of occurrence of Pen type cases (Pen A + Pen B) would be more than that of Super type cases.

Differentiation of Highly Malignant Intramucosal Cancer

Korenaga et al. studied 70 patients with small gastric cancers with intramucosal or minimally submucosal invasion, in terms of DNA ploidy [10]. Patients with high ploidy were found in 34.3% (24/70), and all were cases of differentiated carcinomas. There were two recurrences within 24 cases: one patient with a mucosal lesion died of lung metastasis 6 years after surgery and another with slight submucosal invasion died of multiple bone metastasis 5 years and 7 months after surgery. This finding indicates that cases of the Pen A type cancer detected at the mucosal stage had a 5-year survival rate of 100% and a 10-year survival rate of 91.1%. Considering that only 64.8% of Pen A submucosal cancer cases survived 5 years, detection of the Pen A cancer in the mucosal stage should be a primary goal.

Okamura et al. studied the histologic modes of cancer growth in terms of DNA ploidy in 66 intramucosal gastric cancers and found that 18 lesions with an expansive growth had high ploidy DNA patterns (27.2%) [11]. In addition, the fact that high DNA ploidy is known to be found in about 30% of the small mucosal cancers and also in nearly 50% of differentiated adenocarcinomas is useful in the evaluation of highly malignant cancer in routine examinations.

Kamegawa et al. reported the ploidy and ploidy coincidence of DNA patterns between biopsied materials and the resected specimens to be 93% (39/42) [12]. This study provided evidence that the highly malignant type of early gastric cancer, the Pen A type, could be distinguished on endoscopically biopsied specimens by using DNA analysis.

The Detection of Highly Malignant Cancer in the Mucosal Stage

At present, the only successful way to detect highly malignant cancer, the Pen A type, at an early stage would be to perform periodic examinations at shorter intervals. In mass surveys in the Fukuoka district of Japan which were conducted from 1964 to 1980, 267 gastric cancer cases were detected, of which 196 were found at the first examination (Group A) and another 71 at a subsequent sequential examination after two or more examinations had been done (Group B). The incidence of Super type was 32.9% in Group A, higher than the 7.7% in Group B, while that of the Pen type was 23.1% in Group B, higher than the 11.4% in Group A. The incidence of small mucosal cancer was 51.3% in Group B, higher than the 24.3% in Group A. Although the breakdown of the small mucosal cancer in terms of the DNA ploidy awaits further study, the above data indicate that annual periodical examinations are useful for the detection of the Pen type in the mucosal stage.

Discussion

The initial opportunity to start the present study was the incidental experience starting more than 30 years ago of early gastric cancer cases with extremely slow growth. Subsequent experience of early cancer with rapid recurrence after surgery led us to the concept of categorizing Super and Pen types in gastric cancer. The paradoxical phenomenon according to which slow growing cancers (Super) which are frequently detected at an early stage are less frequently found in an advanced stage, whereas rapid growing cancers (Pen) which are less frequent in the early stage are mostly seen in advanced stages, aroused our interest and has now been explained by the concept illustrated in Fig. 6.

Current advances in sophisticated diagnostic techniques, as well as the prevalence of periodic examinations of the stomach, have considerably enhanced the rate of detection of intramucosal gastric cancer and, accordingly, the distribution figures of growth patterns appear to have changed when compared to previous patterns (Fig. 3). Table 5 indicates chronological trends of early gastric cancer in the Kyushu Cancer Center Hospital during the past 15 years (M. Furusawa, personal communication, 1992). The Super type has decreased and, in its place, intramucosal cancer has increased, while the Pen type shows little change. However, this phenomenon may not be unnatural, since it is thought that cancer of the Super type, which was defined in the present study as being more than 4 cm in size, is detected more frequently before it reaches this definitive size. Presumably, a considerable number of cases of the Super type may be mucosal

Table 5. Chronological tendencies of the detection of early gastric cancer at Kyushu Cancer Center Hospital. (M. Furusawa, personal communication, 1992).

		1972–1974	1975–1979	1980–1984	1985–1989
Super	m	12 ⎫ 21 (46.6)[a]	18 ⎫ 35 (21.3)	26 ⎫ 47 (21.6)	25 ⎫ 46 (17.6)
	sm	9 ⎭	17 ⎭	21 ⎭	21 ⎭
Pen	A	4 ⎫ 11 (24.4)	16 ⎫ 41 (25.0)	18 ⎫ 54 (24.8)	5 ⎫ 40 (15.3)
	B	7 ⎭	25 ⎭	36 ⎭	35 ⎭
Small mucosal		6 ⎫ 13 (28.8)	68 ⎫ 88 (53.6)	87 ⎫ 116 (53.4)	140 ⎫ 175 (67.0)
		7 ⎭	20 ⎭	29 ⎭	35 ⎭
Total		45	164	217	261

[a] Figures in parentheses represent percent of total
m, Mucosa; *sm*, submucosa

cancer, leading to the increase in the number of such cases. Be that as it may, it can be said that the principal idea of our concept of growth patterns of gastric cancer is not influenced by the recent data.

If the term "early cancer" is used to mean "curable cancer", then the early cancer of the Pen A type should be comprised of cases in an intramucosal stage, excluding submucosal cancer, whereas cancers of the Super and Pen B types may include submucosal cancer. Although it may certainly be a triumph of modern medicine that early cancer accounts for over one-half of the gastric cancer patients treated in major hospitals in Japan, and that about one-half of these are of intramucosal cancer, we must still keep in mind that the Pen type constitutes merely about one-fourth of early cancer, with the rate of Pen A (high ploidy) cancer being even less. We must bear in mind that our rough estimation of the rate of high ploidy and low ploidy cancer at initial occurrence is presumed to show equal distribution, but high ploidy cancers are relatively few in the early stage, and are allowed to develop to advanced stages. We must not rest on our laurels from the successful detection of many early cancers, but aim to more effectively detect high ploidy cancer in the mucosal stage.

Acknowledgments. We should like to express our heartfelt thanks to Dr. M. Furusawa of Kyushu Cancer Center Hospital and Professor K. Soejima of Fukuoka Dental College for their cooperation. We also thank Professor J. Patrick Barron for his critical reading of the manuscript.

References

1. Inokuchi K, Inutsuka S, Furusawa M, Soejima K, Ikeda T (1966) Development of superficial carcinoma of the stomach: Report of late recurrence. Ann Surg 64:145–151
2. Inokuchi K, Furusawa M, Soejima K, et al (1966) Reflections on early gastric cancer: Clinicopathological analysis viewed from the growth patterns (in Japanese). Nippon Ijishinpo Issue 2211, pp 3–9

3. Kodama Y, Inokuchi K, Soejima K, Matsusaka T, Okamura T (1983) Growth patterns and prognosis in early gastric carcinoma: Superficially spreading and penetrating growth types. Cancer 51:320–326
4. Inokuchi K, Kodama Y, Sasaki O, Kamegawa T, Okamura T (1983) Differentiation of growth patterns of early gastric carcinoma determined by cytophotometric DNA analysis. Cancer 51:1138–1141
5. Inokuchi K (1986) Early gastric cacinoma: Analysis of its growth patterns. In: Inokuchi K, Murphy GP, Sugano H, Sugimura T, Veronesi U (eds) Gann monograph on cancer research, no. 31. Japan Scientific Societies, Tokyo, pp 87–97
6. Okabe H (1971) Growth of early gastric cancer. Clinical study of growth and invasion patterns of early gastric cancer, its position in the natural history of gastric cancer. In: Inokuchi K, Murphy GP, Sugano H, Sugimura T, Veronesi U (eds) Gann monograph on cancer research, no. 11. Japan Scientific Societies, Tokyo, pp 67–79
7. Kusaba I (1983) Current status of surgery of gastric cancer and reflections on mass examination (in Japanese). Shokaki-shudankenshin 61:26–36
8. Haraguchi M, Okamura T, Korenaga D, Tsujitani S, Marin P, Sugimachi K (1987) Heterogeneity of DNA ploidy in patients with undifferentiated carcinomas of the stomach. Cancer 59:922–924
9. Korenaga D, Haraguchi M, Okamura T, Sugimachi K, Kaibara N, Koga S, Inokuchi K (1986) Consistency of DNA ploidy between primary and recurrent gastric carcinoma. Cancer Res 46:1544–1546
10. Korenaga D, Okamura T, Sugimachi Km Inokuchi K (1985) Prognostic study of intramucosal carcinoma of the stomach with DNA aneuploidy. Jpn J Surg 15:443–448
11. Okamura T, Korenaga D, Haraguchi M, Tsujitani S, Sugimachi K, Mori M, Enjoji M (1987) Growth mode and DNA ploidy in mucosal carcinomas of the stomach. Cancer 59:1154–1160
12. Kamegawa T, Okamura T, Sugimachi K, Inokuchi K (1986) Prognostic detection of a highly malignant type of early gastric carcinoma by cytophotometric DNA analysis. Jpn J Surg, 16:169–174

Staging of Gastric Cancer

B.J. Kennedy[1]

Key words. Gastric—Cancer—Staging—History—Classification—TNM

The TNM system for classification of tumors has become the principal method for determining prognosis for cancer patients and providing a reliable means for reporting results of treatments. Progress in the treatment of stomach cancer required the development and unification of the TNM system for tumor classification. Although a system had already been developed more than 40 years ago, attempts were made to unify and improve the various later emerging ones through a series of international meetings. Through this process of evolution, a unified international system for classification of stomach cancer was developed. It is to be expected that small variations in the classification system may occur that will result from additional data and improvements in technology in the future.

History

In 1966, the Union International Contra Cancer (UICC) published the first classification for stomach cancer. This was clinical by definition. In view of technical advances in diagnostic radiology and endoscopy, a revised clinical classification was published in 1968 [1]. The Japanese investigators contributed heavily to this development.

The American Joint Committee on Cancer (AJCC) was organized in 1959 for the purpose of developing a system of clinical staging of cancer by sites. In 1969, the Task Force on Stomach Cancer was established to develop a classification system for primary carcinoma of the stomach. A protocol for evaluating stomach cancer was developed utilizing a computer-based analysis for the first time by AJCC. Field trials were developed in seven institutions in North America and Hawaii, involving analysis of the records of 1241 patients. Criteria were selected

[1] Box 286, University of Minnesota Hospital and Clinics, Harvard Street at East River Road, Minneapolis, MN 55455, USA

for describing the primary tumor, regional lymph node involvement, and extent of distant metastases. Based on the extent of disease and duration of survival, a meaningful TNM classification was established by the AJCC. The basis for the staging system was the description of the degree of penetration of the stomach wall by the primary tumor at the time of initial diagnosis [2].

The AJCC report contended that stage classification was based on operative and histopathologic findings, and that a clinical classification was not feasible. As a consequence of this position, a round-table conference was held in Ottawa, Canada, where the UICC recommended a meeting to be held in Hawaii in 1975 and consist of representatives of the Japanese Cancer Committee (JCC), the AJCC, and the UICC. This group appeared to have established an amicable solution to the differences in staging systems, but, unfortunately, what was thought to be agreement was not. One of the primary differences was the contention by the Japanese group that a clinical staging system was essential. This was based on the superb gastrointestinal radiographic technique employed by them plus the use of ultrasound endoscopy to demonstrate the levels of penetration in the stomach wall. These sound arguments resulted in the subsequent acceptance of the need to provide a clinical classification as well as a histopathologic one.

In 1977 and 1978, the AJCC published revisions of its staging system in which the term "resected for cure" was introduced [3, 4]. In the subsequent 1983 report, this term was deleted because it was recognized not to be a specific description [5]. The 1983 staging system was further altered by the AJCC Writing Committee with changes in the T4 description and a requirement that for a tumor to be staged, the primary tumor must be removed. The members of the Task Force on Stomach Cancer did not concur with the decision of the Writing Committee and aired their disapproval. If that requirement were to be maintained, 50% of patients from the United States would be eliminated from the staging procedure. Furthermore, the classification became confusing in its terminology. Three phases of staging were developed: (1) clinical, (2) surgical evaluative, and (3) post-gastrectomy resection-pathologic. The linguistic interpretation of the words "gastrectomy" and "resection" had different meanings in different countries. The AJCC Task Force on Stomach Cancer proposed only two classifications, the clinical diagnostic and the anatomic extent-pathologic stages [6].

Using the Surveillance Epidemiology and End Results (SEER) population-based data, an evaluation of the AJCC stomach cancer system was made. These data represented approximately 10% of the United States population and consisted of 4785 patients available for survival analysis [7]. This study added new information to the AJCC system. The findings agreed with previous studies in the United States and Japan which showed the prognostic significance of depth of tumor invasion. A striking feature was the importance of age in the survival of patients. In Japan, 64% of patients with curative resections were under 60 years of age [8], compared with 28% in the SEER. Patients with lesions in the cardia or fundus had a poorer prognosis than those with tumors of the lesser curvature. The SEER findings had a major drawback in that there were no data on the location of lymph nodes with regard to distance from the primary lesion. With the additional information provided by this study and that of the Japanese, the feasibility of attaining an international system was recognized.

In September, 1983 at the First Cologne Symposium on Gastric Cancer, it was stressed that the UICC, AJCC, and JCC needed "to get their acts together and provide uniformity". In December, 1984, representatives of the UICC, AJCC, and JCC met again in Hawaii for the purpose of unification of a TNM classification. Based on 11 572 analyzed cases from 15 584 registered cases from 56 institutions, superb data were presented by the Japanese in support of a new proposal for stage classification [8]. With clarification and compromise, a unified staging system evolved. The clinical and pathologic stages were the same.

In January, 1985, the AJCC approved the revision of the Stomach Cancer Staging System as being unified at the meeting in Hawaii. Two major changes occurred: (1) in the future, the AJCC would have only two types of staging, clinical and pathologic, and (2) it was no longer required that the primary tumor had to be removed as a prerequisite to stage a gastric cancer.

Finally, at a meeting of the UICC in Geneva in May, 1985, agreement was reached to accept the unified staging system as presented [9, 10]. In 1988, both the publications of the UICC and AJCC contained the same staging classification for gastric cancer. The 1992 Fourth Edition of the Manual for Staging of Cancer of the AJCC continues the acceptance of this staging classification [11]. There will be continued debate regarding the International Classification Stage for Gastric Cancer, because the new classification divided Stage I into IA and IB. The IB category contained lymph node metastases (T1N1M0) [12]. However, the current UICC, AJCC, and JCC international agreement is reasonable. The following constitutes a reproduction of the Gastric Cancer Staging Classification System reprinted with the approval of the AJCC and the authors of the Manual for Staging of Cancer [11].

Principles for Classification

The classification defines the extent of disease in terms of three components: (1) the primary tumor, designated by the letter T and expressed in terms of the degree of penetration by the cancer through the stomach wall, (2) the regional lymph nodes, designated by the letter N, which are the perigastric lymph nodes and lymph nodes along the left gastric, common hepatic, splenic, and celiac arteries, and (3) distant metastasis, designated by the letter M.

For clinical classification, the primary tumor is always designated by the letters cT and for pathologic classification, by the letters pT. The description of the primary lesion is similar for the clinical and pathologic classifications. Similarly, the letters c and p are used in classifying the regional lymph nodes. For pathologic stage grouping of distant metastases, M1 may be either clinical (cM1) or pathologic (pM1).

As in most hollow organs, the prognosis of carcinomas of the stomach depends on the extent of penetration of the wall by the tumor and involvement of adjacent organs. Size, location, and the histologic type of cancer have not been found to be as useful for estimating prognosis. The overall prognosis for carcinomas of the stomach is poor. For reasons unknown, the incidence of stomach cancer has been declining since 1930 in most developed countries. Chronic atrophic gastritis is a predisposing factor. Nearly all carcinomas arise from the mucus-secreting cells of the gastric crypts.

Anatomy

Primary Sites

The stomach is the first division of the abdominal alimentary tract. Its first part is the *esophagogastric junction,* which lies immediately below the diaphragm and is often called the *cardia.* The upper part of the stomach is the *fundus,* and the lower

Table 1. Regional lymph nodes.

Inferior (right) gastric
  Greater curvature
  Greater omental
  Gastroduodenal
  Gastrocolic
  Gastroepiploic, right, or NOS
  Gastrohepatic
  Pyloric, including subpyloric and infrapyloric
  Pancreaticoduodenal (anteriorly along first
    part of the duodenum)
  Splenic
    Gastroepiploic, left
    Pancreaticolienal
    Peripancreatic
    Splenic hilar
Superior (left) gastric
  Lesser curvature
  Lesser omental
  Gastropancreatic, left
  Paracardia; cardial
  Cardioesophageal
  Perigastric; NOS
  Celiac
  Hepatic (excluding gastrohepatic)
Distant (all other lymph nodes)
  Retropancreatic
  Hepatoduodenal
  Aortic
  Portal
  Retroperitoneal
  Mesenteric

NOS, Not otherwise specified

part is the *antrum*. The pylorus is continuous with the duodenum. The shorter right border is the *lesser curvature* and the longer border on the left is the *greater curvature*. The *stomach wall* has five layers: mucosal, submucosal, muscular, subserosal, and serosal.

Metastatic Sites

Distant spread to the liver, lungs, and supraclavicular lymph nodes is common, although widespread visceral involvement can also occur. Frequently, there is direct extension to the liver, the transverse colon, the pancreas, or the diaphragm.

Rules for Classification

Clinical Staging

Designated as cTNM, clinical staging is based on evidence acquired before definitive treatment is instituted. It includes physical examination, imaging, endoscopy, biopsy, and other findings. All cases must be confirmed histologically.

Pathologic Staging

Pathologic staging depends on data acquired clinically along with results of surgical exploration and examination of the resected specimen or biopsy. Pathologic assessment of the regional lymph nodes entails removal of nodes adequate enough to validate the absence of metastasis and to evaluate the highest pN category. Metastatic nodules in the fat adjacent to the gastric carcinoma, without evidence of residual lymph node tissue, are considered regional lymph node metastases. If there is doubt concerning the correct T, N, or M assignment, the lower (less advanced) category should be selected. This guideline also applies to the stage grouping.

Table 2. Primary tumor (T): the principal factor is the degree of penetration of the stomach wall by carcinoma.

TX	Primary tumor cannot be assessed
TO	No evidence of primary tumor
Tis	Carcinoma in situ: intraepithelial tumor without invasion of the lamina propria
T1	Tumor invades lamina propria or subucosa
T2	Tumor invades the muscularis propria or the subserosa[a]
T3	Tumor penetrates the serosa (visceral peritoneum) without invasion of adjacent structures[bc]
T4	Tumor invades adjacent structures[bc]

[a] A tumor may penetrate the muscularis propria with extension into the gastrocolic or gastrohepatic ligaments or into the greater or lesser omentum without perforation of the visceral peritoneum covering these structures. In this case, the tumor is classified T2. If there is perforation of the visceral peritoneum covering the gastric ligaments or omenta, the tumor should be classified T3. [b] The adjacent structures of the stomach are the spleen, transverse colon, liver, diaphragm, pancreas, abdominal wall, adrenal gland, kidney, small intestine, and retroperitoneum. [c] Intramural extension to the duodenum or esophagus is classified by the depth of greatest invasion in any of these sites, including the stomach

Definition of TNM

Regional Lymph Nodes (N)

The principal factor is the distance of metastatic nodes from the primary tumor. The regional lymph nodes are the perigastric nodes along the lesser (1,3,5) and greater (2,4a,4b,6) curvatures (Fig. 1) and the nodes located along the left gastric (7) and common hepatic (8), splenic (10,11), and celiac arteries (9) (Fig. 2). Involvement of other intra-abdominal lymph nodes, such as hepatoduodenal (12) (Fig. 2), retropancreatic, mesenteric, and paraaortic, is classified as distant metastasis.

Note: The numerical order corresponds to the proposals of the Japanese Research Society for Gastric Cancer Study in Surgery and Pathology, the Japanese Journal of Surgery, Tokyo 11:127–145, 1982.

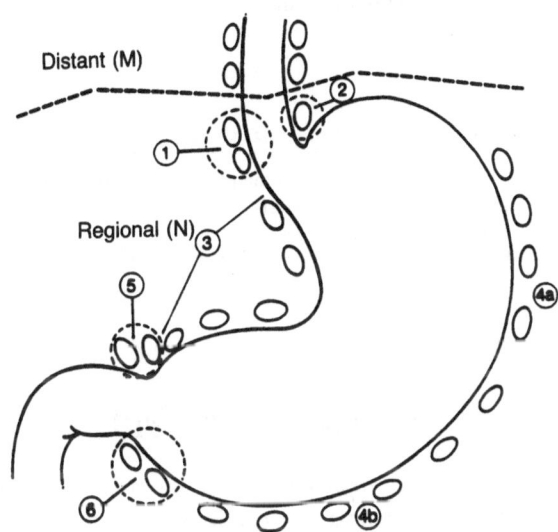

Fig. 1. Gastric regional lymph nodes. For identification of the *circled numbers*, see text. *M*, Metastasis; *N*, node. (From [11] with permission)

Table 3. Regional lumph nodes.

NX	Regional lymph node(s) cannot be assessed
N0	No regional lymph node metastasis
N1	Metastasis in perigastric lymph node(s) within 3 cm of the edge of the primary tumor
N2	Metastasis in perigastric lymph node(s) more than 3 cm from the edge of the primary tumor, or in lymph nodes along the left gastric, common hepatic, splenic, or celiac arteries

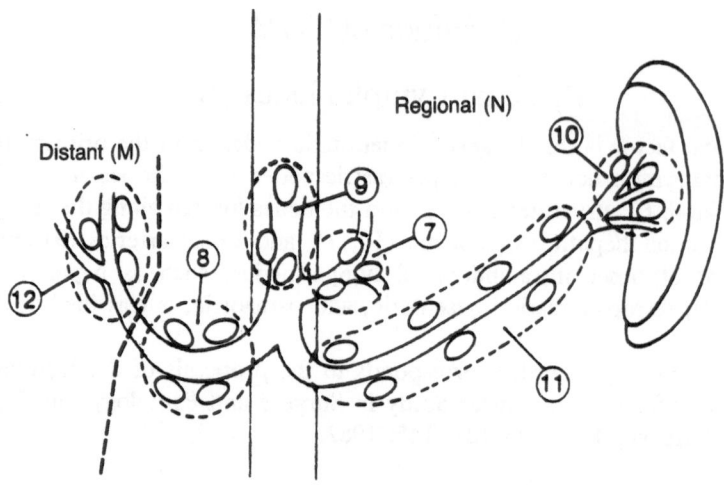

Fig. 2. Gastric regional lymph nodes. For identification of the *circled numbers*, see text. *M*, Metastasis; *N*, node. (From [11] with permission)

Table 4. Distant metastasis (M).

MX	Presence of distant metastasis cannot be assessed
M0	No distant metastasis
M1	Distant metastasis

Histopathologic Type

The staging recommendations apply only to carcinomas and not to other histologic types such as lymphomas, sarcomas, or carcinoid tumors. Adenocarcinomas may be divided into the subtypes intestinal, diffuse, and mixed.

Survival

The Commission on Cancer of the American College of Surgeons sponsored a study of 18 365 patients with gastric cancer treated in 1982 and 1987, based on data from over 700 tumor registries [13, 14]. The pathologic stage was defined in 11 087 patients. The disease-specific survival curve of these patients was recorded (Fig. 3). The survival of patients according to stage demonstrates the reliability of the current staging system. The 1982, 5-year survival of resected patients was compared to corresponding Japanese data [15]. The US study showed that gastric

Table 5. Stage grouping.

Stage 0	Tis	N0	M0
Statge IA	T1	N0	M0
Stage IB	T1	N1	M0
	T2	N0	M0
Stage II	T1	N1	M0
	T2	N1	M0
	T3	N0	M0
Stage IIIA	T2	N2	M0
	T3	N1	M0
	T4	N0	M0
Stage IIIB	T3	N2	M0
	T4	N1	M0
Stage IV	T4	N2	M0
	Any T	Any N	M1

Table 6. Histopathologic types.

Adenocarcinoma
Papillary adenocarcinoma
Tubular adenocarcinoma
Mucinous adenocarcinoma
Signet-ring cell carcinoma
Squamous cell carcinoma
Small cell carcinoma
Undifferentiated carcinoma

Table 7. Histopathologic grade (G).

GX	Grade cannot be assessed
G1	Well-differentiated
G2	Moderately differentiated
G3	Poorly differentiated
G4	Undifferentiated

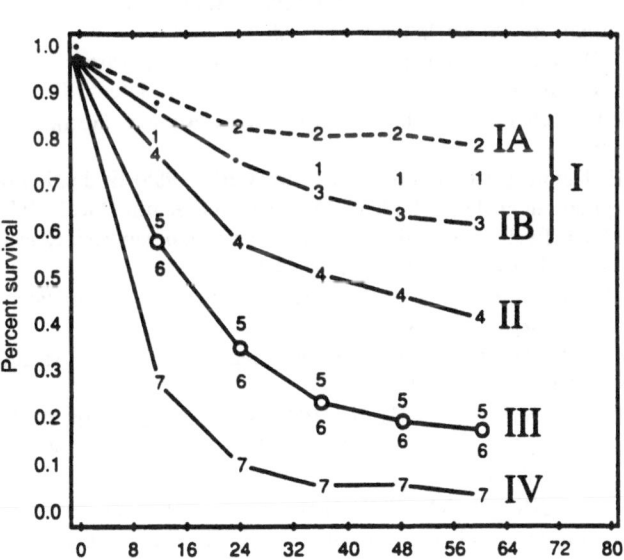

Fig. 3. Disease-specific survival in months according to pathologic stage in Patterns of Care study of the Commission on Cancer, American College of Surgeons Graph symbols: *1*, Stage 0; *2*, Stage Ia; *3*, Stage Ib; *4*, Stage II; *5*, Stage IIIa; *6*, Stage IIIb; *7*, Stage IV. (From [13, 14] with permission)

cancer is a disease of aging. Gastric cancer in the US presents at more advanced stages (76% at Stages III and IV) in contrast to the Japanese (42%). The survival of patients in the United States is poorer than in Japan. Delayed diagnosis, inadequate primary gastrectomy and lymph node dissection, and less detailed pathologic description may account for this impaired stage-related survival [14].

A system for classification of gastric cancer for purposes of staging has been developed. Proper classification and staging of cancer will allow the physician to determine treatment more appropriately, to evaluate results of management more reliably, and to compare worldwide statistics emerging from various institutions on a local, regional, and national basis more confidently. With international agreement regarding the system, investigators are encouraged to use the most recent (1992) definition of staging in reporting end results for gastric cancer.

References

1. UICC (1968) TNM classification of malignant tumors. UICC, Geneva
2. Kennedy BJ (1970) TNM classification for stomach cancer. Cancer 26:971–983
3. American Joint Committee on Cancer (1977) Stomach cancer. Manual for staging cancer. Lippincott, Philadelphia, pp 71–76
4. American Joint Committee on Cancer (1978) Stomach cancer. Manual for staging cancer. Lippincott, Philadelphia, pp 71–76
5. American Joint Committee on Cancer (1983) Stomach cancer. Manual for staging cancer. Lippincott, Philadelphia, pp 67–72
6. Kennedy BJ (1984) Staging problems in patients with gastric carcinoma: Surgical evaluation or anatomic extent. In: Rohde H, Troidl H (eds) Das Magenkarzinom. Methodik klinischer Studien und therapeutischer Ansätze. Georg Thieme, Stuttgart, pp 102–105
7. Curtis RE, Kennedy BJ, Myers MH, Hankey BF (1985) Evaluation of AJC stomach cancer staging: An analysis of 1275 SEER patients. Semin Oncol 12:21–31
8. Miwa K (1984) Evaluation of the TNM classification of stomach cancer for its rational stage-grouping. Jpn J Clin Oncol 14:385–410
9. Kennedy BJ (1987) Evolution of the international gastric cancer staging classification. Scand J Gastroenterol 22:8–10
10. Kennedy BJ (1987) The unified international gastric cancer staging classification system. Scand J Gastroenterol 22:11–13
11. American Joint Committee on Cancer (1992) Stomach cancer. In: Beahrs OH, Henson DE, Hutter RVP, Kennedy BJ (eds) Manual for staging cancer, 4th edn. Lippincott, Philadelphia, pp 63–66
12. Kim JP, Yang HK, Oh ST (1991) Comparison of survival curves of gastric cancer patients according to old, new and modified UICC classification. In: Proceedings of the Tenth Asia Pacific Cancer Conference. International Academic Publishers, Beijing, p 443
13. Kennedy BJ, Wanebo HJ (1991) US National survey of patterns of care for gastric cancer. In: Proceedings of the Tenth Asia Pacific Cancer Conference. International Academic Publishers, Beijing, p 443

14. Wanebo HJ, Kennedy BJ, Chimml J, Winchester D, Steel G (1992) Survey of patterns of care for gastric cancer in the United States. Proc Amer Soc Clin Oncol 11:166
15. Maruzama K, Okabayashi K, Kinoshita T (1987) Progress in gastric cancer surgery in Japan and its limits of radicality. World J Surg 11:418–425

Histogenesis of Gastric Carcinoma and Its Clinicopathological Significance

Kyoichi Nakamura[1]

Introduction

Microcarcinoma of the stomach and the mucosae neighboring it presents an incipient aspect of cancer development. Here, a carcinoma measuring less than 5 mm in diameter is defined as a microcarcinoma, and the neighboring mucosa of the microcarcinoma is defined as the interior area with a radius of 5 mm from center of the microcarcinoma [1–3]. It may be assumed that the histological aspects of microcarcinoma and the adjacent mucosae are simillar to the earliest stage of cancer development.

Histogenesis Deduced from Microcarcinoma

Microcarcinoma Measuring Less than 5 mm in Largest Diameter

Microcarcinomas, 145 in all, were histologically divided into 23 mucocellular and 122 tubular adenocarcinomas (Table 1) [4]. The majority of the microcarcinomas were discovered incidentally by histological examination of the major part of the stomach that was resected for benign lesions or small cancers. Histological examination for microcarcinoma is as follows: slices, 5–8 mm in width, were

Table 1. Histological type of microcarcinoma.

Mucocellular adenocarcinoma	23 foci
Tubular adenocarcinoma	122
Total	145 foci

[1] First Department of Pathology, School of Medicine, Tokyo Medical and Dental University, Yushima 1-5-45, Bunkyo-ku, Tokyo 113, Japan

Table 2. Back-ground lesion of micro-carcin-oma.

Large adenoma of intestinal type	2 foci	(1%)
Ulcer, and ulcer-scar	3	(2%)
Normal or atrophic mucosa	140	(97%)
Total	145 foci	(100%)

made parallel to the lesser curvature in the major part of the resected stomach, and each slice was cut into several compartments (cf. Fig. 10).

The great majority of the microcarcinomas (97%) had been found in the mucosa which was within normal limits or atrophied, and were independent of benign localized lesions such as ulcers or polyps (Table 2). It can be said, from the data obtained, that the great majority of gastric carcinomas arise immediately from normal or atrophic mucosa, independently of ulcers and adenoma [1–6].

Of 140 microcarcinomas independent of ulcers and adenomas, the mucocellular adenocarcinomas were surrounded by proper gastric mucosa, such as the pyloric and fundic gland mucosae, without intestinal metaplasia (Figs. 1–3), and the tubular adenocarcinomas were surrounded by metaplastic mucosa of intestinal type (Figs. 4–6), as shown in Table 3. A Chi-squared (χ^2) test was performed on

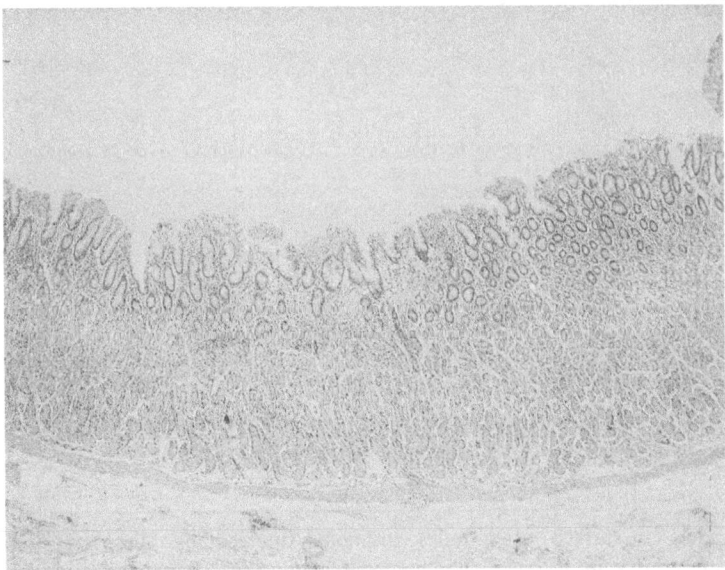

Fig. 1. A cut-surface of microcarcinoma incidentally discovered, measuring approximately 1 mm in diameter. Cancer cells exist in the fundic gland mucosa essentially within normal limits, and are localized on the top half of the mucosa. The major part of the glandular necks disappear. (H&E)

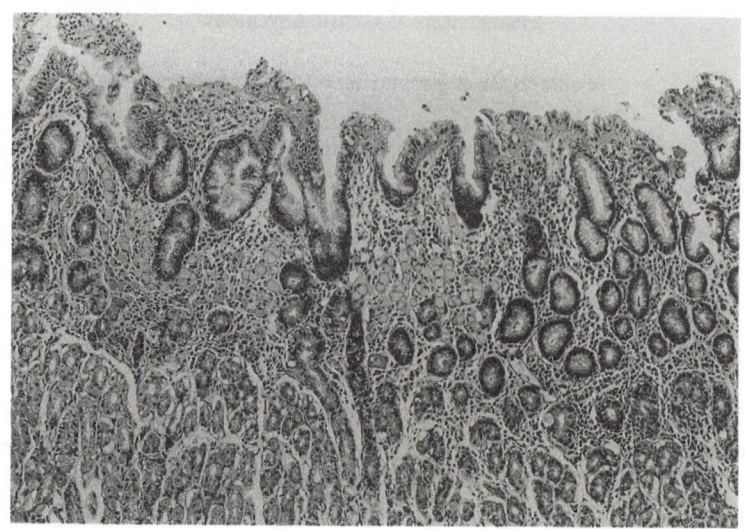

Fig. 2. A high-power view of the microcarcinoma shown in Fig. 1. Histological type is mucocellular adenocarcinoma. Those cells are localized at the propria mucosae. (H&E)

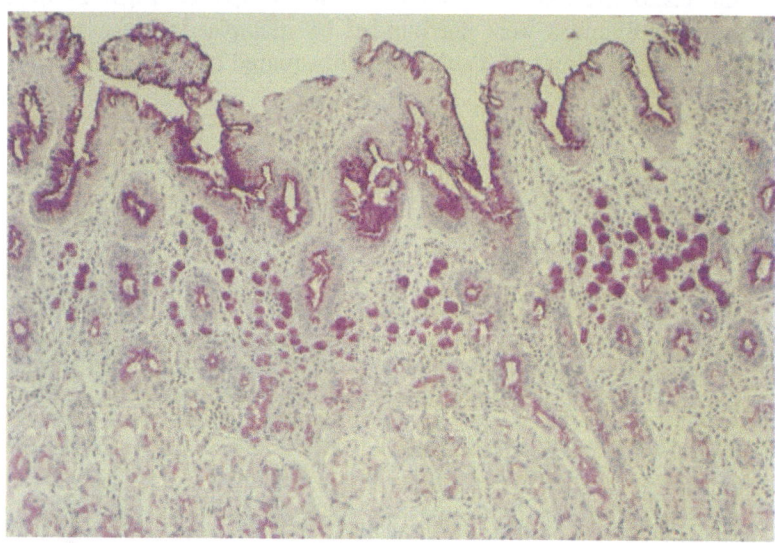

Fig. 3. Periodic acid-schiff (PAS) stain of the mucocellular adenocarcinoma shown in Fig. 2. Cytoplasms of cancer cells are deeply stained with PAS. (H&E)

Fig. 4. The cut-surface of a microcarcinoma incidentally discovered, measuring approximately 1 mm in diameter. The microcarcinoma exists at metaplastic mucosa of the intestinal type. Histological type is tubular adenocarcinoma, and carcinomatous tubules occupy whole layer of the mucosa in thickness. Number of the carcinomatous tubuli situated at lower half of the mucosa is larger than that at the top half. (H&E)

Fig. 5. A high-power view of the tubular adenocarcinoma shown in Fig. 4. Carcinomatous tubules proliferate like tree buds (*arrow*). (H&E)

Table 3. Histological type of microcarcinoma and grade of intestinal metaplasia of the neighboring mucosa.

Grade of intestinal metaplasia	Histological type	
	Tubular adenoca	Mucocellular adenoca
Prominent	97	0 foci
Focal	22	4
None	1	16
Total	120	20 foci

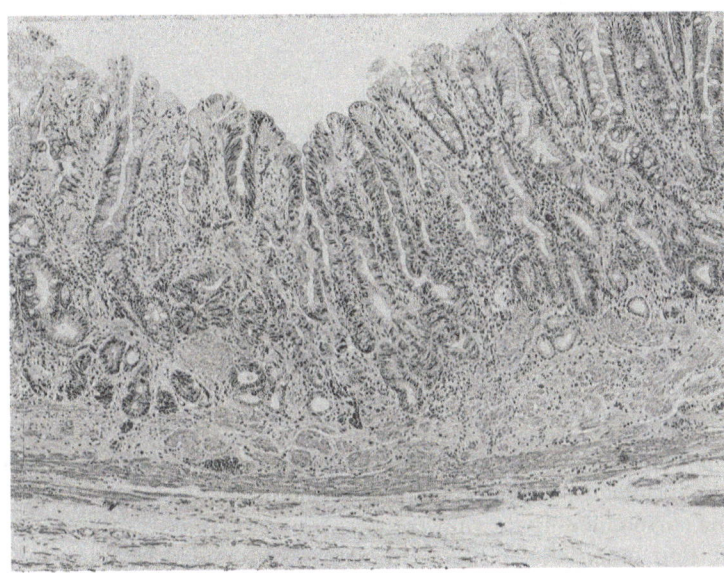

Fig. 4

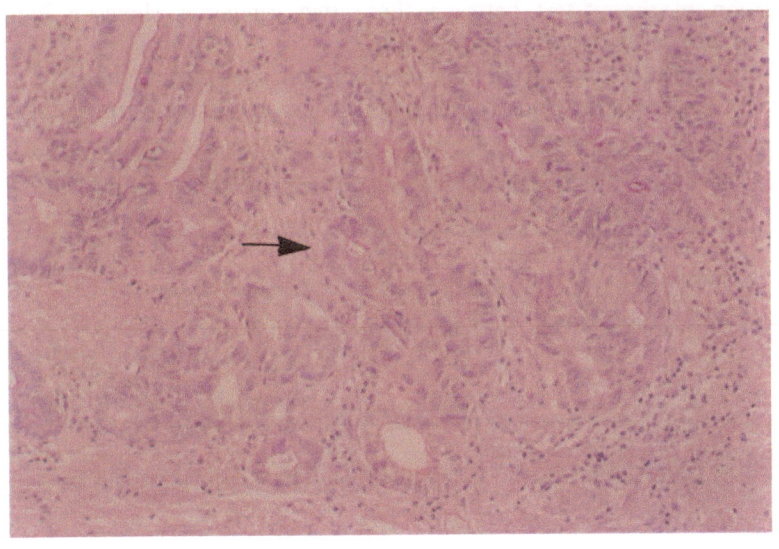

Fig. 5

K. Nakamura

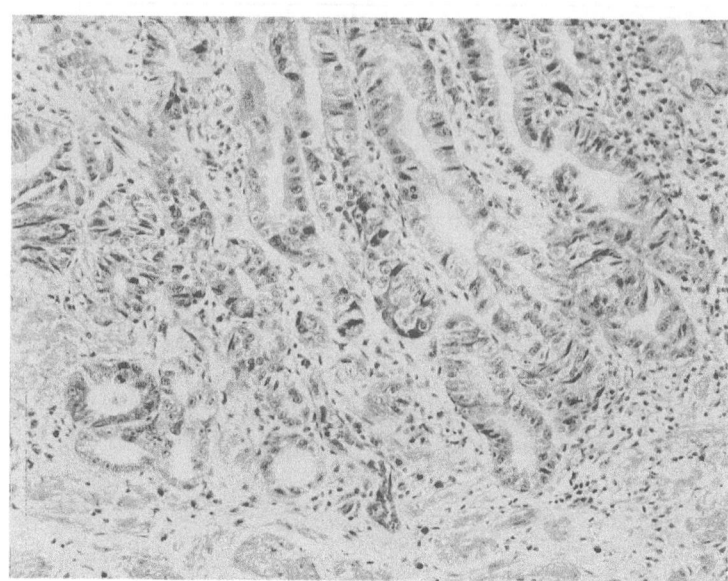

Fig. 6. PAS staining of the tubular adenocarcinoma shown in Fig. 4. Striated border is
seen as red line at free surface of the cancerous tubuli. (H&E)

the relationship between the grade of intestinal metaplasia on the neighboring
mucosae and the histological type of the microcarcinomas in Table 3. One tubular
adenocarcinoma surrounded by the proper gastric mucosa ("None") was added to
"Focal", while four mucocellular adenocarcinomas surrounded by mucosa with
focal metaplasia ("Focal") were added to "Prominent", as shown in Table 4.
Despite those operations where the tendency obtained from Table 3 was worse,
the application of the χ^2-test between those two categories shows a highly
significant difference (P < 0.01) (Table 4) [4].

Cells of mucocellular adenocarcinomas contain mucin in their cytoplasms and
don't have brush borders (Fig. 3). Mucin is generally stained with periodic

Table 4. Application of Chi-squared test between two
categories shown in Table 3.

Grade of intestinal metaplasia	Histological type	
	Tubular adenoca	Mucocellular adenoca
Prominent	97	4 foci
None	23	16
Total	120	20 foci

χ^2 = 28.6 (Yates correction)
χ^2 (1, 0.01) = 6.635
$P = 0$

acid-schiff (PAS) stain and not, or faintly, with Alcian Blue. Mucocellular adenocarcinoma cells are similar to the mucous cells of the foveolar epithelium and the cells of pyloric glands in cell function and structure [2–4, 7]. Meanwhile, cells of tubular adenocarcinomas have brush borders on their free surface, and generally don't produce mucin (Fig. 6). These are similar to absorptive cells of metaplastic epithelium of the intestinal type [3, 4, 7–9]. Based on the findings mentioned previously, it may be concluded that the mucocellular adenocarcinoma arises from the proper gastric mucosa and tubular adenocarcinoma from metaplastic mucosa of the intestinal type [2–5].

Microcarcinoma Measuring less than 2 mm in Largest Diameter

It is clear that cancer cells of the stomach develop from mutations within the mitotic zones of cell renewal in the glandular epithelium. The mitotic zones of cell renewal in the proper gastric glands are situated at the neck portions of the glands, and those of metaplastic tubules of the intestinal type are located at the lower half of the tubule [10, 11]. Therefore, it can be presumed that cells of microcarcinoma having just developed exist mainly around the mitotic zones, since cancer cells develop by mutation in these zones.

Thirty-six microcarcinomas, measuring less than 2 mm in largest diameter, were histologically studied by serial sectioning of paraffin blocks. In addition, their size, measuring less than 2 mm in largest diameter, was estimated as follows: when a microcarcinoma measuring less than 2 mm in largest diameter was revealed by histological examination of the resected stomachs, its size was confirmed by serial sectioning of another paraffin block including it [12].

Twenty-one microcarcinomas out of the 36 were mucocellular adenocarcinomas and the remaining 15 were tubular adenocarcinomas. These microcarcinomas were histologically not erosive. The surface of the mucocellular adenocarcinomas were almost covered with foveolar epithelium, and the tubular adenocarcinomas consisted of carcinomatous epithelium [12–14]. All the mucocellular and tubular adenocarcinomas were situated at the proper gastric mucosa and metaplastic mucosa of the intestinal type respectively (Table 5) [4, 12, 13].

Table 6 shows the location of the 21 mucocellular adenocarcinomas of the

Table 5. Back ground mucosae of micro-carcinoma measuring less than 2 mm in diameter.

Proper gastric mucosa:	21 foci
Fundic gland mucosa	14
Pyloric gland mucosa	7
Metaplastic mucosa of intestinal type:	15
Total	36 foci

Table 6. Location of microcarcinoma measuring less than 2 mm in diameter.

— Mucocellular adenocarcinoma —

Location	Mucosa		Total
	Fundic gland	Pyloric gland	
Superficial half layer	14 (100%)	4 (57%)	18 (86%)
Almost whole layer	0 (0%)	3 (43%)	3 (14%)
Total	14 (100%)	7 (100%)	21 (100%)

Table 7. Ratio of carcinomatous tubuli at the lower half to the top-half of the mucosal layer in tubular adenocarcinoma measuring less than 2 mm in diameter.

Appearance of ca. in cut-surface	Mean of ratio	SD
Flat	3.1	1.2
Slightly depressed	2.3	0.5
Metaplastic mucosa	1.5	

the top half of the proper gastric mucosa (Figs. 1–3), and only 3 foci occupied the top two-thirds or almost the whole layer of the pyloric gland mucosa. These carcinomatous cells existed mainly in the lamina propria mucosae, and those limited to the glands were very rare. Furthermore, the number of neck portions of proper gastric glands at the mucosa affected with carcinomatous cells decreased remarkably in comparison with that of the neighboring mucosa. In other words, cancer cells proliferate at the mucosal layer where the neck portions of the proper gastric glands exist. Based on the findings mentioned previously, it can be concluded that cells of mucocellular adenocarcinomas arise from the neck portions of the proper gastric glands.

On the other hand, the 15 tubular adenocarcinomas completely occupied the whole layer of metaplastic mucosa of the intestinal type, on which carcinomatous tubuli, limited to the lower half of the mucosa, were larger than those limited to the top half, as shown in Table 7 [3, 13, 14]. The ratio of carcinomatous tubuli on the lower half to that on the top half is 2 or 3. Those findings may indicate that carcinomatous tubuli don't proliferate by replacement of preexisting metaplastic tubuli, but do mainly at the lower half of the metaplastic mucosa like tree buds (Figs. 4–6). This is the reason why the ratio of tubular numbers at the lower half to the top half in metaplastic mucosa is 1 or 1.5. Namely, it means that metaplastic mucosa is generally composed of single tubules or that one foveola bifurcates into two tubules.

These findings show that cells of the tubular adenocarcinomas develop at the lower half of metaplastic tubules and proliferate mainly in the lower half of the mucosa by making newly carcinomatous tubuli.

Table 8. Summary of histological findings of microcarcinoma.

	Mucocellular adenoca	Tubular adenoca
Localisation:		
3–5 mm ca.	Proper gastric mucosa	Metaplastic mucosa of intestinal type
less 2 mm ca.	Upper 1/2 layer of proper gastric mucosa	Almost whole layer of metaplastic mucosa
Cancer cells:		
Mucus product	(+)	(−)
Brush border	(−)	(+)

Histogenesis Deduced from Microcarcinomas

Table 8 shows a summary of the histological findings observed in studies of microcarcinomas of the stomach. These findings obtained lead to the following conclusion about histogenesis of gastric carcinoma: mucocellular adenocarcinoma develops from the proper gastric mucosa, and tubular adenocarcinoma from metaplastic mucosa of the intestinal type, independently of ulcers or adenoma (Fig. 7). The major part of the proper gastric mucosae surrounding the mucocellular adenocarcinomas was atrophied or within normal limits. The surrounding mucosae were not affected with inflammatory round cell infiltration of a severe degree, histologically diagnosed as chronic gastritis. The gastric mucosae harboring the microcarcinomas were generally within normal limits, independently of chronic atrophied gastritis [6].

Microcarcinomas are histogenetically classified into two categories, undifferentiated and differentiated carcinomas, in the morphological departure from the structure of the normal mucosa [3–5]. Namely, it is morphologically interpreted that tubular adenocarcinomas are cylindrical cells which are of a tubular structure and are similar to the normal mucosa, and mucocellular adenocarcinomas are small cells individually spread and/or sometimes show cord-like arrangement and are far removed from the normal mucosa in structure. A histological picture of the section is a complicated design made up of cancer cells. When the complicated design is extremely simplified, the design of the undifferentiated and differentiated carcinomas can be shown to be the essential difference. This is because, after such simplification, the undifferentiated

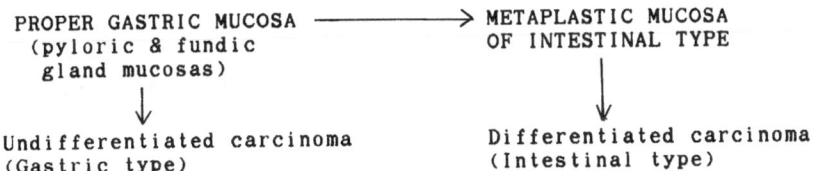

Fig. 7. The histogenesis of gastric carcinoma

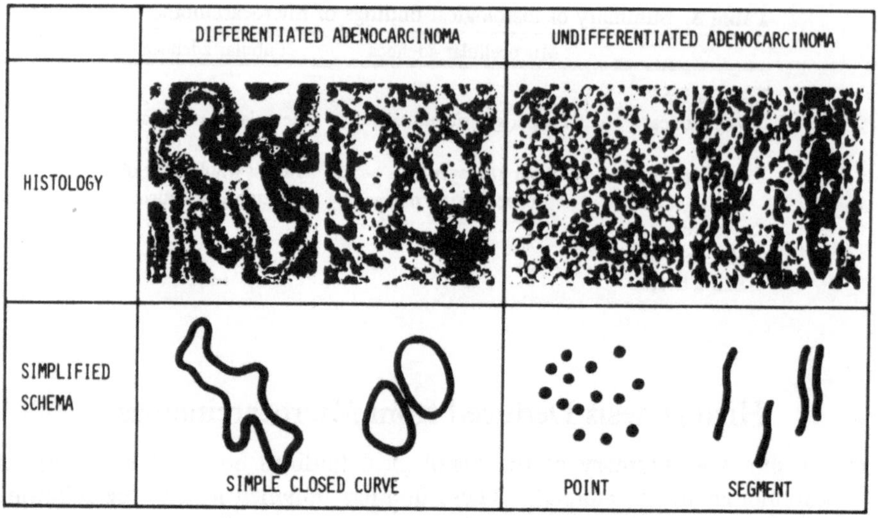

Fig. 8. Extreme simplification of the undifferentiated and differentiated carcinomas

carcinoma can be considered as a point or segment, whereas the differentiated carcinoma can be seen as a simple closed curve (Fig. 8). According to Jordan's theorem in topology, a simple closed curve divides a plane into interior and exterior areas, but a point and segment do not have this character. Carcinoma not forming tubuli in the mucosa is defined as the undifferentiated carcinoma, while carcinoma forming tubuli is refered to as differentiated carcinoma. This histological classification of gastric carcinoma is very simple, and pattern perception is objective and easy for interpreting the histological type.

Evidence Supporting the Histogenesis of Carcinoma of a Common Size

It becomes necessary to examine whether the histogenesis of gastric carcinoma deduced from the microcarcinomas do not conflict with the results of carcinoma of a common size, because the microcarcinoma is a specific state in the development of carcinoma. Here are two pieces of evidence supporting the histogenesis of carcinoma of a common size.

Relationship Between Histological Type of Carcinoma and the Grade of Intestinal Metaplasia in the Stomach Harboring It

The relationship between histological types of carcinomas and grade of intestinal metaplasia has been studied on 293 resected stomachs harboring an intramucosal

Table 9. Grade of intestinal metaplasia and histological type of intra-mucosal carcinoma measuring more than 0.6 cm in diameter.

Grade of intestinal metaplasia	Histological type		Total
	Undifferentiated	Differentiated	
Nil to Slight	69	8	77 cases
	(37.8)	(39.2)	
Moderate to Marked	75	141	216
	(106.2)	(109.8)	
Total	144	149	293 cases

( ): Theoretically expected frequency
$X^2 = 68.62$, $X^2 (1, 0.01) = 6.635$, $P = 0$

carcinoma measuring more than 0.6 cm in diameter (Table 9) [4, 5]. There was a tendency for intramucosal carcinoma in stomachs with mild intestinalization to belong to the undifferentiated type. In cases with moderate to marked intestinalization, intramucosal carcinomas belongs to the differentiated type in many instances. The frequency of mild intestinalization differs little in undifferentiated carcinoma, but is slightly greater than that of the marked intestinalization. The majority of stomachs having the differentiated carcinoma tend to show marked intestinalization. In the relationship between the histological type and the grade of intestinalization, application of the chi-square (χ^2) test yielded a P value of less than 0.01. However, about a half of the undifferentiated carcinomas existed in the stomachs with marked intestinalization. Although this finding seems to conflict with the histogenesis, it is a natural consequence, when the shifting of F-boundary line with increasing age is taken into account. In other words, as time passes, cancer increases in size, and intestinal metaplasia becomes severe. The F-boundary line (F-line) is the border of the fundic gland mucosa area without intestinal metaplasia. The F-line

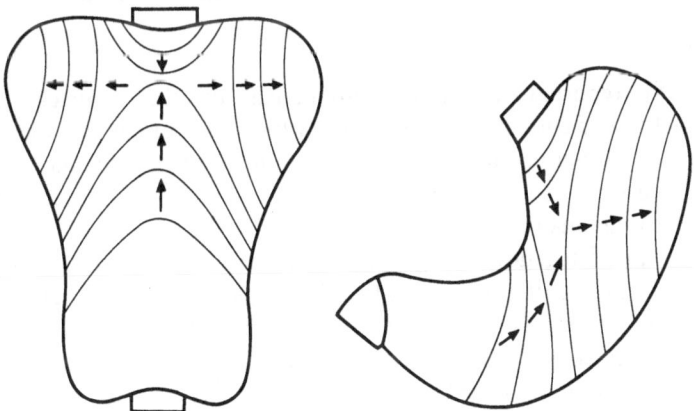

Fig. 9. Shifting of F-boundary line with increasing age

shifts, reducing the interior area it encircles with increasing age, and the shifting of the F-line is generally irreversible (Fig. 9) [5, 6, 15, 16].

Carcinomas from the Fundic Gland Mucosa Without Intestinal Metaplasia

It is clear that carcinomas situated at the interior area of the F-boundary line arose from the fundic gland mucosa, regardless of their size, because the interior encircled by the F-boundary line consists of the fundic gland mucosa without intestinal metaplasia, and shifting of the F-boundary line with increasing age is irreversible. According to the histogenesis deduced from the microcarcinoma, the carcinomas having arisen from the fundic gland mucosa should be histologically of the undifferentiated type.

Table 10. Histological type of carcinoma completely limited to the fundic gland mucosa without intestinal metaplasia.

Mucocellular adenocarcinoma	196 cases (99%)
Tubular adenocarcinoma	2 cases (1%)
Total	198 cases

Table 10 shows the histological type of carcinomas completely limited to the fundic gland mucosa without intestinal metaplasia. Of those carcinomas, 99% were the undifferentiated type, independent of their size (Figs. 10–12). This result decisively demonstrates that the undifferentiated carcinoma arises from the proper gastric mucosa [4, 5, 17].

Review of the Literature on Minute Carcinoma and Histogenesis

Mallory [18] reported 4 minute carcinomas of the stomach measuring approximately 1–5 cm in diameter, in which he discussed ulcer cancer. Murakami [19] reported on a few foci of tubular microcarcinomas that were incidentally encountered by routine histological examination of resected stomachs harboring a carcinoma of common size.

In regard to histogenesis of gastric carcinomas, Järvi and Lauren [8, 7], Morson [20], and Ming et al. [9] have suggested that a certain tubular adenocarcinoma may arises from metaplastic epithelium of the intestinal type. However, they have not been referring to the histogenesis of mucocellular and scirrhous adenocarcinomas. Nakamura, et al. [1, 2] reported on 33 foci of gastric microcarcinomas, and mentioned that carcinomas without and with tubular formation at the mucosa may arise from the proper gastric mucosa and the

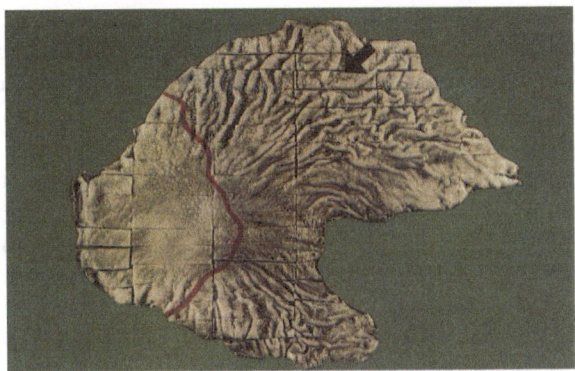

Fig. 10. A resected stomach harboring a carcinoma situated at the fundic gland mucosa without intestinal metaplasia (*arrow*). The carcinoma measures approximately 1x1 cm in dimension. A solid line means F-boundary line limited to the fundic gland mucosa without intestinal metaplasia

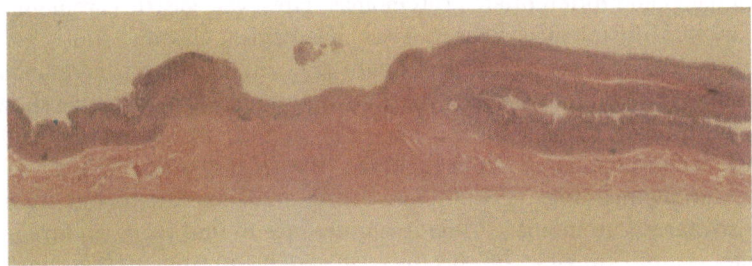

Fig. 11. A cut-surface of the carcinoma shown in Fig. 10. The carcinoma is completely surrounded by the fundic gland mucosa without intestinal metaplasia. Cancer cells infiltrate the submucosa diffusely, proper muscle and subserosa with marked desmoplasia. (H&E)

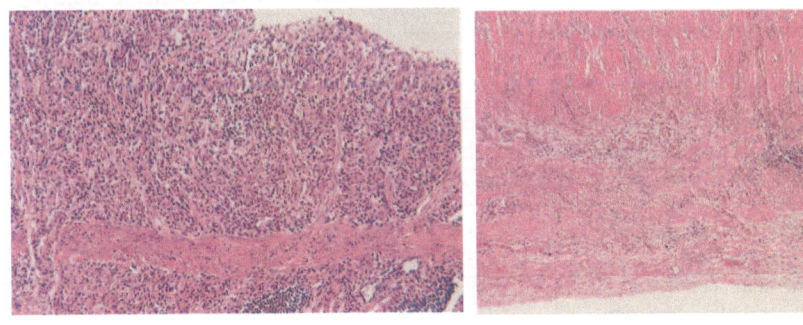

Fig. 12a,b. High-power view of the carcinoma in Fig. 11. Histological type of the carcinoma is undifferentiated carcinoma in the mucosal spreading portion (**a**), and carcinomatous cells infiltrating scirrhously in the submucosa are also seen (scirrhous adenocarcinoma) (**b**). (H&E)

metaplastic mucosa of the intestinal type respectively. Nagayo [21] also studied histogenesis of gastric carcinomas using microcarcinomas, and mentioned that there was a tendency for mucocellular adenocarcinomas to be situated at the proper gastric mucosa and tubular adenocarcinomas to be situated at the metaplastic mucosa of the intestinal type.

Recently, many microcarcinomas of the stomach have been preoperatively diagnosed in Japan [4]. Generally speaking, the majority of them have been discovered as a minute lesion of Type IIc + IIa or Type IIc by endoscopical and radiological examinations and the diagnosis of microcarcinoma has been finally made by biopsy examination.

Histological Typing of Gastric Carcinomas Based on Their Histogenesis

On the basis of the histogenesis deduced from studies of microcarcinomas mentioned previously, the gastric carcinoma is essentially divided into two types, undifferentiated and differentiated carcinomas. However, gastric carcinomas have a large variety of histological figures. Their histological classification is generally done with a predominant histological figure [22, 23]. Advanced carcinomas are histologically classified into several types, but intramucosal carcinomas show only 3 histological types similar to the microcarcinomas, as shown in Table 11. Scirrhous adenocarcinomas, muconodular adenocarcinomas (Figs. 13–16), medullary carcinomas (Figs. 17–20), and adenosquamous carcinomas are usually found as advanced carcinomas, while it is quite rare to find them as intramucosal carcinomas [4, 5]. In view of this fact, it can be presumed that those four histological types are secondarily modified figures which appear as the result of infiltration of carcinoma in tissues other than the mucosa. Those four histological types of advanced carcinomas can be classified into either undifferentiated or differentiated carcinomas in areas where only the mucosa is involved (Table 12) (Figs. 13–20). The majority of scirrhous adenocarcinomas representing 88.2%, shows the undifferentiated type in the mucosal spreading portion (Table 13).

Table 11. Incidence of histological types in advanced and intra-mucosal carcinomas of the stomach.

	Advanced carcinoma	Intramucosal carcinoma
Papillotubular adenoca.	215	40 cases
Tubular adenoca.	238	109
Scirrhous adenoca.	493	—
Mucocellular adenoca.	—	144
Medullary adenoca.	33	—
Muconodular adenoca.	40	—
Adenosquamous ca.	2	—
Total	1021	293 cases

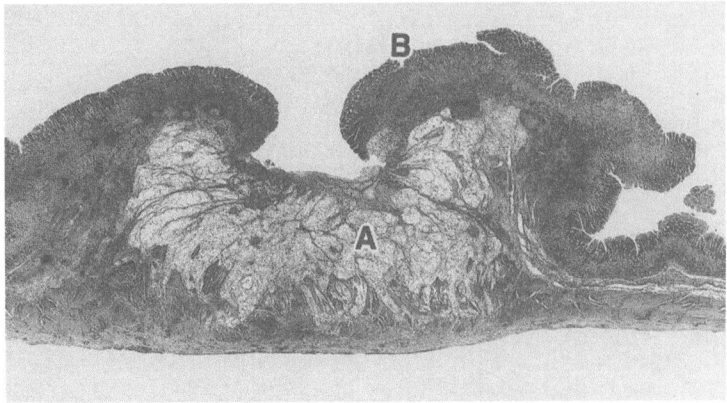

Fig. 13. The cut-surface of muconodular adenocarcinoma. The carcinoma shows histo-logically muconodular type (*A*) in the gastric wall except for the mucosa (*B*). (H&E)

Table 12. Histological types of intramucosal spreading portion of carcinoma classified by predominant figure.

Predominant figure	Histological type in mucosa		Total
	Undifferentiated	Differentiated	
Medullary adenoca.	31 (34%)	60 (66%)	91 cases
Muconodular adenoca.	34 (61%)	22 (39%)	56
Adenosquamous ca.	1 (50%)	1 (50%)	2

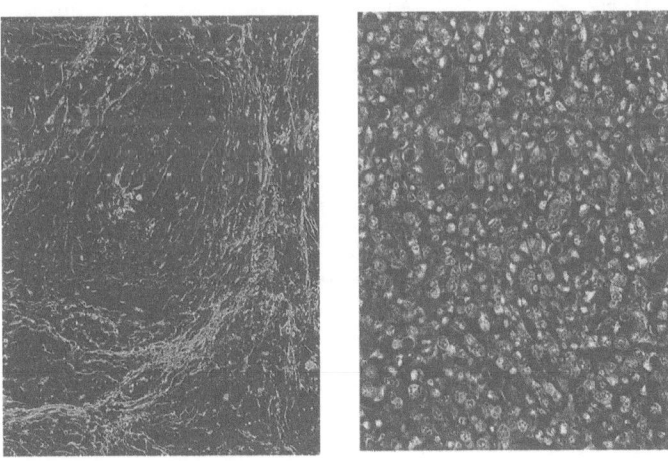

Fig. 14a,b. High-power view of the carcinoma shown in Fig. 13. **a** Muconodular adeno-carcinoma. **b** Undifferentiated carcinoma in the mucosa (mucocellular adenocarcinoma). (H&E)

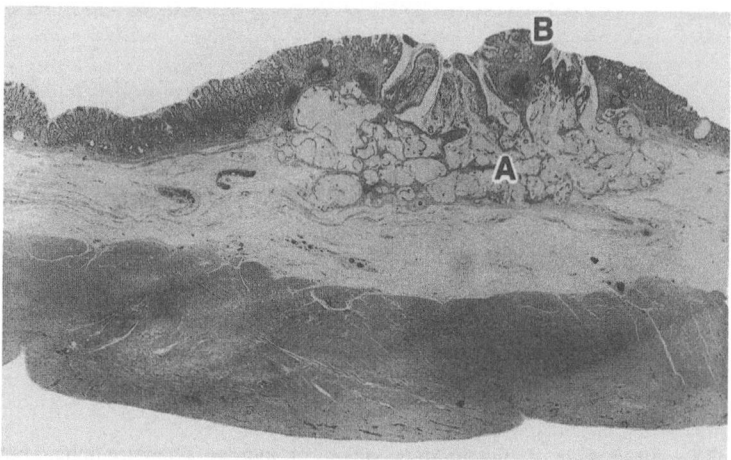

Fig. 15. The cut-surface of muconodular adenocarcinoma. The carcinoma shows histologically muconodular type (*A*) in the gastric wall except for the mucosa (*B*). (H&E)

Table 13. Morphological changes of undifferentiated carcinoma by invasion to the gastric wall other than the mucosa.

Histological type in the mucosa	Predominant figure in the gastric wall		
Undifferentiated ca. 559 cases (100%)	Scirrhous adenoca.	493 cases	(88.2%)
	Muconodular adenoca.	34	(6.1%)
	Medullary adenoca.	31	(5.5%)
	Adenosquamous ca.	1	(0.2%)

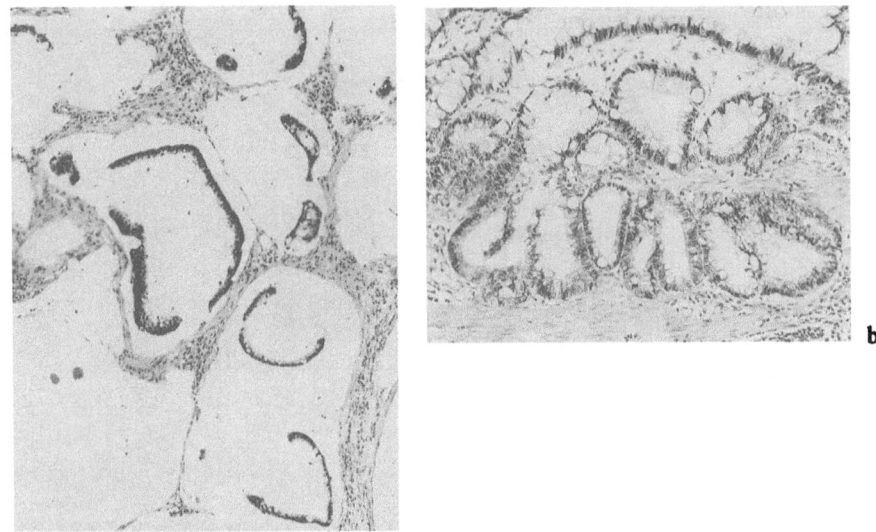

Fig. 16a,b. High-power view of the carcinoma shown in Fig. 15. **a** Muconodular adeno-carcinoma, **b** differentiated carcinoma in the mucosa (tubular adenocarcinoma). (H&E)

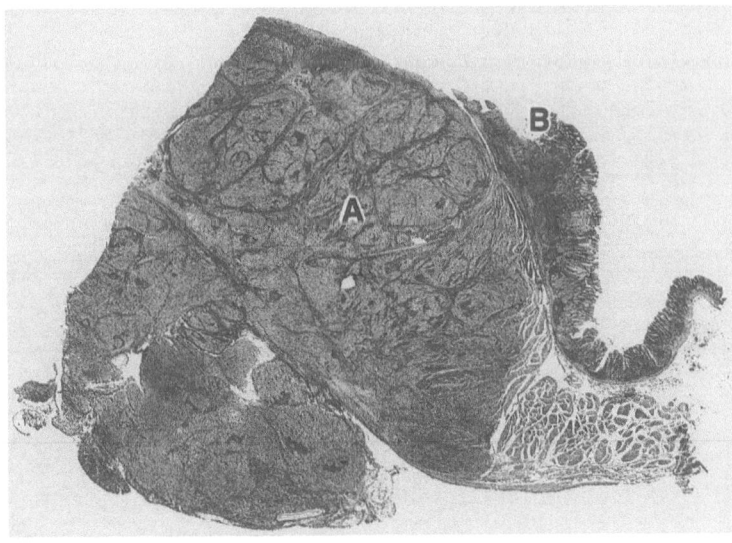

Fig. 17. The cut-surface of medullary carcinoma. Histological figure is medullary carcinoma (*A*) in the gastric wall except for the mucosa (*B*). (H&E)

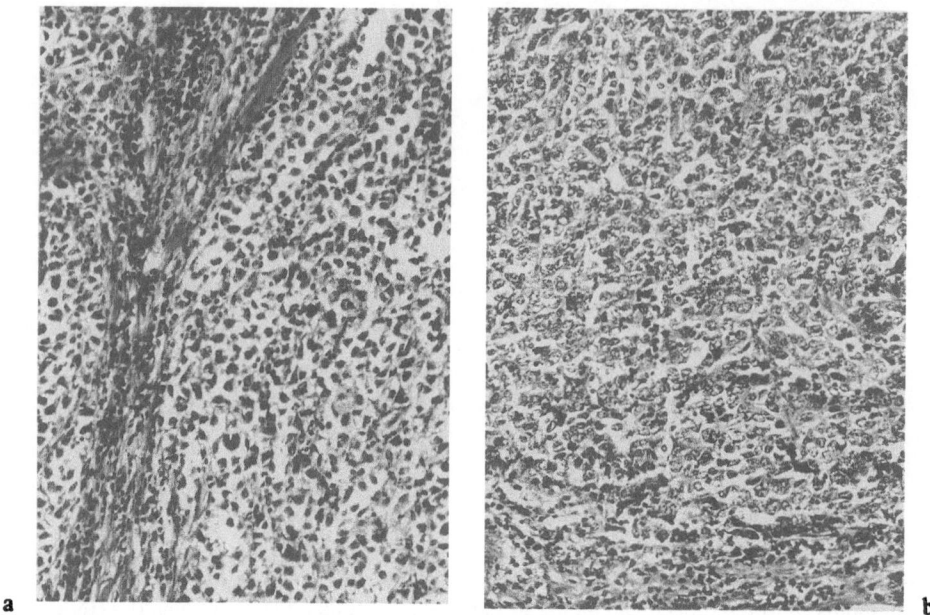

a   b

Fig. 18a,b. High-power view of the carcinoma shown in Fig. 17. **a** Medullary carcinoma, **b** undifferentiated carcinoma in the mucosa (mucocellular adenocarcinoma). (H&E)

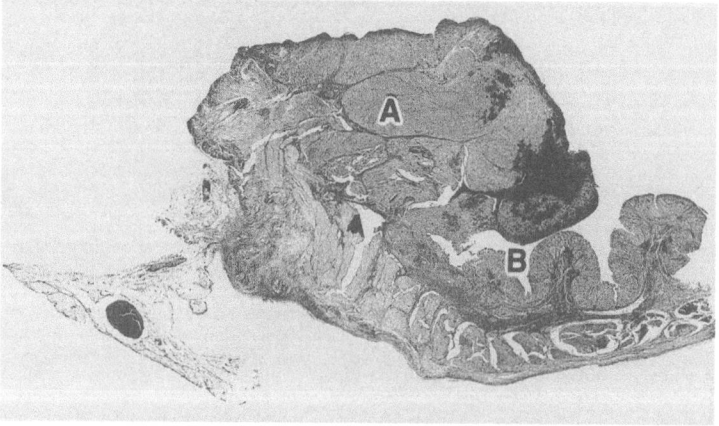

Fig. 19. The cut-surface of medullary carcinoma. Histological figure is medullary carcinoma (A) in the gastric wall except for the mucosa (B). (H&E)

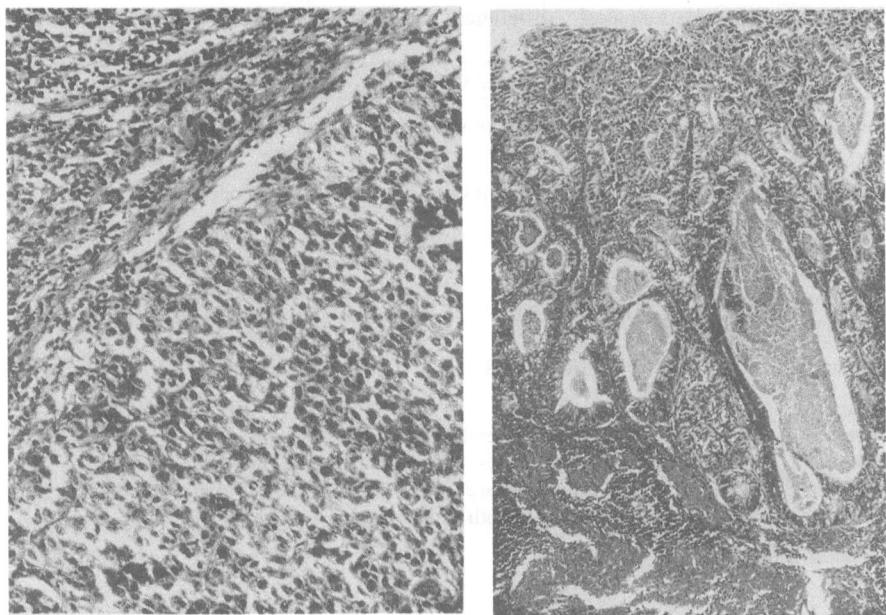

a   b

Fig. 20a,b. High-power view of the carcinoma shown in Fig. 19. a Medullary carcinoma, b differentiated carcinoma in the mucosa (tubular adenocarcinoma). (H&E)

From the histogenesis view point, histological typing of the gastric carcinoma should be classified into two types of carcinoma spreading the mucosa, undifferentiated and differentiated types. Because, if the histological typing of the gastric carcinoma is done with a predominant figure, the histological type of a certain carcinoma is renamed with cancer growth, despite of the same carcinoma. That is a strange logic in the histological classification of the gastric carcinoma.

Biopsy specimens of gastric carcinomas are generally taken from their mucosal spreading portion, and the majority of their histological types can be classified into undifferentiated and differentiated carcinomas. Furthermore, clinico-pathological differences between them are found in various points, as shown in Table 14. Therefore, histological typing of the gastric carcinoma should be principally classified in its mucosal spreading portion into the two categories.

Generally speaking, undifferentiated carcinomas and differentiated carcinomas that have been histogenetically divided by the studies of the microcarcinomas correspond respectively to the mucous cell carcinoma and intestinal cell carcinoma according to Mulligan and Rember [24], to diffuse carcinoma and intestinal-type carcinoma by Järvi and Lauren [7, 8, 25], and to infiltrating carcinoma and expanding carcinoma by Ming [26] (Table 15). However, expression of their nomenclatures is not adequate for carcinoma in the early phase, because spreading of the carcinoma in the mucosa neither infiltrates diffusely, nor develops expansively.

Table 14. Clinicopathological differences of undifferentiated and differentiated carcinoma [4, 5].

	Undifferentiated Carcinoma	Differentiated Carcinoma
Histogenesis	arising from the proper gastric mucosa	arising from mucosa of intestinal type
Histological figure in the mucosa	Mucocellular adenoca.	Tubular adenoca.
Macroscopic type:		
Early	Depressed (IIc, IIc + III)	Depressed or protruded (IIc, IIc + III, IIc + IIa) (IIa, IIa + IIc, I)
Advanced	Borrmann IV, III	Borrmann II, I, III
Macroscopic appearance of IIc, IIc + III:		
Area	Erosive with several islets	Smooth
Depth	Deeper	Shallow
Margin	Suddenly depressed, clear, relatively smooth	Gradually depressed, unclear, serrated
Metastasis to the liver:		
	Less frequent, Diffuse, Via periportal lymphatics	More frequent, Multiple nodular, Via portal vein
Metastasis to the lung:		
	Lymphangitis carcinomatosa, Lymphogenous spread (Via peribronchial lymphatics)	Disseminated nodules, Hematogenous spread (Via left vein angle)
Peritoneal carcinomatosis	(+)	(−)
Jaundice	Slight	Severe
Ascites fluid	Severe (caused by peritoneal carcinomatosis)	Slight (caused by portal hypertension)
Age, Sex	Younger, Female	Older, Male
Post-operative 5-year survival rate:		
Early	95%	85%
Advanced		
Up to 4 cm size and the subserosa involved	85%	60%
Up to 4 cm size and the serosa involved	58%	50%
More than 4 cm size and the subserosa involved	78%	65%
More than 4 cm size and the serosa involved	27%	38%

Table 15. Histological typing of gastric carcinoma.

Histological typing of gastric carcinoma

Järvi, O. and Lauren, P. (1951, 1965):
1) Intestinal-type carcinoma
2) Diffuse carcinoma
3) Undifferentiated solid carcinoma without mucous production

Mulligan, R. M. and Rember, R. R. (1954):
1) Intestinal cell carcinoma
2) Pylorocardiac carcinoma
3) Mucous cell carcinoma

Nakamura, K. and Sugano, H. (1968):
1) Differentiated carcinoma (Intestinal type)
2) Undifferentiated carcinoma (Gastric type)

Ming, Si-C. (1977):
1) Expanding type
2) Infiltrative type

References

1. Nakamura K, Sugano H, Takagi K, Fuchigami A (1966) Back-ground, mucosa of carcinoma of the stomach in incipient phase (abstract). 25th Japanese Cancer Congress, Osaka p 125
2. Nakamura K, Sugano H, Takagi K (1968) Carcinoma of the stomach in incipient phase: Its histogenesis and histological appearances. Jpn J of Cancer Res (Gann) 59:251–258
3. Nakamura K, Sugano H (1983) Microcarcinoma of the stomach measuring less than 5 mm in largest diameter and its histogenesis. 13th International Cancer Congress, Part D: Research and Treatment, Alan R Liss Inc, New York, pp 107–116
4. Nakamura K (1990) The structure of gastric carcinoma, 2nd Edition (in Japanese). Igaku-shyoin, Tokyo
5. Nakamura K (1984) Histogénesis de Cáncer Gastrico y su Aplicación Clinico-Patologica. In Llorens P, Nakamura K (eds) Diagnostico de las Afecciones Gastricas. Hospital Paula Jaraquemada, Santiago pp 289–330
6. Nakamura K, Takizawa T (1985) Pathological aspects of chronic gastritis: Definition and relationship with cancer. International Congress Series No. 713, Excerpta Medica, pp 52–63
7. Järvi O (1974) Histogenesis of gastric cancer. XI International Cancer Congress, Abstracts I, Florence p 105
8. Järvi O, Lauren P (1951) On the role of heterotopias of the intestinal epithelium in the pathogenesis of gastric cancer. Acta Pathol Microbiol Scand 29:26–44
9. Ming Si-C, Goldman H, Freiman DG (1967) Intestinal metaplasia and histogenesis of carcinoma in human stomach: Light and electron microscopic study. Cancer 20:1418–1429
10. Lipkin M, Sherlock P, Bell B (1963) Cell proliferation kinetics in the gastrointestinal tract of man. II. Cell renewal in stomach, ileum, colon and rectum. Gastroenterology 45:721–729

11. McDonald W, Trier JS, Evertt NB (1964) Cell proliferation and migration in the stomach, duodenum, and rectum of man: Radioautographic studies. Gastroenterology 46:405–417
12. Saitoh Y, Nakamura K, Makino T, et al (1987) Proliferative mode of undifferentiated carcinoma of the stomach following cancer cell development (in Japanese). Stomach and Intestine 22:1061–1071
13. Nakamura K (1990) Histogénesis del cáncer gástrico. Las etapas iniciales de su desarrollo. Gastroenterología Latinoamericana 1:71–90
14. Shinohara, Nakamura K, Klkuchi M, et al (1985) Growing mode of the gastric microcarcinoma in incipient phase of cancer development (in Japanese). Stomach and intestine 20:431–439
15. Nakamura K (1970) Histogenesis of cancer in the upper segment of the stomach (in Japanese). Stomach and Intestine 5:1111–1119
16. Llorens P (1984) Diagnostico Diferencial. II. Lesiones deprimidas o ulceradas In: Llorens P and Nakamura K (eds) Diagnostico De Las Afecciones Gastricas. Hospital Paula Jaraquemada, Santiago, pp 251–265
17. Nakamura K, Sugano H (1974) Stomach cancer arising from the fundic gland mucosa; Its histological type and clinical behavior. XIth International Cancer Congress, Abstract, Florence p 473
18. Mallory TB (1940) Carcinoma in situ of the stomach and its bearing on the histogenesis of malignant ulcers. Arch Path 30:348–362
19. Murakami T, Nakamura S, Suzuki T (1953) On the histogenesis of adenocarcinoma of the stomach. Gann 44:33–38
20. Morson BC (1955) Carcinoma arising from areas of intestinal metaplasia in the gastric mucosa. Brit J Cancer 9:377–385
21. Nagayo T (1975) Microscopical cancer of the stomach. A study on histogenesis of gastric carcinoma. Int J Cancer 16:52–60
22. Japanese Research Society for Gastric Cancer (1981) The General Rules for the Gastric Cancer Study in Surgery and Pathology. Jpn J Surg 11:127–145
23. Oota K, Sobin LH (1977) International Histological Classification of Tumors. No. 18, Histological Typing of Gastric and Esophageal Tumors, WHO, Geneva
24. Mulligan RM, Rember RR (1954) Histogenesis and biologic behavior of gastric carcinoma: Study of one hundred thirty-eight cases. Arch Path 58:1–25
25. Lauren P (1965) The two histological main types of gastric carcinoma: Diffuse and so-called intestinal-type carcinoma. An attempt at a histo-clinical classification. Acta Pathol Microbiol Scand [A] 64:31–49
26. Ming Si-C (1977) Gastric carcinoma. A pathological classification. Cancer 39:2475–2485

Biopsy Interpretation in Diagnosis of Gastric Carcinoma

Yo Kato, Akio Yanagisawa, and Haruo Sugano[1]

Key words. Biopsy interpretation—Gastric carcinomna—Group classification

Introduction

The interpretation of biopsy specimens from clinically obvious carcinomas, whether they appear in early or advanced stages, does not usually present any great problem. However, it is sometimes extremely difficult to evaluate changes because of the limited amounts of tissue available when small specimens are taken from so-called "borderline lesions", i.e., neoplasias that are difficult to define as benign or malignant even when complete (surgically removed), or when artifacts are present due to the sampling process. Here, we present the histological criteria (group classification) widely used for diagnosis of gastric carcinoma in Japan and discuss how to manage problematic cases as well as several changes easily mistaken for carcinoma in routine examinations.

Group Classification for Diagnosis of Gastric Carcinomas

The group classification proposed by the Japanese Research Society for Gastric Cancer (JRSGC) [1] divides the variety of changes found in gastric biopsy specimens into five groups according to structural and cellular atypia in the epithelia and to standardize the interpretation of biopsy specimens. However, since the latter is not always easy because of the reasons described above, groups such as III and IV include several categories and require explanatory notes as indicated below:

Group I: Normal epithelium and changes involving metaplastic and hyperplastic processes without atypia

---

[1] Department of Pathology, Cancer Institute, 1-37-1 Kami-Ikebukuro, Toshima-ku, Tokyo, 170 Japan

Group II: Atypical changes interpreted as regenerative or reparative processes
Group III: Atypical changes corresponding to benign neoplasia (adenoma), neoplasia, or dysplasia, in which the determination of malignancy is difficult, i.e., borderline lesions and changes in which it is difficult to distinguish between regenerative atypia and very well-differentiated carcinoma
Group IV: Changes strongly suggestive of carcinoma
Group V: Overt carcinoma

Groups III and IV are categories necessitating follow-up care including the examination of biopsy samples to establish a definite diagnosis and the most appropriate treatment.

In a paper published by an international gastric cancer study group [2], as well as in the WHO blue book [3] and several textbooks from European countries and the United States, the term "dysplasia" refers to precancerous epithelial lesions with changes in architecture and aberrant differentiation as well as cytological disturbances and to indicate mostly adenomatous changes. In our sense, the concept of dysplasia corresponds to changes encompassing what we call "atypical epithelium [4, 5] (in a wide sense)" or several types of adenoma. However, the features of "dysplasia" or "atypical epithelium" are fairly different from book to book, from author(s) to author(s), and from school to school. Actually, an appreciable discrepancy in concept exists between European or American and Japanese pathologists. The former favor a wider interpretation than the latter, which in some cases seems to match the changes in group II to group IV of our biopsy interpretation: Mild, moderate, and severe dyplasia correspond roughly to groups II, III, and IV, respectively.

Group II Lesions

In active regenerative processes, the epithelium becomes variously basophilic and may present as simply flat, straight tubular, or fairly distorted; it is also associated with various degrees of inflammatory cell infiltration in the interstitium. The tubular structures are in general regularly distributed with some differentiation from bottom to top of the tubules (Fig. 1). Furthermore, a gradual transition between basophilic epithelium in the upper regions and completely benign glandular epithelium at the bottom is usually noticed somewhere in the affected area.

Group III Lesions

Among several changes in this category, the most frequent is the one corresponding to so-called "ATP (atypical epithelium)" [4, 5] or flat adenoma [3, 6]. The lesion is usually of the flat, elevated type, consisting of immature, intestinal-type tubules. It can be divided into two subtypes according to the presence of structural and cellular atypias: (1) low-grade atypia and (2) high-grade (severe) or

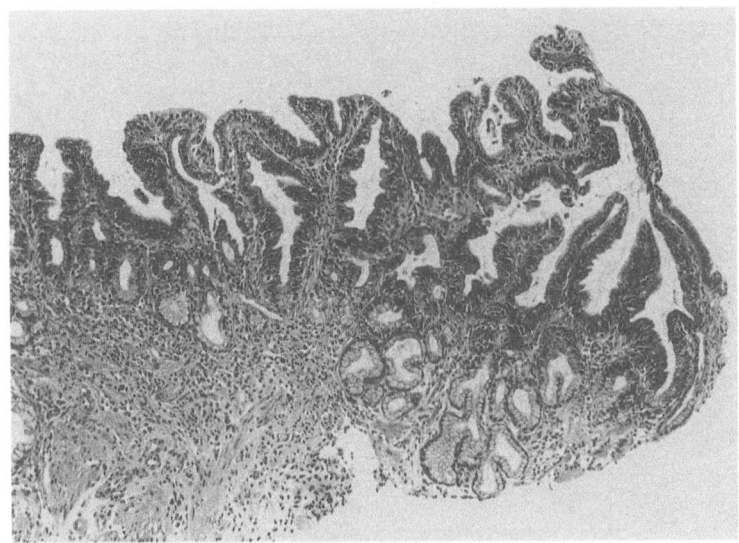

Fig. 1. Group II. Regenerative atypia

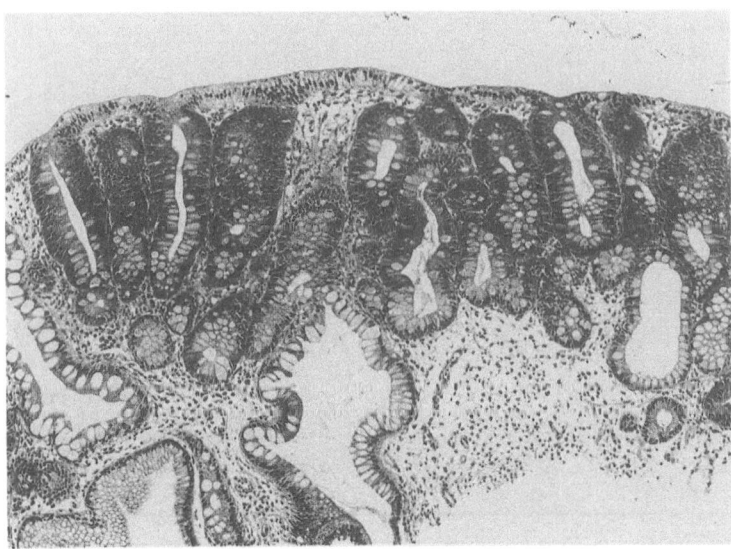

Fig. 2. Group III. So-called ATP or flat adenoma, with low-grade atypia

borderline atypia (borderline lesion). In the former, homogeneous straight or round tubules densely proliferate to produce variously dilated neoplastic or non-neoplastic glands. The epithelium is tall and columnar and the nuclei are long and slender, particularly in the upper part of the lesion, being located adjacent to the basement membrane (Figs. 2, 3). In the latter lesion, the tubules

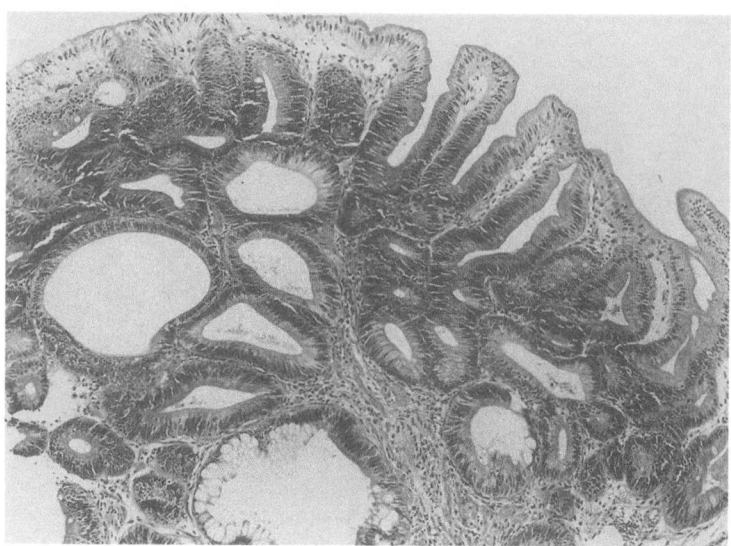

Fig. 3. Group III. So-called ATP or flat adenoma, with low-grade atypia

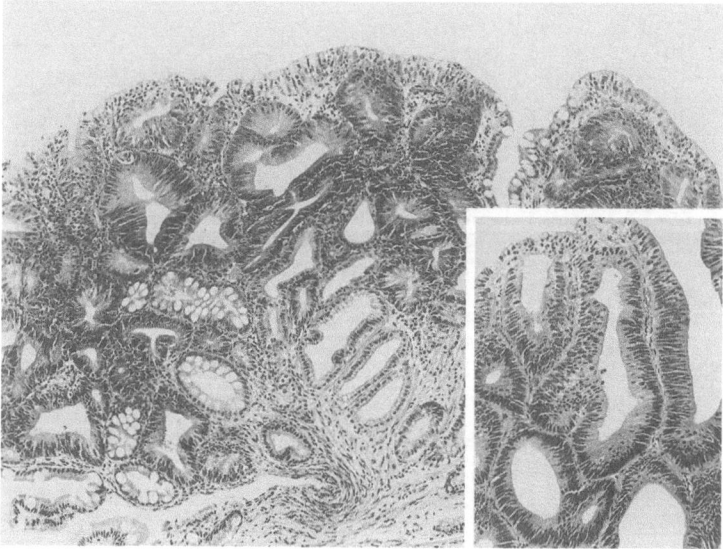

Fig. 4. Group III. ATP or flat adenoma, with high-grade or borderline atypia. The sizes and shapes of the glands are slightly irregular, and loss of polarity of the nuclei (*inset*) is rather prominent

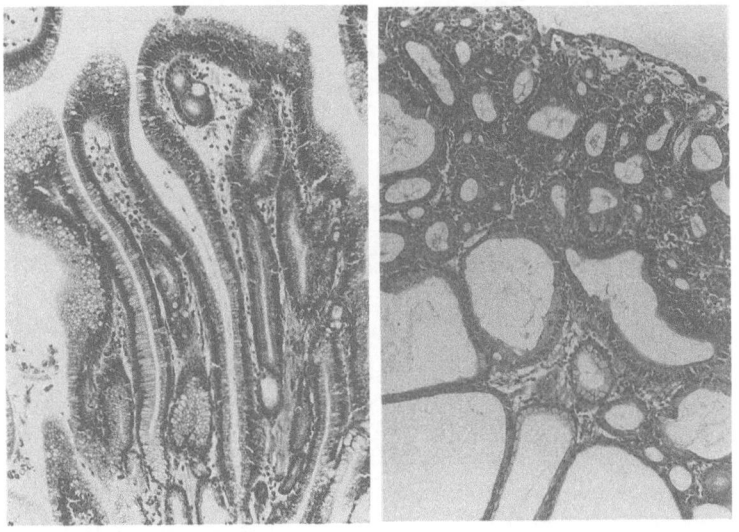

a   b

Fig. 5a,b. Group III. Gastric type ATPs or adenomas. **a** Foveolar type. **b** Glandular type

are slightly irregular in size and shape and the nuclei are conspicuously detached from the basement membrane (loss of polarity or pseudostratification of the nuclei) (Fig. 4). Other findings, such as papillary structures and plump nuclei, can be counted as diagnostic points for the "borderline lesion".

Polypoid or depressed-type changes are rather rare. The former is also called colonic-type because of its macroscopic resemblance to adenomas commonly found in the colorectum [6]. The latter is problematic, since this type of change is often difficult to differentiate from regenerative atypia or very well-differentiated carcinoma. In addition, extremely rare lesions composed of gastric-type epithelium (foveolar or glandular-type) exist in this category (Figs. 5a, 5b). It should be remembered that foveolar-type atypical epithelium is quite often associated with a carcinoma in the same legion [7].

Group III lesions that are difficult to differentiate from regenerative atypia and well-differentiated carcinomas will be described again later.

Very Well-Differentiated Carcinoma (VWDC)

The carcinomas described here are tumors basically belonging to the well-differentiated category. However, since the lesions are mostly limited to the mucosa and can be cured by endoscopic resection (ER), it is of value to separate them from overt carcinomas. The common characteristics for VWDCs are well-developed tubular or papillary structures with columnar or cuboidal epithelium and relatively small nuclei. However, the nuclei are more round than those in regenerative or hyperplastic epithelium, and loss of nuclear polarity is in general

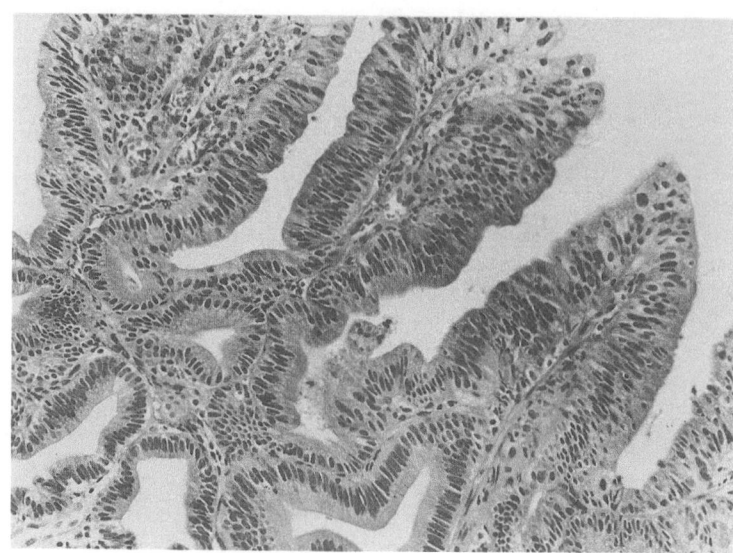

Fig. 6. Very well-differentiated carcinoma (VWDC). Although tubular or papillary structures are simple and regular and the nuclei are slender, loss of polarity of the nuclei is prominent, particularly in the upper part

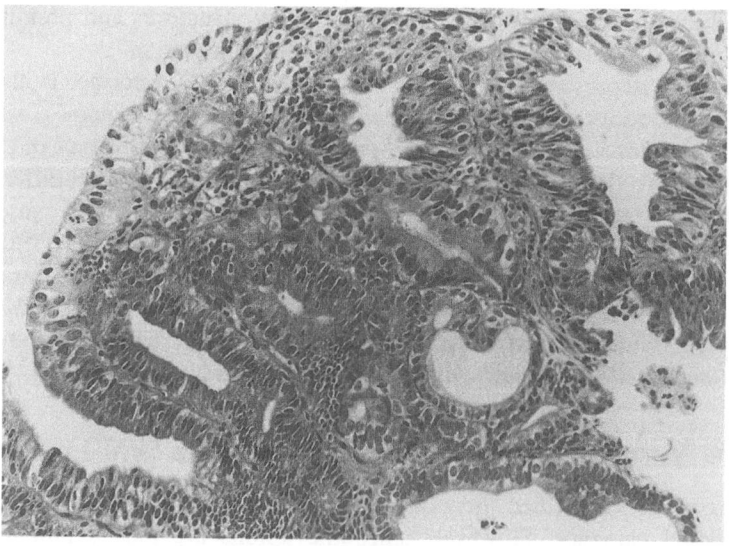

Fig. 7. Very well-differentiated carcinoma (VWDC). Tubular patterns are well-developed, but the nuclei are round and plump

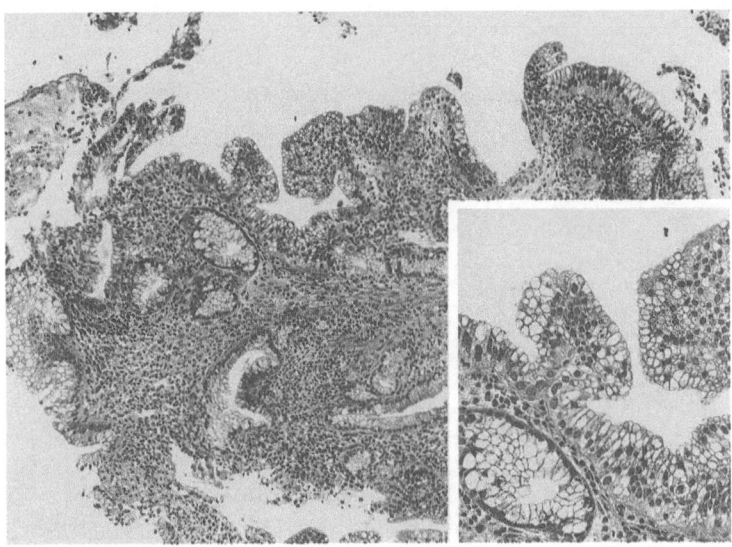

Fig. 8. Very well-differentiated carcinoma (VWDC). The level of atypia is often overlooked, leading to diagnosis as a hyperplastic change. Note slightly swollen nuclei and loss of their polarity (*inset*)

more evident than in adenomas (Figs. 6, 7). Papillary or tubular structures composed of clear mucinous cells should be differentiated from hyperplastic foveolar or glandular epithelia (Fig. 8). When only one specimen, particularly at the first biopsy, is positive for such atypical glands or it is difficult to make a definite diagnosis of malignancy, Group IV would be the best choice for decisions necessitating a rebiopsy within a few weeks.

Carcinoma with Anastomosing Glands: "WHYX Lesion"

Irregularly anastomosing or fusing glands with little cellular atypia are characteristic of this lesion (Fig. 9). Since the glands resemble certain English letters such as W, H, Y, X, etc. (Fig. 10), we often call the change a "WHYX lesion" [8]. This type of change is mostly very superficial in the mucosa and grossly flat and ill-defined (sometimes being so inconspicuous as to be classified as IIb according to JRSGC). Therefore, there is a controversy on whether the change is neoplastic or regenerative in nature. However, one should remember that the change is quite often associated with more obvious carcinomas such as tubular or signet-ring cell carcinoma with a greater potential for submucosal invasion. In the case of a small change in a specimen, however, it should preferably be classified as group IV, since a similar but very focal change can take place in reparative processes.

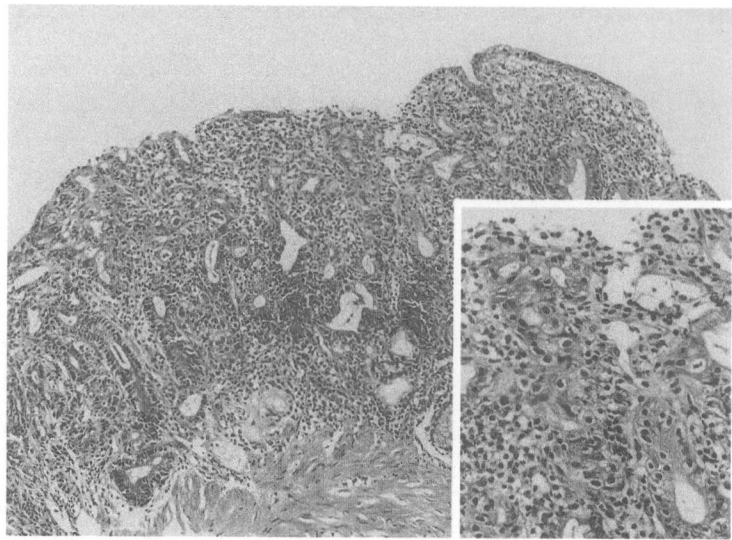

Fig. 9. Carcinoma with anastomosing glands (WHYX lesion). Irregularly anastomosing or fusing glands with little or no cellular atypia (*inset*) are seen mainly in the upper part of the mucosa

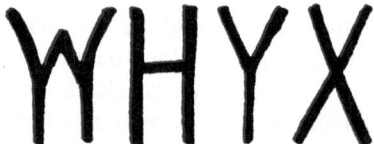

Fig. 10. Schematic representation of irregularly anastomosing or fusing carcinoma with little cellular atypia: WHYX lesion

Recommendation of PAS or AB-PAS Staining for Routine Examination

It is sometimes difficult to diagnose signet-ring cell carcinoma, particularly when the amount of available tissue is very limited. To overcome this hurdle, periodic acid-Schiff (PAS) or alcianblue (AB)-PAS staining for routine biopsy examination is recommended, since mucin droplets or intracytoplasmic microcysts in the tumor cells are positive with these procedures, and this also allows discrimination from xanthoma cells, which are usually negative (Fig. 11). These approaches are particularly useful in the detection of linitis plastica, where a few signet-ring cells are often involved in a deeper part of the mucosa (Fig. 12).

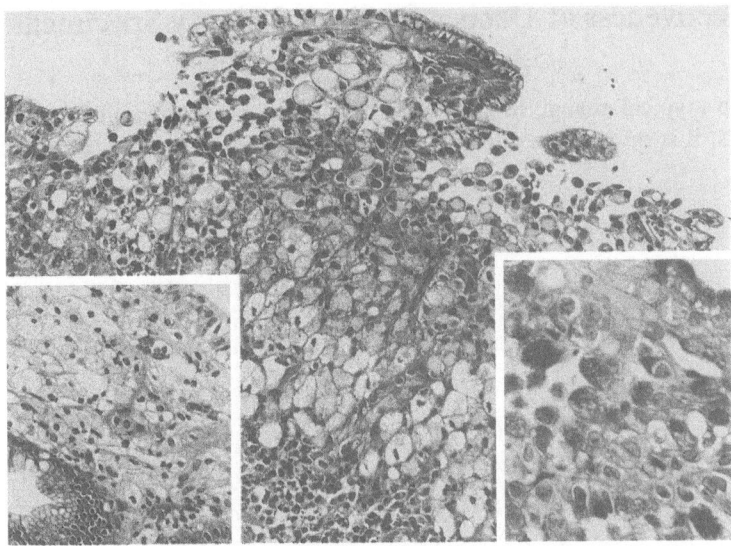

Fig. 11. Signet-ring cell carcinomas are usually positve for PAS reaction (*right lower inset*). In contrast, xanthoma cells with small nuclei in the cell centers (*left lower inset*) are generally negative for the reaction

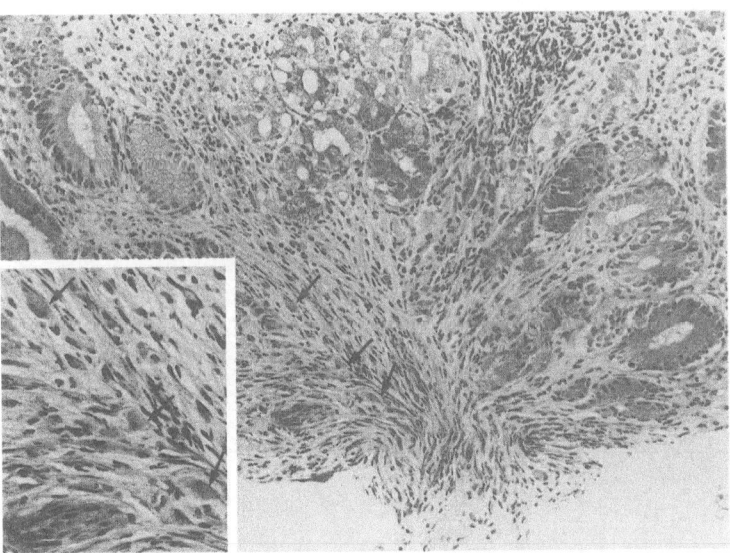

Fig. 12. Signet-ring cell carcinoma (*arrows*) detected by the PAS reaction. Inset is high-power magnification of the area with arrows

Effectiveness of Deeper Cutting of Biopsy Specimens for Diagnosis of Carcinomas

When an atypical change in the biopsy specimens is insufficient for unequivocal diagnosis, it is quite often effective to perform deeper cutting of the specimen. In

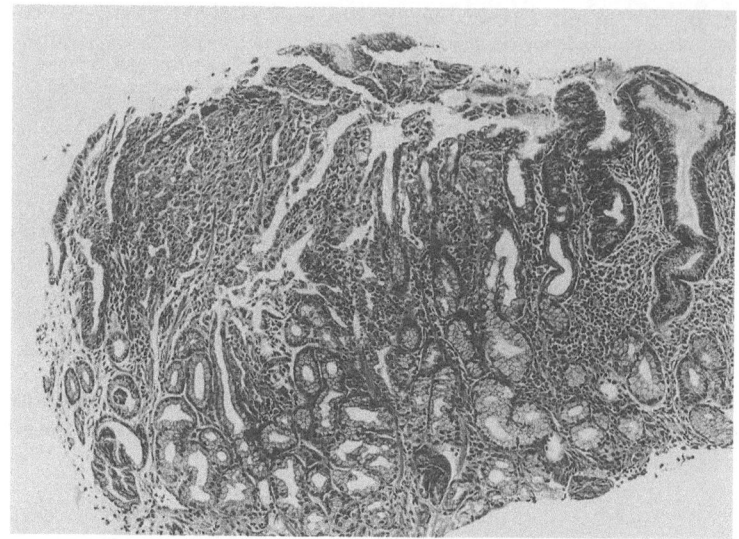

a

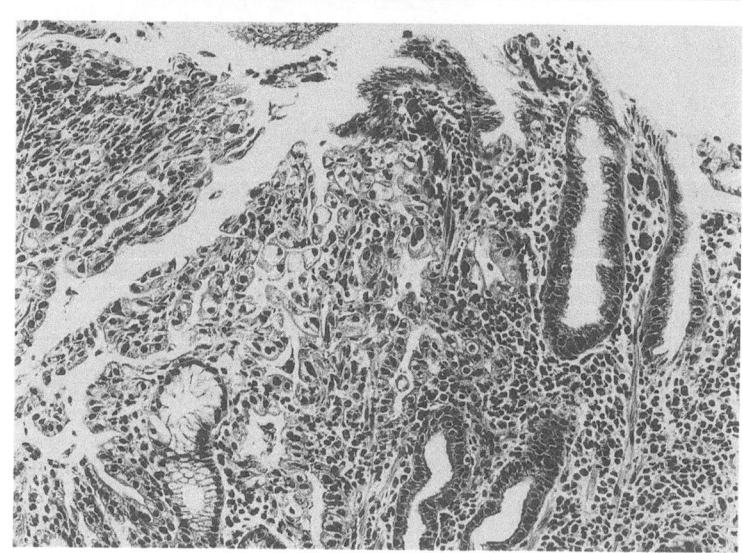

b

Fig. 13a,b. Difference in histology between **a** original and **b** deeper-cut sections from the same biopsy specimen. The original slide (**a**) was classified as group III because of the difficulty in distinguishing carcinoma from regenerative changes or artifacts. However, a moderately to poorly differentiated adenocarcinoma was disclosed after deeper sampling of the specimen (**b**)

the case illustrated in Fig. 13, a group III diagnosis was made after examination of the original slide because of difficulty in determining with such a small amount of atypical cells whether the change was carcinomatous, regenerative, or an artifact (Fig. 13a). Deeper cutting of the specimen, however, disclosed an obvious carcinoma (Fig. 13b). In the case of Fig. 14, a small cluster of atypical glands suggestive of malignancy (the first slide was therefore classified as group IV [Fig. 14a]) proved to be an overt tubular carcinoma upon examination of a deeper section of the block (Fig. 14b).

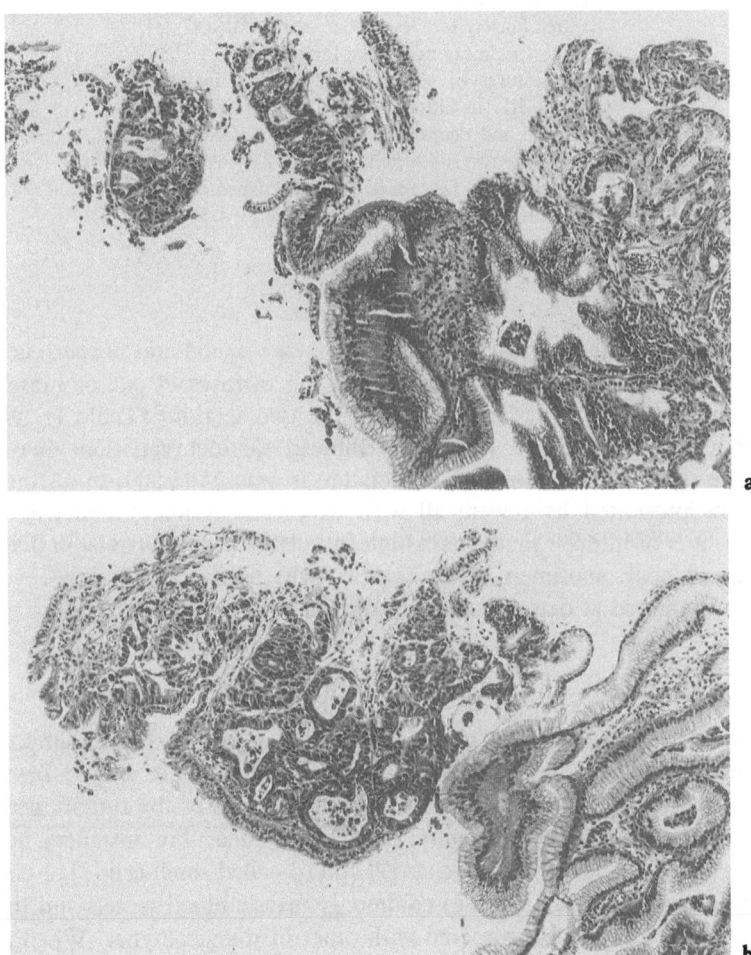

Fig. 14a,b. Difference in histology between **a** original and **b** deeper-cut sections from the same biopsy specimen. The original slide (**a**) was classified as group IV because of insufficient amounts of atypical glands suggestive of carcinoma. A deeper cut section (**b**) established its identity as a moderately differentiated adenocarcinoma

Table 1. Comparison of group classification[a] between original and deeper-cut slides from the same biopsy specimens[b].

Reclassification	No. of specimens[c] ($n = 653$)
$0 \longleftrightarrow V$	7 (1%)
$I \longleftrightarrow III$	2 (0.3%) 76 (12%)
$I \longleftrightarrow IV,V$	67 (10%)
$III \longleftrightarrow IV$	10
$IV \longleftrightarrow V$	19

[a] Group classification for diagnosis of gastric carcinoma by biopsy according to the Japanese Research Society for Gastric Carcinoma (JRSGC) [1].
[b] The specimens used were limited to those showing features of one or more groups, including group III, in either or both of two specimens, original and deeper-cut. The level difference between the two slides compared was 250 to 500 μm.
[c] Upgrading was found in approximately 2/3 of the specimens; the remaining 1/3 were downgraded.

Our studies of histological changes compared original and deeper-cut sections from the same block using specimens showing features of one or more groups, including group III, in either or both of the two sections (Table 1). We found that 76 (12%) out of 653 specimens showed distinct variations between the two. The difference in the two section levels was 250~500 μm. Although the specimens presented here were all with neoplastic lesion(s) somewhere in the stomach, it is of interest that such a high frequency of discrepancy in diagnosis of the same biopsy specimen exists, particularly when considering that certain biopsies are aimed at determining the surgical resection margin.

Diagnosis of Gastric Carcinomas of Special Types

As mentioned above, the interpretation of biopsy specimens from clinically overt carcinomas is usually not difficult. In this situation, care should be taken to determine whether further information on the nature of the tumor, particularly regarding the grade of malignancy, can be obtained. For instance, both AFP (α-fetoprotein)-producing carcinomas [9] and so-called small-cell [3] or endocrine-cell carcinomas [10] are known to commonly invade blood vessels and thus show an unfavorable prognosis compared with other histological types. When papillary and solid structures composed of clear or slightly eosinophilic cells with occasional bizarre giant nuclei are revealed, the possibility of AFP-producing carcinoma should be considered (Fig. 15). Furthermore, solid nests of cells with a high N/C (nucleocytoplasmic) ratio and hyperchromatic nuclei could indicate endocrine-cell carcinoma (Fig. 16).

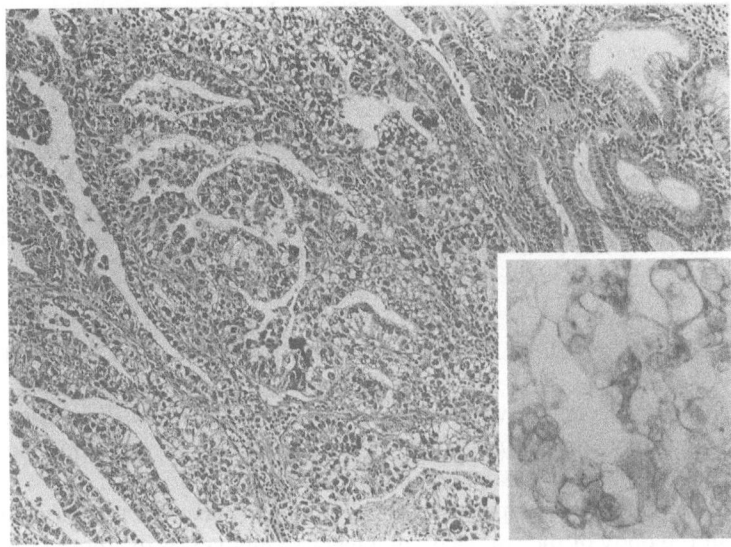

Fig. 15. AFP (α-fetoprotein)-producing carcinoma. Cytoplasm is irregularly positive for AFP with immunostaining (*inset*)

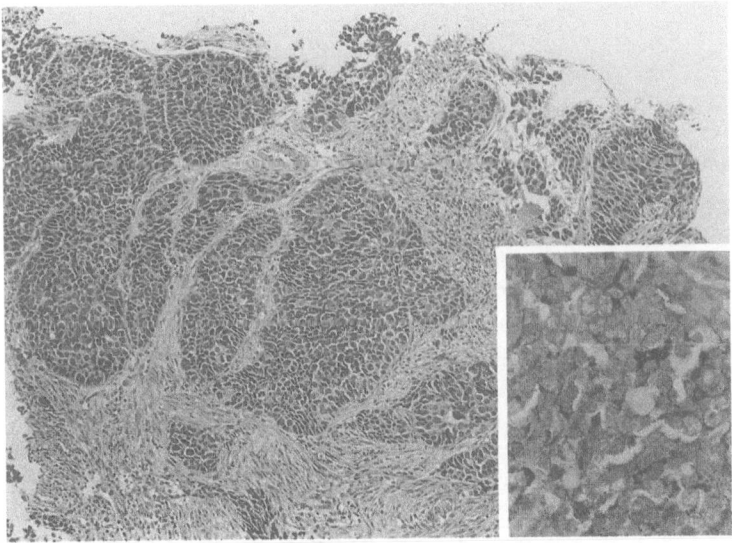

Fig. 16. Small-cell or endocrine-cell carcinoma. Cytoplasm is strongly positive for Grimelius' stain (*inset*)

Diagnosis of Carcinoid

Carcinoid diagnosis is relatively simple when trabecular or solid nests of equal-sized cuboidal cells with small round and hyperchromatic nuclei (Fig. 17) are found. Most of these tumors are positive for Grimelius' argyrophilic reaction, and mitotic figures are rare. However, when the nuclei are swollen and pleomorphic and, further, mitotic figures are apparent, this may indicate atypical carcinoid, which has a poorer prognosis. The features of anaplastic endocrine-cell tumors, i.e., endocrine-cell carcinomas, have already been presented (Fig. 16).

Benign Processes Leading to Misdiagnosis of Carcinoma

There are many occasions where one might be misled into diagnosing malignancy. Here, some representative cases are presented, illustrating lesion types other than the reparative changes already discussed.

In the case of Fig. 18, a specimen taken from a 26-year-old man with multiple erosions in the body of the stomach, an adenocarcinoma was diagnosed because of the appearance of irregularly anastomosing glands. If consideration had been given to the rarity of this tumor in individuals in their twenties and the presence of parietal cells in certain glands, this misinterpretation could have been avoided.

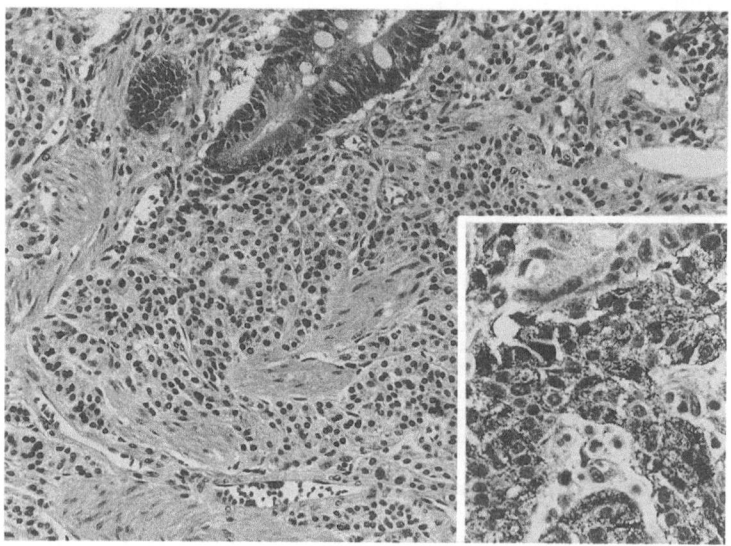

Fig. 17. Typical carcinoid with trabecular or solid nests composed of equal-sized cuboidal cells with small, round, and hyperchromatic nuclei. This case was strongly positive for Grimelius' argyrophilic reaction (*inset*)

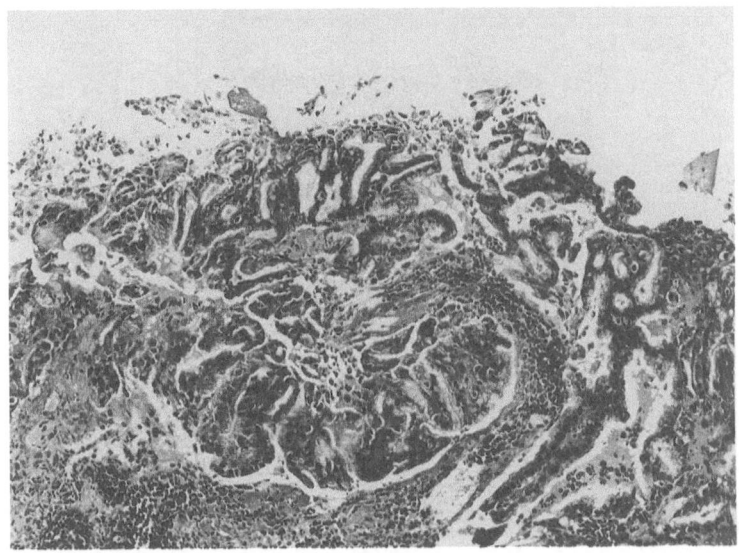

Fig. 18. Irregularly distorted glands in tangentially cut surface mucosa from a 26-year-old man with an acute gastric mucosal lesion. The change is often mistaken for carcinoma

Furthermore, care should have been taken to examine a tangentially cut specimen.

Exfoliated foveolar epithelia from ulcer edge tissue can sometimes be perplexing because of the similarity to signet-ring cell carcinoma (Fig. 19). Here, the absence of nuclear atypia and the gradual transition of scattered mucinous cells from unequivocally benign epithelia become clues to resolving the question. Activated histiocytes in granulation tissue can also be mistaken for signet-ring cell carcinoma (Fig. 20). A demonstration of fine reticular networks in slightly basophilic cytoplasm and negative PAS reaction can facilitate diagnosis in this situation.

Granulation tissue consisting of capillaries with remarkably swollen endothelium also constitutes a change which can lead pathologists to misdiagnosis (Fig. 21). This change often occurs in rather prolonged cases of granulation, such as with chronic ulcers and syphilitic gastritis, and is characterized by regularity in the assembly of trabecular or acinar structures, with occasional small spaces containing red corpuscles, and the uniformity of round or ovoid nuclei, with finely dispersed chromatin and prominent round nucleoli.

Degenerative or deformed glands appearing in lymphoproliferative disorders are also changes to be differentiated from carcinoma (Fig. 22). The mixed presence of mucinous (ballooning) and non-mucinous cells in small cell cords surrounded by increased lymphoid cells can help in the interpretation of such specimens as reflecting lymphoproliferative disorders.

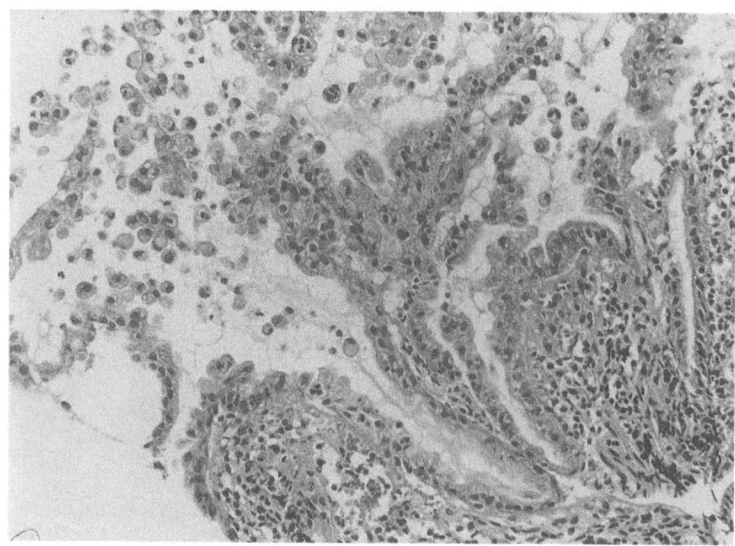

Fig. 19. Exfoliated foveolar epithelia in a biopsy specimen from the edge of an ulcer. Signet-ring cell carcinoma should be ruled out

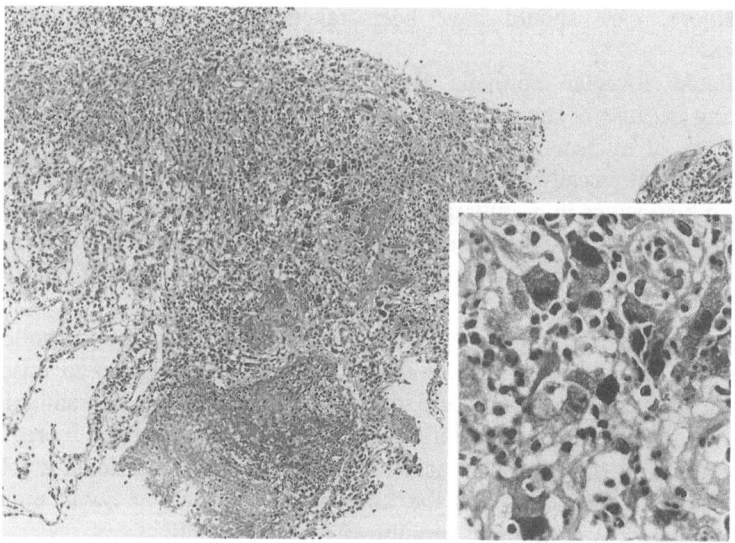

Fig. 20. Granulation tissue with activated histiocytes (bizarre giant cells, *inset*). Signet-ring cell carcinoma should be ruled out

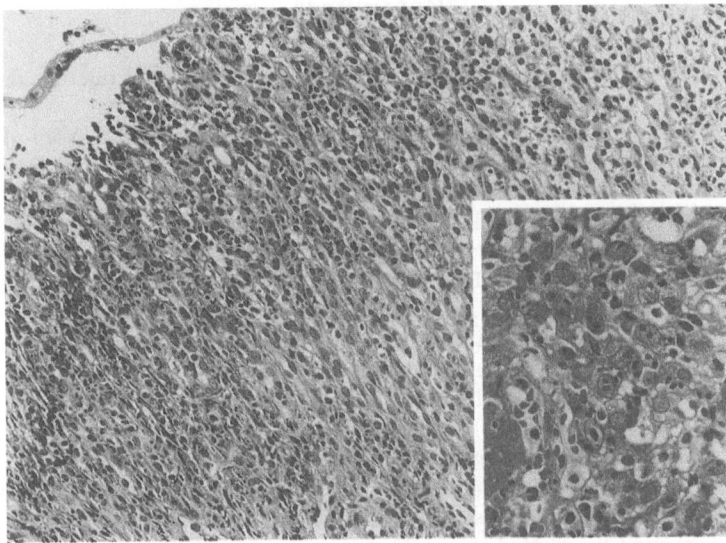

Fig. 21. Granulation tissue with swollen endothelial cells. Chromatin in enlarged nuclei is finely dispersed and nucleoli are prominent and round (*inset*). Poorly differentiated carcinoma should be ruled out

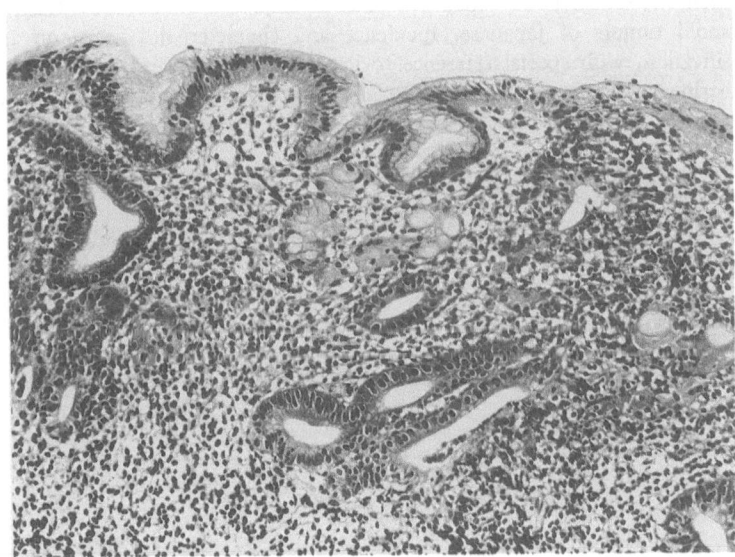

Fig. 22. Degenerative glands (*arrows*) in the stomach caused by a lymphoproliferative disorder. The change resembles a signet-ring cell carcinoma

References

1. Japanese Research Society for Gastric Cancer (1985) The general rules for the gastric cancer study, 11th edn. (in Japanese). Kanehara, Tokyo
2. Morson BC, Grundmann E, Johansen A, Nagayo T, Serck-Hansen A (1980) Precancerous conditions and epithelial dysplasia in the stomach. J Clin Pathol 33:711–721
3. Watanabe H, Jass JR, Sobin LH (1990) Histological typing of esophageal and gastric tumours, 2nd edn. International histological classification of tumours (WHO). Springer, Berlin Heidelberg Hong Kong
4. Sugano H, Nakamura K, Takagi K (1971) An atypical epithelium of the stomach. A clinico-pathological entity. GANN Monograph on Cancer Research 11:257–269
5. Kato Y, Yanagisawa A, Sugano H (1981) Borderline lesions (ATP) of the stomach (in Japanese). Saishin-Igaku 36:21–30
6. Nakamura K, Kino I (1980) Histopathology of the gastrointestinal tract. Biopsy interpretation (in Japanese). Igaku-Shoin, Tokyo
7. Hirota E, Harada M, Itabashi M (1983) Biopsy interpretation and management of "borderline lesions" in the esophagus and stomach (in Japanese). Byori to Rinsho (Pathology and Clinical Medicine) 1:33–52
8. Kato Y, Kawabuchi B, Yanagisawa A, Mernyei M (1992) Interpretation of gastric biopsy specimens (in Japanese). Shokaki-Naishikyo (Endoscopia Digestiva) 4:753–762
9. Ishikura H, Kurimoto K, Shamoto M et al. (1986) Hepatoid adenocarcinoma of the stomach. An analysis of 7 cases. Cancer 58:119–126
10. Iwafuchi M, Watanabe H, Noda Y, Ajioka Y, Enjoji M, Ito M (1989) Gastrointestinal carcinoid tumors of Japanese. Incidence and characteristics based on anatomocal classification, with special reference to the difference between carcinoid tumor and endocrine cell carcinoma (in Japanese). I to Cho (Stomach and Intestine) 24:869–882

Endocrine Cell Tumor of the Stomach

Hisao Ito[1] and Eiichi Tahara[2]

Key words. Stomach—Endocrine cells—Carcinoid—Mucocarcinoid—Endocrine cell carcinoma

Introduction

The gastrointestinal (GI) tract is rich in neuropeptides and amines of which at least 25 types have been identified as existing in both gut endocrine cells and in nervous systems [1, 2]. As a rule, different types of gut peptides are detected in endocrine cells and nervous systems, with a few exceptions such as CCK, enkephalin, motilin, and somatostatin [3, 4]. They play an important role on the regulation of gastrointestinal functions including digestion, absorption, motility and growth in the form of endocrines, paracrines, and neuroendocrines.

The representative tumor related to GI peptides is carcinoid, but its concept or definition has been altered with the identification of various types of distinct endocrine cells of the GI tract. Confusion has arisen from the needless abuse of the term "carcinoid" and the occurrence of a few neuroendocrine cells in ordinary adenocarcinomas. In addition, many authors have reported gastric endocrine cell tumors histologically showing poorly differentiated appearances which are referred to variously in reports as "diffuse argentaffinoma" [5], "argentaffin cell adenocarcinoma" [6], "atypical carcinoid" [7], or "argyrophil cell carcinoma" [8] (Table 1). Consequently, the classification of endocrine cell tumors of the GI tract varies extensively among the authors [4, 9–11].

The following is a description of the pathological and clinical properties of gastric endocrine cell tumors, as well as the mixed endocrine-epithelial tumors according to the recently introduced classification by Tahara [9] (Table 1). The

[1] Department of Pathology, Tottori University School of Medicine, 86 Nishi-machi, Yonago, Tottori, 683 Japan
[2] Department of Pathology, Hiroshima University School of Medicine, 1-2-3 Kasumi, Minami-ku, Hiroshima, 734 Japan

Table 1. Classification of gastrointestinal endocrine tumors.

Tahara (1989) [9]	Soga (1971) [10]	WHO (1980) [11]	Others (synonyms)

I. Carcinoid	Types A and B	I. Carcinoid
		   A. EC cell
		   B. G cell
		   C. Other
			Typical or classical
			   carcinoid

II. Mucocarcinoid	Type C	II. Mucocarcinoid	Microglandular goblet cell carcinoma Crypt cell carcinoma Goblet cell carcinoid Adenocarcinoid Mucinous carcinoid

III. Endocrine cell carcinoma
   A. Medullary type
      1. Well-differentiated
      2. Poorly differentiated
      3. Undifferentiated
   B. Scirrhous type
	Type D	III. Mixed carcinoid-
		   adenocarcinoma
			Atypical carcinoid
			   large cell type
			Undifferentiated
			   carcinoid small cell
			   type
			Scirrhous argyrophil
			   cell carcinoma

preceding review of the distribution of endocrine cells containing peptides and amines in the human stomach will provide a better understanding of gastric endocrine cell tumors.

Endocrine Cells in Normal Gastric Mucosa and Pathological Conditions

The gastrointestinal endocrine cells are confined to the mucosa, being distributed diffusely between the epithelial cells existing as single cells or in small clusters, and occasionally within the lamina propria in some pathological conditions [4, 12–15]. They were originally described by Nicholas [16] and Kultschitzky [17] as basigranulated cells, situated in the intestinal crypts and characterized by small infranuclear eosinophilic granules. Heterogeneity and multiplicity of gut endocrine cells were not recognized at that time; a variety of names had been given to them, such as clear, yellow, or enterochromaffin cells, and they were also divided into two cell types based on their silver-reducing power, argentaffin and argyrophil, which were originally considered to be one cell in different stages of secretion [4].

In the human stomach, gastrin-containing G cells are located exclusively in the middle one-third of the antral and intermediate zone mucosa [13] (Fig. 1a). Somatostatin-containing D cells and serotonin-containing EC cells are sparsely distributed in the lower one-half of the gastric mucosa in both the antral and fundic mucosa [15]. Distribution is highest for G cells, followed by EC and then D cells. Conversely, in fetal gastric mucosa the number of D cells exceeds that of

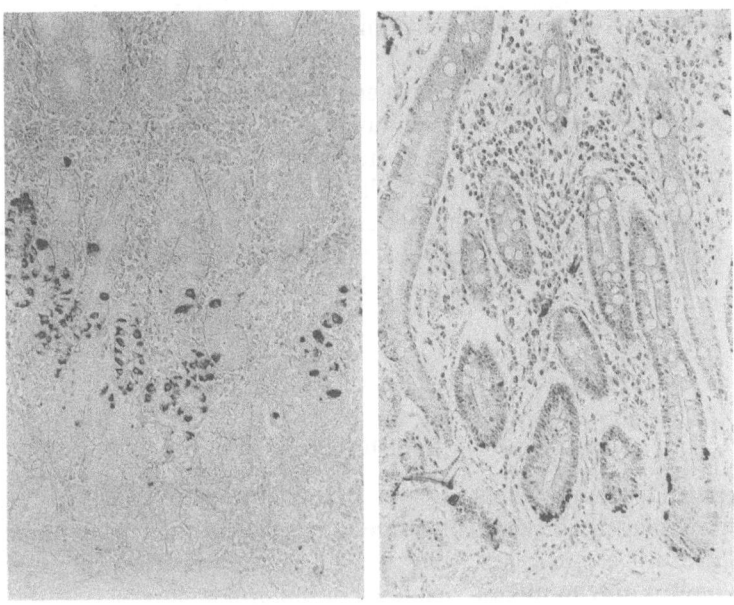

Fig. 1a,b. a Gastrin-containing G cells in antral mucosa with mild atrophic gastritis. **b** Glicentin-containing L cells in intestinal metaplastic glands of stomach. Immunostaining, ×150

G and EC cells [18]. With the progress of chronic atrophic gastritis, the number of these endocrine cells gradually decreases, but intestinal-type EC cells appear in intestinalized gastric mucosa [15]. Glicentin-containing L cells first occur in intestinalized gastric mucosa [12, 14] (Fig. 1b). They frequently show hyperplasia or micronodules in the budding area of the deeper metaplastic glands, but decrease remarkably in completely intestinalized mucosa. Glicentin might play an important role in the development of intestinal metaplasia of the gastric mucosa by means of a trophic action on intestinal epithelia and inhibition of gastric acid secretion. Other types of endocrine cell include an enterochromaffin-like (ECL) cells containing histamine in the fundic mucosa and D_1 cells containing a VIP-like peptide [2]. A small amount of ACTH and calcitonin might be presented in G cells [19].

It is common to find an endocrine cell micronodule (ECM) composed of five or more endocrine cells in a variety of pathological conditions. Endocrine cell types of EMC include G or EC cells in the gastritis mucosa [13, 15] and L cells in the intestinal metaplastic mucosa [14].

Endocrine cell hyperplasia is defined as an increased cell mass, but the diagnosis is difficult in practical terms because of the dispersed nature of the cells and technical problems in quantification [4]. Moreover, serum levels of a variety of gastrointestinal hormones do not correlate with the number of given endocrine cells [4, 20]. Hyperplasia of gastric endocrine cells are extremely rare except for gastrin-containing G cells associated primarily with Zollinger-Ellison syndrome type I or duodenal ulcer [4, 21] and secondarily with hypocholorhydria, both conditions resulting in hypergastrinemia and fundic ECL cell hyperplasia. G cell hyperplasia also occurs in a few conditions, such as excluded gastric antrum, postvagotomy, acromegaly, and hyperparathyroidism [4]. It is less common in subsequent neoplastic transformation in the vast majority of cases with endocrine cell hyperplasia except for ECL hyperplasia in type A gastritis with pernicious anemia which may occasionally be associated with carcinoids [4, 22–24]. Hyperplasia has not been well documented in other endocrine cells.

Endocrine Cell Tumor of the Stomach

Carcinoids

Gastric carcinoids occupy about 27% of the total of gastrointestinal carcinoid tumors reported in the Japanese literature [25], whereas they make up between 2% to 7% of European and American cases [4, 26–28]. Histologically, the term should be limited only to tumors composed of uniform endocrine cells which are arranged in nests (Fig. 2a) and infiltrating strands, or having trabecular, ribbon (Fig. 2b), or acinar patterns. A mixed growth pattern is common. Nuclear pleomorphism and mitotic figures are essentially absent. In their ultrastructure,

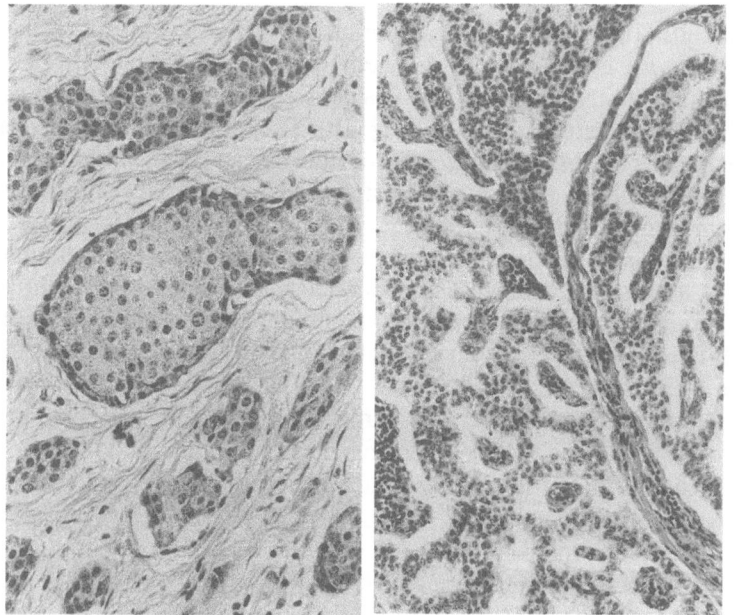

a   b

Fig. 2a,b. Classical gastric carcinoid showing **a** solid nest and **b** trabecullar or ribbon patterns. H and E staining, ×300

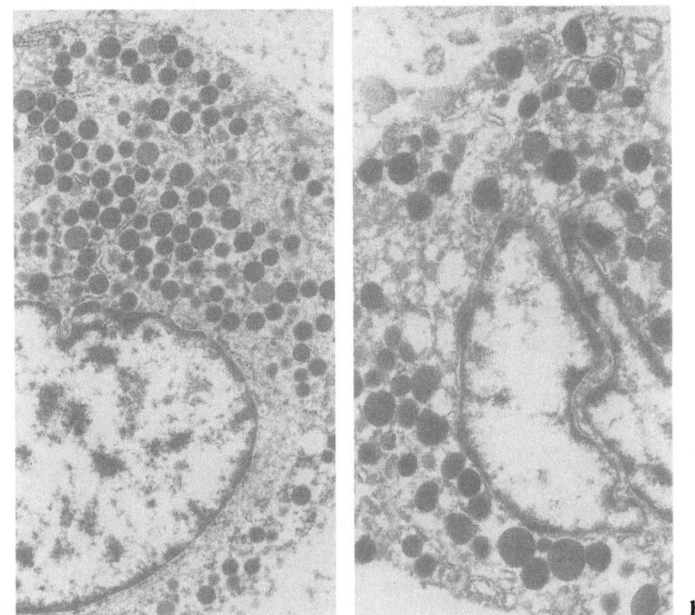

Fig. 3a,b. Endocrine secretory granules in the cytoplasm of the same gastric endocrine carcinoma. **a** Round and electron-dense granules measuring 240–320 nm and **b** 400–480 nm. ×11 000

tumor cells contain endocrine granules of various shapes and sizes in the cytoplasm (Figs. 3, 4.c). The stroma is loose and abundant in blood vessels and fibrous tissue. The majority of gastric carcinoids are argyrophilic and rarely argentaffin positive [4, 9, 29].

In terms of histogenesis, typical gastric carcinoids might be classified into two types, one arising de novo and another associated with type A gastritis confined to fundic mucosa. In de nove carcinoids with or without ulceration, tumor cells usually arise from the deep mucosa and infiltrate into the submucosa from an early stage. A large tumor is indistinguishable from an ulcerated ordinary carcinoma. It may be yellowish or grey in color and appear solid on the cut surface.

Type A gastritis, also called autoimmune gastritis associated with or without pernicious anemia, causes multifocal proliferation of ECL cells in the fundic mucosa, including intraglandular hyperplasia (Fig. 4.a), endocrine cell micronodule, and carcinoids (Fig. 4.b). Among patients with pernicious anemia, the prevalence of gastric carcinoids is 2%–9% [24, 29, 30]. Most cases remain subclinical, but a frequency in association with gastric adenocarcinoma was also pointed out, 3% being a high frequency in this area [30]. Histologically, there are myriads of endocrine cell nests in which it is occasionally difficult to discriminate between non-neoplastic lesions and microcarcinoids [31]. Itsuno et al. [32] defined a neoplastic microcarcinoid as follows; (1) endocrine cell micronodule (ECM)

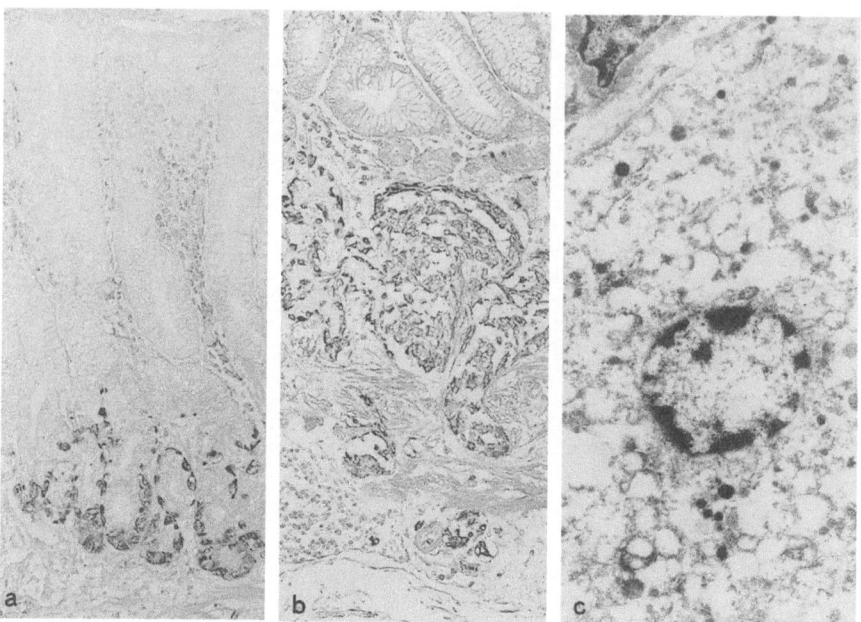

Fig. 4a–c. Fundic gland mucosa in type A gastritis. **a** Endocrine cell hyperplasia in the deeper zone of fundic mucosa and **b** a microcarcinoid infiltrating into the muscularis mucosae and submucosa. Grimelius staining, ×180. **c** Numerous round secretory granules measuring 75–450 nm with variable density in the microcarcinoid. Same case as **a** and **b**. ×6000

measuring more than 0.1 mm in the largest diameter, (2) ECM, even if it is less than 0.1 cm in diameter, infiltrating into the muscularis mucosae or submucosa, or showing carcinoid-like structures such as trabecular or ribbon-like ones without stroma, or (3) ECM, even if it is less than 0.1 mm in diameter, composed of large atypical cells.

Mucocarcinoids

Mucocarcinoids, also called mucinous or adenocarcinoids, show a quite different histological appearance from carcinoids and endocrine cell carcinomas. The tumor is composed predominantly of small clumps, strands, or glandular collections of mucin-producing cells looking like goblet cells (Fig. 5a) or signet-ring cells, and intermingled with endocrine cells in a variable number (Fig. 5b) and occasionally with Paneth's cells. The admixed endocrine cells comprise a variety of cell types, such as EC, ECL, and D [4]. They are often sparse and, in about 10% of cases, difficult to find. The tumor was originally considered to be a variant of a carcinoid. The frequent paucity of endocrine cells and more aggressive clinical nature are not consistent with such speculation. Mucocarcinoids are a variant of adenocarcinomas showing differentiation to both mucin-producing cells and

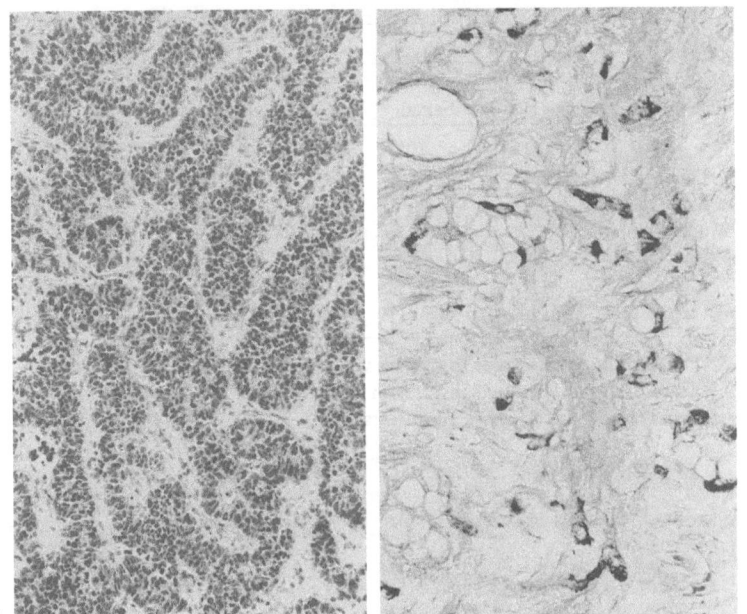

a   b

Fig. 5a,b. Gastric mucocarcinoid. **a** Tumor cells resembling goblet cells forming acinar and trabecullar patterns. H & E staining ×140. **b** same case as in **a**; serotonin-positive tumor cells intermingled with goblet-type tumor cells. Immunostaining, ×300

endocrine cells. [4, 9]. They occur most frequently in the appendix, but rarely in stomach [4, 33]. We have treated only one case in the last 10 years (Table 2).

Endocrine Cell Carcinoma (ECC)

Endocrine cell carcinoma is diagnosed when histological findings fulfill the following two criteria: (1) the vast majority of tumor cells are endocrine cells with cellular atypia, pleomorphism, and many mitoses, and (2) these endocrine cells are present with diffuse distribution throughout the tumor tissue [4]. Most of the ECC cells are argyrophilic. ECCs are divided into two types according to the amount of stromal connective tissue, both medullary and scirrhous. The incidence of gastric medullary ECC occurs in about 0.1% of all gastric cancer, while scirrhous ECC is seen in about 30% of gastric scirrhous carcinomas which correspond to Borrmann's type IV carcinoma [8].

Medullary ECC

Medullary ECCs are subdivided into three types according to the grade of cellular and structural atypicality, well-differentiated, poorly differentiated, and undifferentiated. Of these, the frequency is highest for the well-differentiated type,

Table 2. Case and 5-year survival rate of endocrine cell tumors of the stomach.

Histological type	Number of cases	Femal	Male	Mean age (years)	5-Year survival[a] (cases)
Carcinoid					
De novo	9	3	6	67.1 ± 10.8	50.0% (6)
Multiple	7	3	4	61.5 ± 8.4	100.0% (6)
Mucocarcinoid	1	0	1	78	Unknown
ECC					
Medullary	16	6	10	60.5 ± 7.5	45.7% (10)
Scirrhous	14	8	6	47.2 ± 18.2	11.2% (10)

Multiple, Multiple carcinoids associated with type A gastritis
[a] 5-Year survival is analyzed in cases of stages III and IV, except for multiple carcinoids which are all classified into stage I

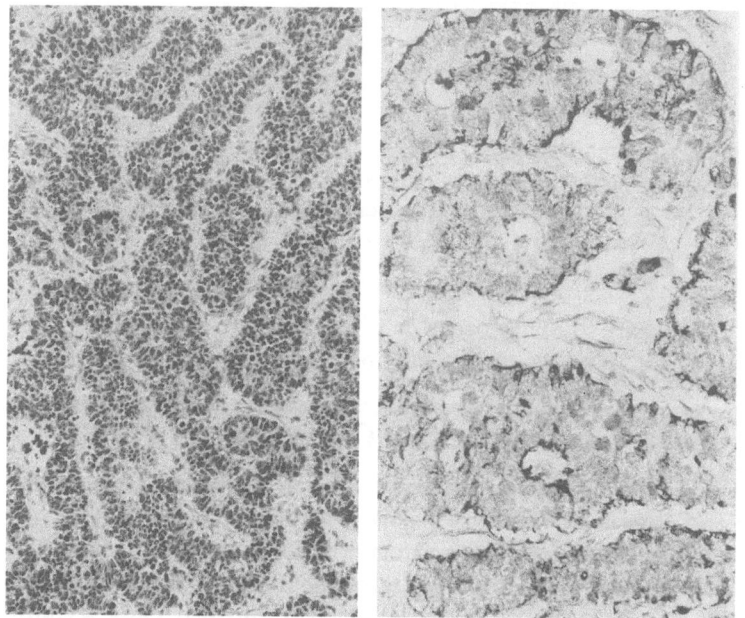

a   b

Fig. 6a,b. Medullary endocrine cell carcinoma of the stomach. **a** Tumor cells showing a few mitoses and apparent atypia form a solid nest or trabecullar pattern. H and E staining, ×140. **b** Tumor cells are diffusely positive with argyrophil reaction. Grimelius staining, ×300

followed by the undifferentiated type of medullary ECCs of the stomach. The poorly differentiated type occurs in the colon and rectum, but is exceedingly rare in the stomach [4]. An ECC of the well-differentiated type usually shows polypoid carcinomatous growth corresponding to Borrmann's type I, and is

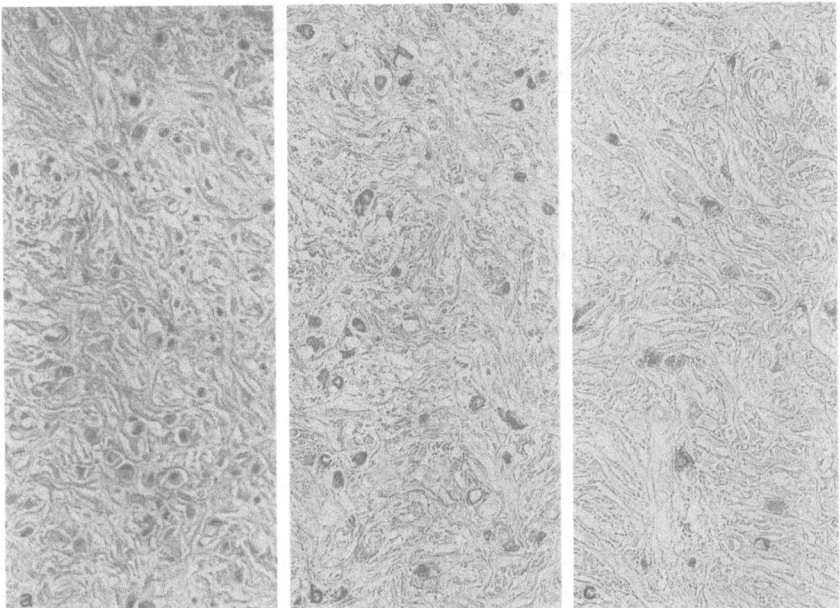

Fig. 7a–c. Scirrhous endocrine cell carcinoma of the stomach. **a** The tumor shows productive fibrosis. H and E staining, ×200. **b** and **c** A good number of tumor cells show gastrin- (**b**) and calcitonin- (**c**) immunoreactivity. Immunostaining, ×200

especially more common in the fundus than in the antrum. Microscopically, the tumor cells have solid islands or trabecular patterns (Fig. 6a,b), resembling carcinoids but also having remarkable cellular atypia and a few mitoses. The undifferentiated type cannot be distinguished marcoscopically from ordinary gastric carcinomas. The tumor cells show histological pleomorphism, including such varieties as small cell, intermediate cell, and large cell types.

Scirrhous ECC

Scirrhous ECC evidently occurs in younger patients (30–40 years of age, Table 2) compared to those with medullary ECC (50–60 years of age). It frequently develops in the fundus, and often manifests as a diffuse infiltrative carcinoma or Borrmann's type IV carcinoma. Microscopically, the tumor cells resemble poorly differentiated adenocarcinoma with abundant fibrosis (Fig. 7a). Careful observation reveals fine eosinophilic granules in the cystoplasm of many tumor cells. A few signet-ring cells may intermingle with the tumor cells.

Function of Endocrine Cell Tumors of the Stomach

Endocrine cell tumor is well known to produce both amines and a variety of peptides. Gastric endocrine cell tumors have only rarely been associated with

Table 3. Serotonin and peptide immunoreativity in endocrine cell tumor of the stomach.

Histological type	Number of case	Argyro-philia[a]	Immunoreativity[b]							
			5-TH	Gas	Som	Glu	Gli	PP	Cal	ACTH
Carcinoid										
De novo	9	8	1	2	0	0	0	0	0	0
Multiple	7	7	6	1	1	0	0	0	0	0
Mucocarcinoid	1	1	1	0	0	0	0	0	0	0
ECC										
Medullary	16	16	6	1	1	0	3	0	0	0
Scirrhous	14	14	9	4	5	2	5	2	4	0

Multiple, Multiple carcinoids associated with type A gastritis

[a] Argyrophilia determined by Grimelius staining

[b] *5-HT* Serotonin; *Gas*, gastrin; *Som*, somatostatin, *Glu*, glucagon; *Gli*, glicentin; *PP*, pancreatic polypeptide; *Cal*, calcitonin, *ACTH*, adrenocorticotropic hormone

systemic effects of carcinoid syndrome when metastasis occurs, the incidence being less than 8% in gastric carcinoids [25, 26, 34]. Thus, they are commonly endocrinologically silent. Rare modes of presentation are Cushing's syndrome due to ACTH production [35] and a gastric carcinoid associated with multiple endocrine neoplasia syndrome [28, 36, 37]. Zollinger-Ellison syndrome occurs due to gastrinomas which commonly arise from the pancreas.

Immunohistochemically, gastric endocrine cell tumors frequently contain serotonin, with its incidence of 64% being highest in scirrhous ECC (Table 3; Fig. 8a,b). In cases with multiple endocrine cell micronodules and carcinoids associated with type A gastritis, a few serotonin-immunoreactive cells are frequently detected, in contrast to the lower incidence in de novo carcinoids. It is of interest that gastric carcinoids show a lower incidence or almost an absence of peptide-immunoreactivity [9, 29], although negative immunoreactivity does not necessarily imply the total absence of the antigen examined. In fact, endocrine granules of variable types and numbers are electron-microscopically detected in all gastric carcinoids examined. On the contrary, gastric ECCs show a broad array of peptide-immunoreactivity, such as gastrin, somatostatin, glucagon, glicentin, PP, and calcitonin (Fig. 7b,c). Synchronous production of these peptides is not a rare phenomenon and is frequently associated with serotonin, especially in scirrhous ECCs.

The reason for the less frequent association with paraendocrine syndome and paucity or lack of immunoreactivity in the majority of tumor cells seems to be as follows [4, 9]: (1) the amount of peptides within the tumor is too low to be detected immunohistochemically, (2) peptides produced by tumor cells are in atypical molecular forms or prohormones resulting from post-transcriptional changes in hormone synthesis, (3) extracellular secretion of peptides from tumor cells is small, especially into the blood vessels, and (4) simultaneous production of multiple peptides shows mutual competition.

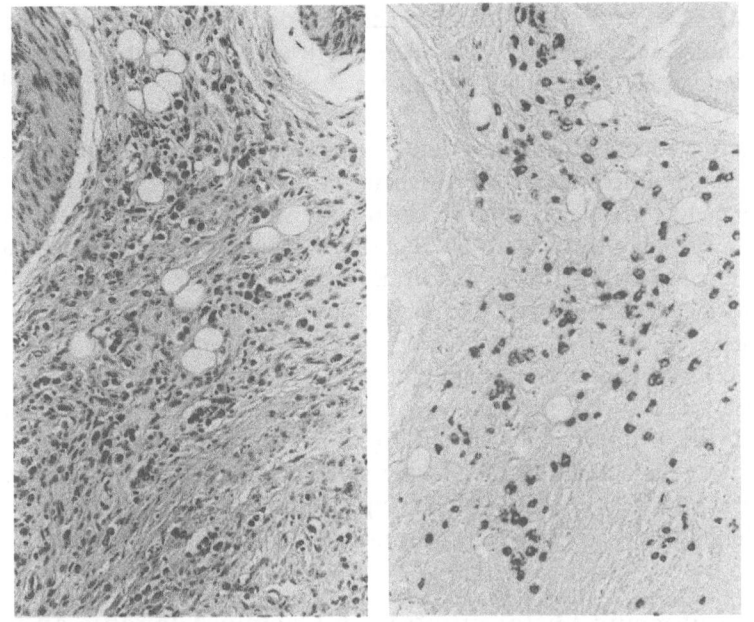

a b

Fig. 8a,b. Diffuse serotoninoma of the stomach. **a** Tumor cells resembling poorly differentiated adenocarcinoma infiltrating fibrotic submucosa. H and E staining, ×150. **b** A
majority of tumor cells show sertonin immunoreactivity. Semiserial section of Fig. 8a.
Immunostaining, ×150

Biological Behavior and Treatment of Endocrine Cell Tumors

All gastric carcinoids are typically slow-growing, but these potential malignancy,
which is compatible with prolonged survival despite the occurrence of metastases.
In 368 patients with gastric carcinoids reported in the Japanese literature, 130
(35.3%) had metastases, and these were most frequently to the regional lymph
nodes and liver [25]. The average 5-year survival for gastric carcinoids has been
reported to be approximately 50%–70% in the worldwide literature [4, 28, 38].
In our cases, the 5-year survival rate is 50% in de novo carcinoids of Stages III
and IV (Table 3), while all seven patients with multiple carcinoids associated with
type A gastritis are alive at 5 years after undergoing surgical procedures. The
latter are all classified into Stage I. The unpredictable behavior of carcinoid
tumors also mades their management difficult, especially when they are multiple.
Management of these tumors is based on the following generalization. Tumors
exceeding 2 cm in diameter have a significant potential for metastases, over 50%,
while those that are less than 2 cm in diameter have a lower risk for metastases [4,
25, 39]. The incidence of metastasis is reported to be 8.5% in gastric carcinoids
under 2 cm in diameter and 10.2% in early gastric cancer invading into the
submucosa [25]. Tumors less than 0.5 cm in diameter remain stable for many

years, often with no progress in size and never metastasizing, according to the Mayo Clinic study [39]. On the basis of these findings, it is recommended that lesions larger than 2 cm in diameter should be resected immediately after diagnosis. Lesions in the range of 1–2 cm could be treated by polypectomy, circumscribed local resection, or the usual procedure for gastrectomy. For the smaller and multiple lesions of less than 0.5 cm in diameter, one must choose between endoscopic polypectomy or strip biopsy and periodic endoscopic surveillance [4, 39, 40]. Antrectomy by abolishing hypergastrinemia might cause the arrest or regression of fundic endocrine micronodules or even carcinoids associated with type A gastritis [24]. The effectiveness of antrectomy remains to be confirmed.

Gastric ECCs appear to be highly invasive and to have a greater potential for metastases. The 5-year survival rates in our patients with Stages III and IV is 45.7% in the medullary type and 11.2% in the scirrhous type (Table 2). Thus, gastric ECCs biologically reveal a higher grade of malignancy than do carcinoids. There are, however, insufficient follow-up data on the prognosis of gastric ECCs. They should be removed even if the tumor is under 1 cm in diameter.

Endocrine Differentiation in Gastric Adenoma and Adenocarcinoma

Since the report of Hamperl in 1927 [41], it has been known that neoplastic argentaffin and/or argyrophil cells are frequently observed in gastric adenomas and adenocarcinomas [5, 42–44]. They are considered to be an integral part of the tumor, but the role in the development and growth of gastric tumors has not been adequately elucidated.

Gastric adenoma, a benign tumor of glandular epithelium, is now regarded as a precancerous or borderline lesion with the recent introduction of the concept of gastric dysplasia [45–47]. In 54 gastric tubular adenomas, a variety of endocrine cells was detected in 43 (79.6%) lesions with mild to moderate atypia. Both the frequency and distribution density are highest for EC cells (75.9%) (Fig. 9a), often showing hyperplasia followed in descending order by L cells (66.7%), D cells (35.2%), Mo cells, PYY cells, and PP cells [45]. Most of these endocrine cells are located in deeper zones of the adenoma glands. The number of endocrine cells is almost inversely proportional to the grade of epithelial atypicality in tubular adenomas, and there are no endocrine cells in the foci of carcinoma within some adenomas. The rates of occurrence of these endocrine cells in gastric tubular adenomas are similar to those for intestinal metaplasia, suggesting a close relationship between the two lesions. Paucity of endocrine cells, on the other hand, characterizes gastric papillary adenoma which is an exceedingly rare lesion [46].

The frequency of endocrine cells in ordinary gastric adenocarcinoma varies considerably in individual studies, ranging from 1.7% to 30% of all gastric adenocarcinomas [5, 42, 44, 48, 49] (Fig. 9b). We observed serotonin-containing

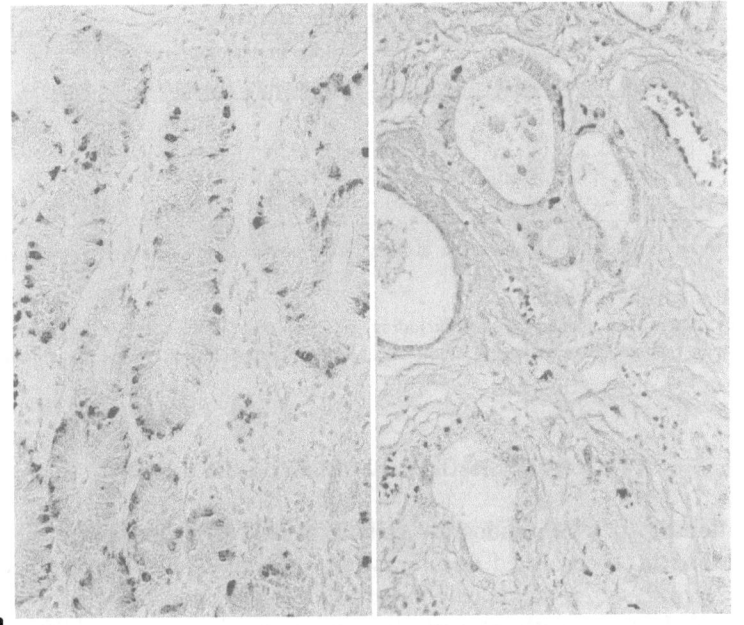

Fig. 9.a Tubular adenoma of the stomach containing numerous adenoma cells with serotonin immunoreactivity. Immunostaining, ×270. **b** Gastric tubular adenocarcinoma infiltrating submucosa. A few tumor cells show argyrophil reaction. Grimelius staining, ×270

tumor cells in more than 30% of all gastric adenocarcinomas, regardless of their histological type [48]. In most cases, endocrine cells are scattered or restricted to a small area of the tumor. The variably reported frequency of the endocrine cells in the tumor might be accounted for by the techniques used for analyzing these cells. Apparently, immunohistochemical techniques are the most sensitive and specific for detecting serotonin [48] as well as a variety of peptides.

Table 4 shows the incidence of endocrine cells containing various peptides adenocarcinomas of the stomach [9]. In early gastric cancer, there is no significant difference in the incidence of endocrine cells between well-differentiated and poorly differentiated adenocarcinoma. In advanced cancer, on the other hand, the incidence of argyrophil cells is significantly higher in the poorly differentiated type (48%) than in the well-differentiated type (26.7%). Immunohistochemically, the incidence of gastrin and somatostatin immunoreactivity in well-differentiated adenocarcinoma is fairly identical in early cancer (18.2%) and in advanced cancer (17.2%). Glicentin-immunoreactive tumor cells occur more frequently in the well-differentiated type than in the poorly differentiated type, the incidence being from 7% to 12%. The occurrence of glicentin might be regarded as an expression of an intestinal or fetal phenotype. On the contrary, calcitonin immunoreactivity is demonstrated only in advanced, poorly differentiated adenocarcinoma.

Table 4. Endocrine cells in adenocarcinoma of the stomach.

Stage	Histological type	Number of Cases	Peptide Immunoreactivity				Argyrophil Cells
			Gastrin	Somat	Glicentin	Calcitonin	
Early	Well	44	8 (18.2)[a]	8 (18.2)	3 (6.8)	0	10 (22.7)
	Poor	21	3 (14.3)	2 (9.5)	1 (4.8)	0	4 (19.0)
Advanced	Well	58	10 (17.2)	10 (17.2)	7 (12.1)	0	12 (26.7)[b]
	Poor	94	12 (12.7)	19 (20.2)	8 (9.6)	12 (12.7)	39 (48.1)[b]

[a] Values in parentheses represent incidence of cases with peptide-immunoreactivity or argyrophil cells (percentages)

[b] Significantly different ($p < 0.01$)

Well, Well-differentiated adenocarcinoma including papillary and tubular; *Poor*, poorly differentiated adenocarcinoma including signet-ring cell carcinoma and mucinous carcinoma; *Somat*, Somatostatin

Histogenesis of Endocrine Cell Tumor

The relationship between endocrine cells in the GI tract and endocrine cells to other tumors can be analyzed as follows: (1) classical carcinoid of endocrine cell origin, (2) ECC, often showing poorly differentiated adenocarcinoma, and (3) endocrine cell clones with a scattered appearance in a tumor [49]. Classical carcinoid occurs from mucosal endocrine cells whose endodermal origin was recently disclosed. This is well supported by the fact that some gastric carcinoids occur in association with endocrine cell hyperplasia, e.g., in cases of type A gastritis [31]. The histogenesis of endocrine cell clones in ordinary gastric carcinomas is thought to be similar to that of other gastric adenocarcinomas composed of several cell lines, namely, to arise from immature multipotential stem cells [4]. Thus, endocrine cell clones in the tumor may not originate from endocrine cells, but may be based on differentiation of some tumor cells into endocrine cells. Meanwhile, Warner and Seo [50] proposed the theory of "cell hybridization", which implies that hybridization of a neoplastic epithelial cell with an endocrine cell will progress to a tumor with a mixed cell population. It is possible that tumor cells might fuse with endocrine cells in the gastric mucosa adjacent to a carcinoma and then infiltrate into the submucosa as an endocrine cell clone [48]. On the other hand, there are several possible origins of ECC, including epithelial stem cells, endocrine cells, carcinoids, and endocrine cell clones within adenocarcinomas. In view of the morphological and functional heterogeneity of ECC, multipotent stem cells and endocrine cell clones in an adenocarcinoma may be the most closely related to the development of ECC.

Conclusions

Gastric endocrine cell tumors occur more frequently in Japan than in Europe and America. They have only rarely been associated with systemic effects of paraendocrine syndrome, and they are generally endocrinologically silent. Histologically, they show a broad spectrum but are divided into two types, well-differentiated (classical carcinoid) and poorly differentiated (endocrine cell carcinoma; ECC). Gastric ECC seems to have remained less familiar to both clinicians and pathologists, so its incidence might be estimated lower than it actually is. However, subclassification of gastric endocrine cell tumors should be essential for their clinical management because of their different biological behavior and prognosis. Attention, therefore, should be paid to the existence of gastric ECC, which might have been previously classified as poorly differentiated adenocarcinoma or scirrhous carcinoma.

Alterations of various oncogenes and suppressor genes have never been examined systematically in the gastric endocrine cell tumors and remain to be elucidated in the future.

References

1. Solicia E, Creutzfeldt W, Falkmer S, Fujita Y, Greider MH, Grossman MI, Grude D, Håkanson R, Larsson LI, Lechago J, Lewin KJ, Polak JM, Rubin W (1981) Human gastroenteropancreatic endocrine-paracrine cells: Santa Monica 1980 classification. In: Grossman MI, Brazier MAB, Lechago J (eds) Cellular basis of chemical messengers in the digestive systems. Academic Press New York, pp 159–165

2. Ito H, Tahara E (1987) Gut hormone: Distribution. Annual Review, Gastrointestinal Tract 1987 (in Japanese). Chugai-Igakusha, Tokyo, pp 17–23

3. Burnstock G (1982) Studies of autonomic nerves in the gut: Past, present and future. Scand J Gastroenterol [Suppl] 71:135–138

4. Lewin KJ, Riddell RH, Weinstein WM (1992) Endocrine cells. In Gastrointestinal pathology and its clinical implication. Igaku-Shoin, Tokyo, pp 197–257

5. Kubo T, Watanabe H (1971) Neoplastic argentaffin cells in gastric and intestinal carcinomas. Cancer 27:447–454

6. Soga J, Tazawa K, Aizawa O, Wada K, Tuto O (1971) Argentaffin cell adenocarcinoma of the stomach: An atypical carcinoid? Cancer 28:999–1003

7. Sweeney EC, McDonnell L (1980) Atypical gastric carcinoids. Histopathology 4:215–224

8. Tahara E, Ito H, Nakagami K, Shimamoto F, Yamamoto M, Sumii K (1982) Scirrhous argyrophil cell carcinoma of the stomach with multiple production of polypeptide hormones, amine, CEA, lysozyme, and HCG. Cancer 49:1904–1915

9. Tahara E (1988) Endocrine tumors of the gastrointestinal tract: Classification, function and biological behavior. Dig Dis Pathol 1:121–147

10. Soga J, Tazawa K (1971) Pathologic analysis of carcinoid. Histologic re-evaluation of 62 cases. Cancer 28:990–998

11. World Health Organization (1980) Histological typing of endocrine tumours. In: International histological classification of tumours, 23. WHO, Geneva

12. Tsutsumi Y, Nagura H, Watanabe K, Yanaihara N (1983) A novel subtyping of intestinal metaplasia of the stomach, with special reference to the histochemical characterizations of endocrine cells. Virchows Arch [A] 401:73–88

13. Ito H Tahara E (1983) Immunohistochemical study on G and D cells in human resected stomach with peptic ulcer diseases. In: Miyoshi A (ed) Gut peptides and ulcer. Biomedical Research Foundation, Tokyo, pp 180–187

14. Ito H, Yokozaki H, Hata J, Mandai K, Tahara E (1984) Glicentin-containing cells in intestinal metaplasia, adenoma and carcinoma of the stomach. Virchows Arch [A] 404:17–29

15. Ito H, Yokozaki H, Tokumo K, Nakajo S, Tahara E (1986) Serotonin-containing EC cells in normal human gastric mucosa and in gastritis. Immunohistochemical, electron-microscopic and autoradiographic studies. Virchows Arch [A] 409:313–323

16. Nicholas A (1891) Recherches sur l'epithelium de l'intestine Grele. Int Monatschr Anat Physiol 8:1–62

17. Kultschitzky N (1897) Zur Frage über den Bau des Darmkanals. Arch Mikrosk Anat 49:7–35

18. Yokozaki H (1986) Epithelial phenotypic expression of human foetal gastrointestinal mucosa: An immunohistochemical analysis. HIJM 35:207–222

19. Ito H, Hata J, Yokozaki H, Tahara E (1986) Calcitonin in human gastric mucosa and carcinoma. J Cancer Res Clin Oncol 112:50–56

20. Tahara E, Ito H (1983) Study on changes in G and D cells and serum gastrin levels in patients with peptic ulcer. In: Miyoshi A (ed) Gut peptides and ulcer. Biomedical Research Foundation, Tokyo, pp 164–170

21. Lewin, KJ, Elashoff JD, Yang K, Walsh J, Ulich T (1984) Primary gastrin cell hyperplasia. Report of five cases and a review of the literature. Am J Surg Pathol 8:821–832

22. Rode J, Dhillon AP, Papadaki L, Stockbrügger R, Thompson RJ, Moss E, Cotton PB (1986) Pernicious anaemia and mucosal endocrine cell proliferation of the non-antral stomach. Gut 27:789–798

23. Müller J, Kirchner T, Müller-Hermelink HK (1987) Gastric endocrine cell hyperplasia and carcinoid tumors in atrophic gastritis type A. Am J Surg Pathol 11:909–917

24. Borch K (1989) Atrophic gastritis and gastric carcinoid tumours. Ann Med 21:291–297

25. Soga J (1990) Pathology of gastrointestinal carcinoid. (1) Statistical analysis. Clin Gastroenterol 5:1661–1667

26. Sanders RJ (1973) Carcinoids of the gastrointestinal tract. Charles C. Thomas, Spring-field, Ill

27. Hajdu SI, Winawer SJ, Myers WPL (1974) Carcinoid tumors. A study of 204 cases. Am J Clin Pathol 61:521–528

28. Creutzfeldt W, Stöckmann F (1987) Carcionids and carcinoid syndrome. Am J Med 82 [Suppl 5B]:4–16

29. Iwafuchi M, Watanabe H, Yanaihara N, Ito S (1983) Immunohistochemical and ultrastructural characteristics of gastric carcinoids. Biomed Res 4 [Suppl]:307–314

30. Sjöblom S-M, Sipponen P, Miettinen M, Karonen S-L, Järvinen HJ (1988) Gastro-scopic screening for gastric carcinoids and carcinoma in pernicinous anemia. Endoscopy 20:52–56

31. Solcia E, Bordi C, Creutzfeldt W, Dayal Y, Falkmer S, Grimelius L, Havu N (1988) Histopathological classification of nonatral gastric endocrine growths in man. Digestion 41:185–200

32. Itsuno M, Watanabe H, Iwafuchi M, Ito S, Yanaihara N, Sato K, Kikuchi M, Akiyama N (1989) Multiple carcinoids and endocrine cell micronests in type A gastritis. Cancer 63:881–890

33. Issacson P (1981) Crypt cell carcinoma of the appendix (so-called adenocarcinoid tumor). Am J Surg Pathol 5:213–224

34. Cheek RC, Wilson H (1971) Carcinoid tumors. In: Wilson H, Cheek RC, Sherman RT (eds) Carcinoid tumors, current problems in surgery. Year Book Medical, New York, pp 4–31

35. Olurin EO, Sofowaora EO, Afonja AO, Kolawole TM, Junaid TA (1973) Cushing's syndrome and bronchial carcinoid tumor. Cancer 31:1514–1519.
36. Solcia E, Capella C, Fiocca R, Rindi G, Rosai J. (1990) Gastric argyrophil carcinoidosis in patients with Zollinger-Ellison syndrome due to Type I multiple endocrine neoplasia. Am J Surg Pathol 14:503–513.
37. Rode J, Dhillon AP, Cotton PB, Wodf A, O'Riordan JLH (1987) Carcinoid tumour of the stomach and primary hyperparathyroidism: A new association. J Clin Pathol 40:546–551
38. Godwin JD (1975) Carcinoid tumors, an analysis of 2837 cases. Cancer 36:560–569
39. Moertel CG (1987) An odyssey in the land of small tumors. J Clin Oncol 5:1503–1522
40. Stolte M, Ebert D, Seifert E, Schulte F, Rode J (1988) Zur Prognose der Karzinoidtumoren des Magens. Leber Magen Darm 18:246–256
41. Hamperl H (1927) Über die "gelben (chromaffinen)" Zellen im gesunden und kranken Magen-Darmschlauch. Virchows Arch [A] 266:509–548
42. Azzopardi JG, Pollock DJ (1963) Argentaffin and argyrophil cells in gastric carcinoma. J Pathol Bacteriol 86:443–451
43. Watanabe H (1972) Argentaffin cells in adenoma of the stomach. Cancer 30:1267–1274
44. Tahara E, Ito H, Shimamoto F, Taniyama K, Iwamoto T, Sumiyoshi H, Kajihara H, Yamamoto M (1982) Argyrophil cells in early gastric carcinoma: An immunohistochemical and ultrastructural study. J Cancer Res Clin Oncol 103:187–202
45. Ito H, Hata J, Yokozaki H, Nakatani H, Oda N, Tahara E (1986) Tubular adenoma of the human stomach. An immunohistochemical analysis of gut hormones, serotonin, carcinoembryonic antigen, secretory component, and lysozyme. Cancer 58:2264–2272
46. Ito H, Yokozaki H, Ito M, Tahara E (1989) Papillary adenoma of the stomach. Pathologic and immunohistochemical study. Arch Pathol Lab Med 113:1030–1034
47. Ito H, Yasui W, Yoshida K, Nakayama H, Tahara E (1990) Depressed tubular adenoma of the stomach: Pathological and immunohistochemical features. Histopathology 17:419–426
48. Ito H, Hata J, Oda N, Miyamori S, Tahara E (1986) Serotonin in tubular adenomas, adenocarcinomas and endocrine tumours of the stomach. An immunohistochemical study. Virchows Arch [A] 410:239–245
49. Tahara E, Haizuka S, Kodama T, Yamada A (1975) The relationship of gastrointestinal endocrine cells to gastric epithelial changes with special reference to gastric cancer. Acta Pathol Jpn 25:161–177
50. Warner TFCS, Seo IS (1979) Goblet cell carcinoid of appendix. Ultrastructural features and histogenic aspects. Cancer 44:1700–1706

Remnant Stomach and Gastric Cancer

Lennart Domellöf[1]

Key words. Peptic ulcer disease—Partial gastrectomy—Carcinogenesis—Micro-organisms—Pathology—Stomach neoplasms—Diagnosis

Introduction

Before the modern era of H2-receptor antagonists and proton pump inhibitors, gastric surgery was the sole effective treatment for ulcer disease. Successful partial gastrectomy with gastroduodenostomy was first performed by Theodor Billroth in 1881 for distal gastric carcinoma; 1 year later Ludwik Rydygier performed a similar operation for ulcer disease with gastric outlet obstruction. Over the next few decades the Billroth I- operation was extensively attempted and modified. In 1885 Billroth introduced another anastomotic principle, using closure of the duodenum and a gastrojejunostomy (Billroth II). Parallel with the introduction of partial gastrectomy, Wölfler designed a gastrojejunostomy which was favored by most surgeons, being an easier, more rapid, and thus safer method. However, due to the high frequency of postoperative complications this method was abandoned in the 1920s and partial gastrectomy according to Billroth I or Billroth II became the method of choice. The latter operation took over as the standard procedure in peptic ulcer disease, reaching its peak of popularity in the mid 1950s. Later Billroth I regained popularity but was soon taken over by proximal gastric vagotomy.

In 1970 peptic ulcer surgery was performed on 71.1 per 100 000 British men and about 60 per 100 000 Americans [1, 2]. The classical ulcer operations were highly effective and protected the patients from ulcer recurrence, but were not rarely complicated with postcibal symptoms. About 10% of patients with remote Billroth II gastrectomy suffer from severe postoperative distress. The recent introduction of potent antisecretory drugs and the decline in duodenal ulcer disease has markedly reduced the need for ulcer surgery. However, the number

---

[1] Department of Surgery, Örebro Medical Center Hospital, S-70185 Örebro, Sweden

of formerly-resected patients is large and the related morbidity not negligible. The most severe complication is the late development of neoplastic changes in the remnant mucosa and this has received much attention during the last few decades.

Gastric Stump Carcinoma

The gastric remnant, stump, or residue is that part of the stomach remaining after partial resection generally performed for benign ulcer disease. The remnant usually comprises 20%–50% of the stomach mucosa. In order to reduce gastric acidity adequately, males with duodenal ulcer were subjected to more extensive resections according to Billroth II than females or gastric ulcer patients, who generally were subjected to Billroth I resections.

In 1922, Balfour [3] reviewed 1280 patients who had undergone partial gastrectomy for gastric ulcer at the Mayo Clinic, and published the first report of an increased risk of death from cancer of the gastric remnant. In 1954 Freedman and Berne [4] collected several cases of gastric cancer after remote surgery from the literature, 23 cases after partial gastrectomy and 35 after simple gastroenterostomy. Two years later, Helsingen and Hillestad [5] defined gastric stump carcinoma as cancer developing in the remnant mucosa more that 5 years after surgery for benign gastroduodenal disease. This limitation was chosen in order to eliminate gastric cancer already present at the time of ulcer surgery. Up to 1979, Peitsch [6] reported about 3000 published cases of stump cancer and today this has increased to about 4000 cases from all over the world.

Pathogenesis of Stump Cancer

From epidemiological studies we know that there is an excessive incidence of gastric cancer in Japan, Chile, and Venuzuela, while in other countries there is a medium or low risk. At present, no comparable studies exist regarding stump cancer. However, there may be a geographic variance in risk, pointing to a decreased risk ratio in Japan contrary to that in Europe and the United States [7]. A number of environmental and dietary factors have been incriminated; the remnant mucosa is particularly sensitive to various noxious or protective agents that act locally, e.g, exo- and endogenous detergents, carcinogens, and vitamins C and E, and these determine the course of events.

It is well known that human gastric cancer never develops in a healthy mucosa. Partial gastrectomy leads to several chronic changes in the stomach residue that separately, or in combination, may promote cancer development in the relatively, low risk area that the upper part of the stomach normally constitutes compared with the antrum. Thus, the gastric remnant may be regarded as a clinical model for studying carcinogenic factors responsible for malignant change in the stomach mucosa.

Gastric Peptides

Over the last decade it has become clear that gastric function is regulated by peptides that act as hormones, neurotransmitters, and paracrine agents [8]. Partial gastrectomy with removal of the gastrin-producing antrum is followed by reduced serum gastrin levels. Gastrin is an important trophic factor and controls the growth of corpus mucosal cells in general, and enterochromaffin cells in particular. Low gastrin levels have been proposed to be responsible for postgastrectomy gastritis. However, no correlation was found between serum gastrin and gastritis or between endoscopic reflux gastritis and dysplasia late after Billroth II resection [9, 10]. Animal studies have shown that increased serum gastrin levels reduce the incidence of N-methyl-N'-nitro-N-nitrosoguanidine (MNNG)-induced adenocarcinoma in the intact stomach as well as in the gastric remnant after a Billroth II procedure [11].

The local endocrine effects following partial gastrectomy and their possible relevance for cancer development are more speculative. However, growth factors and the paracrine interplay between the mucosal cells will probably be influenced, leading to impaired local host defence mechanisms. Consequently, the surrounding cells may not manage to restrain initiated or neoplastic cells from proliferating in the presence of sufficient stimuli.

Duodenogastric Reflux

Bile reflux was early suggested as an important etiological factor in the development of gastritis and chronic gastric ulceration. Experimental duodenogastric reflux was shown to produce reversible gastric mucosal alterations such as epithelial proliferation and pseudopyloric metaplasia. Atrophic gastritis followed, characterized by a loss of chief and parietal cells, which were replaced by mucus-secreting cells in tortous glands and by the appearance of cysts in the lamina muscularis mucosa [12]. We postulated that duodenogastric bile reflux induces hyperplastic polyps or adenomas in humans [13] and promotes the initiation of gastric cancer [14]. Reflux of bile and pancreatic juice from the small intestine into the stomach is known to cause mucosal damage and has also been implicated in the genesis of gastric stump cancer. By studying gastric aspirates from a group of patients with remote partial gastrectomy we found a mean pH of 7.3 and the concentration of total bile acids to be 2.6 ± 2.0 mg/ml (about 6 mM), 23% of which were deconjugated. Deoxycholic acid, known to promote carcinogenesis in animals, amounted to 27% of the total bile acids [15]. As recently shown [16], these concentrations cause inhibition of the cytoprotective gastric carbonic anhydrase activity in rat (20%–40%) and human (10%–90%) gastric mucosa. Inhibition of gastric carbonic anhydrase might be one mechanism contributing to mucosal damage caused by bile reflux.

We also found fecal type flora, mostly *E. coli*, klebsiella, and *Chlostridium perfringens* in 85% of these patients, bacteria that were responsible for the deconjugation of bile salts to promoting, (co)mutagenic free bile acids. Lysolecithin is endogenously formed from the hydrolysis of biliary lecithin by pancreatic phospholipase. It is highly cytotoxic and has been identified in gastric aspirates after partial gastrectomy in greater concentrations than after other forms of gastric surgery [17]. In rats, partial gastrectomy has been shown to increase the susceptibility to cancer induction by the mutagen MNNG [18]. This is in line with the known promoter effect of bile acids in gastrointestinal carcinogenicity studies. However, it has also been shown that surgically-induced duodenogastric reflux alone causes gastric cancer within 9 months [19]. In this case, promotion of dietary or endogenously-formed carcinogens has taken place. It is also known that sodium cholate in the diet promotes MNNG-induced carcinogenesis in the remnant mucosa in rats with Roux-en- Y anastomosis that has been performed in order to prevent duodenal reflux [20]. Others have claimed that pancreatico-duodenal juice rather than bile is responsible for the cancer promotion [21]. However, this is not contradictory, as activated pancreatic enzymes, bile acids, and other intraluminal agents probably act synergistically. Mucosal proliferation, as measured by determining DNA content and crypt cell proliferation rate, is increased in animals exposed to reflux and in humans [22], and this could promote gastric carcinogenesis.

Most clinical studies, including our own, have found that the duodeno-gastric reflux is most pronounced after Billroth II resections and that the anastomotic area opposite the afferent loop is a special target site [23].

Gastric Bacterial Flora

Correa and coworkers [24] proposed the hypothesis that gastric carcinogenesis started with atrophy, progressing to chronic atrophic gastritis, reduced acid secretion, and an established resident bacterial flora in the nonoperated stomach. These bacteria were responsible for reducing nitrate to nitrite and they catalyzed the formation of N-nitroso compounds. The intraluminal carcinogens were assumed to initiate cancer of the intestinal type through intestinal metaplasia and severe dysplasia [24]. A wide range of bacterial species are capable of reducing nitrate to nitrite. It is known that E. coli, Pseudomonas aeruginosa, and Neisseria spp. strains are particularly able to catalyze the N-nitroso reaction, and N-nitroso compounds have been demonstrated in the gastric juice of nonoperated ulcer patients and after partial gastrectomy [25]. It is likely that the endogenous production of these mutagenic compounds includes other classes of organotropic carcinogens; this would explain why partial gastrectomy has been associated with cancers at sites other than the gastric mucosa [10, 26]. Our findings regarding the mainly colonic remnant microflora have been confirmed by others [27]. These authors also found elevated gastric juice nitrite concentrations in aspirates with a pH of 4–8, correlating with the presence of nitrate-reducing bacteria (E. coli, Staphylococcus aureus, and Veillonella spp). The detergent effect of free bile acids and lysolecithin on the mucosal barrier and the epithelial cells exposes the stem cells to luminal carcinogens. The multiple biochemical reactions induced by the duodenogastric reflux seem to play a distinct role in the carcinogenesis of the gastric remnant.

Helicobacter Pylori

Campylobacter pylori(dis) was discovered, isolated, and characterized by Marshall and Warren in 1983 from the mucosa of patients with chronic active gastritis [28]. The name has recently been changed to *Helicobacter pylori*. It is a transmissible, gram negative bacterium which adheres to the gastric epithelial surface cells and is protected from the gastric acid by the mucous barrier. A definite relationship between colonization with *H. pylori* in the gastric mucosa and gastric pathology was recently established. *H. pylori* has also been considered as a possible factor in gastric carcinogenesis. To determine this relationship, serum samples were analyzed from patients with confirmed gastric cancer in different sites, nongastric cancer, and benign gastric neoplasms [29]. In this study antibodies to *H. pylori* were detected in 65% of patients with noncardia gastric cancer compared with 38% in patients with cardia cancer. A significant association was found between *H. pylori* infection and noncardia cancer (odds ratio, 2.67) and there was a nonsignificant tendency for patients with intestinal type cancer compared with diffuse type cancer to have *H. pylori* infection. This supported the hypothesis of a relationship between *H. pylori* infection and noncardia gastric cancer. However, in a comparative study of the influence of postoperative bile reflux, Offerhaus and coworkers [30] found *H. pylori* present in the preoperative biopsies of all 17 patients examined. After Roux en Y gastrectomy, this was still the case but after Billroth II resection the *H. pylori* infection was eradicated in about half the cases. In patients cleared from *H. pylori* infection, the reflux gastritis score was significantly higher, suggesting that bile reflux may play a role in eradicating this infection. The mucous layer and superficial epithelial cells with the adherent bacteria were sloughed off by the detergent effect of bile acids. This argues against *H. pylori* playing a role in the etiology of stump cancer.

Gastroscopic and Histological Changes in the Remnant Mucosa

The precursor lesions of gastric cancer start as reversible changes of the normal mucosa, e.g., atrophic gastritis, dysplasia, or adenoma, and these may irreversibly change into cancer. Initiation leads to mucosal atrophy with severe atypia and intestinal metaplasia of the colonic type. Promotion leads to dysplasia and adenoma. All these mucosal alterations are acknowledged precancerous changes that are found in gastric diseases that are recognized as clinically precancerous conditions. The gastric remnant, gastric polyps, and chronic gastric ulcer belong to the latter category.

Chronic Atrophic Gastritis

Chronic atrophic gastritis is a progressive disease that leads to total atrophy in a small proportion of patients [31]. Ever since the basic studies of Konjetzny [32–34] this has been associated with gastric carcinoma and is now recognized as a premalignant change. Chronic atrophic gastritis is a significant postoperative alteration in the remnant mucosa that is found within a few years of and more frequently after Billroth II than after Billroth I resections [30, 35]. We have shown that duodenal ulcer patients, with no histological atrophy and about 30% chronic gastritis in the proximal border of the resection specimen, developed atrophy in 30% and chronic gastritis in 90% of the remnant mucosa within 3 years postoperatively [35]. The loss of mucosal glands in atrophic gastritis is combined with the growth of metaplastic intestinal and so-called pseudopyloric glands. In healthy unoperated individuals, the frequency of atrophic gastritis, including intestinal metaplasia, increases with age [36]. This aging process is markedly accelerated by partial gastrectomy, most dramatically in young subjects operated for duodenal ulcer. In these patients, the histological picture of the mucosa becomes decades older within the 1st postoperative year.

It has been clearly shown that atrophic gastritis precedes stomach cancer, and as many as 10% of patients with severe atrophic gastritis may develop later cancer. The cumulative risk of developing gastric carcinoma is highest in subjects who are young when the mucosal atrophy starts and is twice as high in males with severe atrophic gastritis than in females [31]. This is in agreement with the finding that young males partially gastrectomized of duodenal ulcer, run a significantly higher risk of developing stump cancer [37].

Cystic Dilatation of the Gastric Tubules

This is a histopathological change that has been reported as an early change in experimental gastric carcinogenesis in the rat, but has also been observed close to early gastric cancer in humans. It is a common finding in the gastric remnant, being present in about 70% of stomal biopsies late after Billroth II gastrectomy [23, 35]. The occurrence is slightly more common when the operation is performed for gastric ulcer than for duodenal ulcer (77.5% and 58.5%, respectively). Polyp patients have cystic dilatation of the gastric glands in 85% of cases and it is found in 90% of biopsies from the vicinity of stump cancer [23]. These cysts may play a role in the pathogenesis of gastric cancer, as traps for transformed cells which otherwise would have been shed from the surface like benign epithelial cells [38]. Such transformed cells could rest as dormant cells or progress to neoplasm.

Intestinal Metaplasia

Intestinal metaplasia (IM) is a common finding in gastric biopsies (20%–30%); it increases with age and is more prevalent in high risk gastric cancer areas compared to low risk areas. Evidence which suggests a close relationship between intestinal-type gastric carcinoma and IM associated with chronic atrophic gastritis has accumulated in the literature. Three main types of IM have been found; type I (also termed mature, complete, or small intestinal) is the most common, found in about 70% of cases, followed by type II IM (incomplete) found in about

20%, and type III IM (immature, incomplete, or colonic) representing 10% of IM-positive biopsies. The third, non-sulfated phenotype, is significantly more associated with gastric cancer of the intestinal type than types I and II [39].

Partially-gastrectomized patients develop IM postoperatively. This is most obvious in duodenal ulcer patients with no IM in the resected operation specimen who have almost the same frequency of IM after 1–3 years as operated gastric ulcer patients [35]. The severity of IM is correlated with its extent and with the severity of dysplasia [40]. Occasionally IM is found close to stump carcinomas.

Dysplasia

The criteria for classifying dysplasia of the gastric mucosa are based on the descriptions given by Nagayo in 1971 and adopted by a WHO pathology group in 1980 [41]. Several endoscopic investigations have demonstated varying degrees of dysplasia in the remnant mucosa [10, 40]. The prevalence varies from 5.7% to 59.3%. The severity of dysplasia is reported to vary by time in the few longitudinal studies performed. In 87 subjects who had had gastric surgery more than 20 years previously, Savalgi and coworkers found that the severity of dysplasia was correlated with its extent [40]. Previous Billroth II operation was more strongly associated with dysplasia (85%) than other operations. Furthermore, they found moderate and severe dysplasia more commonly at the stoma (37%) than in the body (10%). The finding that there is a relationship between the severity and extent of the two precancerous lesions, i.e., dysplasia and intestinal metaplasia, suggests a widespread mucosal instability. Sampling error and the number of evaluated endoscopic biopsies may play a role in explaining differences in results from different studies. This was shown by Graem and coworkers [42], who reported that the incidence of dysplasia doubled when the number of biopsies increased from 4 to 16. In a recent follow-up of the clinical value of dysplasia in the remnant mucosa, 13% of patients with moderate dysplasia and 41% of those with severe dysplasia were found to have stump cancer within a few years [10]. Dysplasia is not rarely found in the mucosa surrounding gastric carcinoma. The finding of marked dysplasia in gastric biopsies is a recognized indicator of malignancy and close endoscopic surveillance should be performed.

Lipid Islands

These changes are easily visualized at endoscopy as well-demarcated white or yellow-white, slightly irregular patches. They are flat, or sometimes elevated. Microscopically, they are composed of accumulations of lipid-filled macrophages beneath the surface epithelial cells [43]. The occurrence of lipid islands was previously linked to high age, atherosclerosis, and diabetes mellitus or hypertension. In an extensive survey we found no such correlations in nonoperated or partially-gastrectomized patients [43]. Lipid islands were never found in normal gastric mucosa. In nonoperated patients, lipid islands were found in 6.3% and approximately the same prevalence was found early after partial gastrectomy. However, the prevalence increased with time after surgery and more than 20 years after Billroth II resection, 65% of patients had single or multiple lipid islands at endoscopy compared with 40% after Billroth I operations. There was no difference with regard to gender, previous ulcer disease, or age. No correlation was found with regard to the absence or presence of previous cholecystectomy. The localization of lipid islands to areas exposed to intestinogastric reflux suggested lipid absorption, perhaps in combination with impaired elimination, as the most plausible explanation of the accumulation of lipid-filled scavenger cells in the diseased remnant mucosa. A similar microscopic picture is present in the gallbladder wall in cholesterolosis. The relevance of lipid islands in the development of cancer may be that lipid-soluble carcinogens can be absorbed and temporarily stored in these areas.

Polyps

Sessile or pedunculated polyps are most often found close to the anastomotic area, showing histological features similar to "gastritis cystica polyposa" or "gastric stomal polypoid hyperplasia".

In a long-term follow up of partially-gastrectomized patients, we found polyps at gastroscopy in 8.9% of 336 cases compared to 4.9% in 407 symptomatic, nonoperated subjects [13]. Four of the operated patients had severe dysplasia and four had stump carcinoma (1.2% each). In an extended study, 63 out of 544 patients (11.6%) have had one or several polyps in the gastric remnant at screening endoscopy. Six of these polyps were adenomas, in two cases with severe dysplasia. Similar results were found in an endoscopic and morphological study from Finland [44]. These investigators found gastric polyps in 454 out of 13 200 consecutive gastroscopies (3.4%) performed in nonoperated patients. Adenomas were encountered in 8% of the polyp cases, and foveolar hyperplasia, hyperplastic polyps, and inflammatory polyps in 21%, 34%, and 36%, respectively. Carcinoma was found in 38% of adenoma patients and in 5% of patients with other polyps. We have early claimed that gastric polyps should be regarded as markers of cancer anywhere in the remnant mucosa, not necessarily only in proximity to the polyp [13].

Risk of Developing Carcinoma After Partial Gastrectomy

Chronic gastric ulcer is a recognized precancerous condition; in patients with this condition, there is an increased risk of developing gastric cancer. Duodenal ulcer, in contrast, has a significantly lower risk of cancer development in the generally hypersecretory, but otherwise histologically normal, stomach mucosa [45].

During the last few decades there has been an increasing number of retrospective cohort studies in the literature with sufficient follow up time to judge the incidence or mortality of gastric cancer after partial gastrectomy. The large

L. Domellöf

Table 1. Selected cohort studies of stomach cancer after ulcer surgery.

Study	Year	No of patients	Observed cancer cases	Expected cancer cases	O/E cases	95% Ratio	Follow up conf. limits	End point (years)
Helsingen and Hillestad [5]	1956	222	11	5.2	2.12[a]	1.06, 3.79	10–35	Mortality
Krause [52]	1958	361	25	11.3	2.21[a]	1.43, 3.27	25–50	Mortality
Liavaag [53]	1962	616	9	9	0.94	0.43, 1.78	15–29	Mortality
McLean Ross et al. [54]	1982	779	8	10.4	0.77	0.33, 1.52	15–33	Mortality
Fischer et al. [9]	1983	1000	13	10.6	1.23	0.65, 2.10	22–30	Incidence
Tokudome et al. [55]	1984	3827	34	100.6	0.34	0.23, 0.47	10–33	Mortality
Caygill et al. [56]	1986	4466	80	50.7	1.58[a]	1.25, 1.96	20–40	Mortality
Viste et al. [57]	1986	3470	87	41.4	2.10[a]	1.68, 2.59	25–45	Incidence
Lundegårdh et al. [26]	1988	6459	102	106.8	0.96	0.78, 1.16	25–33	Incidence
Offerhaus et al. [30]	1988	2619	52	36.5	1.80	0.80, 2.10	15–46	Incidence
Present report	1990	1049	26	20.8	1.25	0.82, 1.84	19–36	Incidence
Stael von Holstein et al. [10]	1992	1317	43	25.7	1.67[a]	1.22–2.27	29–59	Mortality

O/E, observed/expected; *conf.* confidence
[a] Significant change

number of patients also allows for the analysis of subgroups according to initial ulcer disease, operation method, and gender (Table 1).

Starting in 1973 we have performed a follow up of all patients operated during the period 1952–1969 at the department of surgery in Umeå, Sweden. All patients with benign ulcer disease who were less than 76 years of age were offered surveillance with repeated endoscopies. In 1977 we reported a significantly increased risk for stump carcinoma 12 years or more after ulcer surgery, but only in males (observed/expected [O/E], 11/4; $P = 0.006$). At a later evaluation in 1986 [46], we found no gastric cancer during the first 9 years, but a significant increase in the male O/E ratio after 17 years (16/5.2; $P = 0.0002$). The estimated annual incidence of gastric carcinoma was ten times higher in operated males aged 50–55 than in the general male population in the region. This was due to the significantly increased proportion of stump cancer in males younger than 40 at partial gastrectomy. No increased incidence was found in females. The last evaluation was performed after the closing date of the study, on December 31, 1988, and included 1049 patients with a follow up of 6 years or more and operated for verified gastric or duodenal ulcer.

Radiologically-verified non-operated ulcer patients from 1960–1969, served as controls. This was the earliest period of record-keeping in the Department of Radiology. A total of 857 patients remained after exclusion of those who had died

Table 2. Cohort study—partial gastrectomy versus nonoperated controls

Group	Number	Males	Females	Gastric ulcer	Duodenal ulcer	Mean age at op	Follow up years (mean)	Person years at risk
Billroth II	300	187	113	151	149	51.2	20.1	5410
Billroth I	749	577	172	245	504	46.9	25.0	15679
Non-operated	857	524	333	404	453	78.4	20.9	17649

within 5 years after diagnosis (Table 2). Comparisons were also made with age; and sex-matched municipality controls.

Stomach cancer was diagnosed in 26 operated patients (23 males). Fifteen of these, including 5 early gastric cancers, were found at endoscopy, 7 were diagnosed radiologically, and 4 at autopsy. Nine gastric carcinomas (seven males) were found in the nonoperated controls. Moreover, we performed endoscopic polypectomies in several cases, including six adenomas of 0.5–2 cm in size. Naturally interventions like this will influence future risk evaluations. Stratified analyses showed a significantly increased risk for males who had undergone duodenal ulcer surgery before the age of 40 compared with municipality controls (standardized incidence ratio [SIR]: 5.13, confidence limits 1.88–11.18; $P = 0.02$). At a univariate comparison of the operated and nonoperated cohorts, a significantly increased relative risk for cancer, by 7.45 times, was found in operated individuals ($P = 0.0251$) and a 9 times increased risk was found for those operated for duodenal ulcer ($P = 0.011$). The relative risk in males operated for duodenal ulcer was 7.45 ($P = 0.0215$), but the risk for males with gastric ulcer was not significantly increased, being 1.66 ($P = 0.2736$). Multivariate analysis of the two cohorts revealed three significant risk variables, namely, surgery, ulcer type, and gender. Thus, when comparing the operated versus nonoperated cohorts, relative risk (RR) was increased by 2 to 3 times after ulcer surgery (RR = 2.29, $P = 0.0315$), in gastric ulcer patients (RR = 2.47; $P = 0.0083$), and in males (RR = 2.95; $P = 0.025$). This is in line with the results of a recent multivariate analysis from Holland [47], in which there was an overall excess risk from gastric cancer of 1.5. Their patients operated on for gastric ulcer were at a 2.6 times higher risk than duodenal ulcer patients, although both groups were at higher risk than the general population. Contrary to Lundegårdh [26], neither they nor we could find any increased cancer risk for females or after Billroth II gastrectomy. The reason for this may be the greater number of patients in their cohort.

Recently, the importance of time since ulcer surgery, originally shown by Stalsberg and Taksdal [48] and later by others, has been amply confirmed. After adjustment for potential confounding by subgroups, the average adjusted risk was increased 28% for each successive 5-year interval after operation [26]. The relative risk was 9.4 after 15–24 years, and 55.6 after 25–46 years [47]. Even though different opinions exist with regard to the risk of development of stump cancer, most recent studies agree that there is a moderate overall excess risk. This risk of gastric cancer increases with time and faster than would be expected from aging in the general population.

It is important to emphasize that all these comparisons have been made without risk adjustment for the size reduction of the mucosal area at risk after partial gastrectomy. We have previously demonstated the effect on relative risk after such adjustments [46]. Finally, it is generally agreed upon that the interval between gastrectomy and the detection of stump carcinoma must be 5 years, in order to eliminate the possibility that the cancer already existed at the time of surgery, but was overlooked. However, with the present knowledge of the slow progression from severe dysplasia to early and finally advanced cancer we would like to extend the exclusion time to the first 10 years postoperatively, in order to include only true operation sequel carcinomas.

Diagnosis of Remnant Carcinoma

Most patients with stump cancer lack specific symptoms, even when they are in advanced stages of the disease, and neither radiological examinations nor laboratory tests can be used for early diagnosis. However, since some centers have introduced endoscopic surveillance of the gastric remnant, combined with multiple biopsies, early detection of precancerous lesions and early gastric cancer has been achieved to a greater extent than we have previously experienced in Europe. Especially after Billroth II gastrectomy, the anastomosis and the remnant mucosa exposed to intestinogastric reflux has been shown to be the site of most

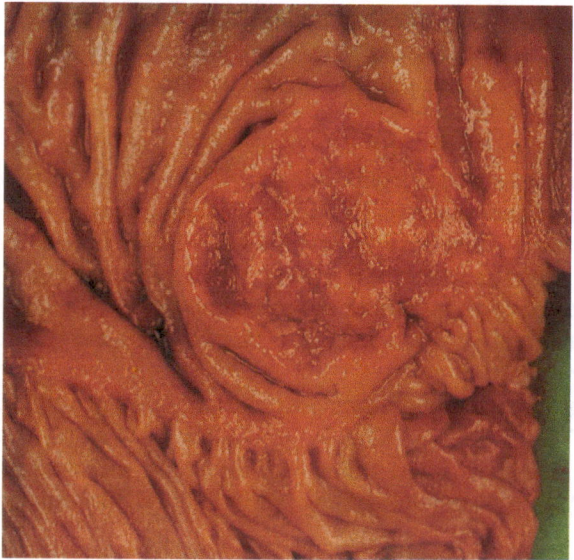

Fig. 1. Early gastric cancer type III at a Billroth II stoma, localized to the area of maximal intestinogastric reflux, i.e., facing the afferent loop. This cancer was diagnosed and resected by total gastrectomy 20 years after the initial ulcer surgery

macro- and microscopic lesions (Fig. 1). The diagnostic (bioptic) accuracy may be further improved by using vital staining of the remnant mucosa at endoscopy.

The conclusion from most surveillance studies, including our own, has confirmed the late increase in stump cancer risk after ulcer operations and recommended endoscopic surveillance from about 15 years postoperatively. Others have questioned the rationale for this, from a cost benefit point of view, although they find it convincingly shown that stump cancer is initiated by the surgical procedure. Admittedly, the total number of stump cancers is low in comparison with the major killers of these patients, e.g., benign cardiopulmonary disease and cancer of the respiratory tract. Consequently, some authors have advocated that greater efforts should be made to persuade partially-gastrectomized patients to stop smoking and to adopt a more prudent lifestyle, rather than offer them endoscopic follow ups [10].

The results obtained from endoscopic screening over 17 years for gastric stump cancer have recently been published [49]. This was a nonrandomized trial with basically incongruent screening and control groups. The authors concluded that "regular endoscopic screening does not significantly reduce gastric cancer mortality and cannot be recommended in asymptomatic patients". They arrived at this conclusion despite the fact that they had diagnosed and successfully operated 17 early gastric cancers (4.8%) in the screening group compared to 2 (0.4%) in the controls.

In a recent review, the 5-year survival rate was reported to be as low as 6% in 1690 patients with gastric stump cancers [50]. However, thanks to the early detection of these cancers, is Japanese studies have shown the prognosis to be comparable to operated primary cancers stage by stage [51]. Results in the same direction have also been achieved in Europe by others and ourselves. There is a general agreement to recommend radical resection as the method of choice in surgery of stump cancer.

Endoscopic screening limited to Billroth II subjects has recently been recommended [37]. If biopsies were taken only from the stoma, the endoscopic workload could be reduced by 85%, with only a small reduction (15%) in the detection of marked dysplasia. We cannot presently accept the negative attitude to endoscopic surveillance of populations at high risk for stump cancer. However, it is certainly not acceptable to conduct meaningless screening in elderly patients who cannot benefit from the early detection of stump cancer. Consequently, we support selected screening of high-risk patients, but suggest an upper age limit of 70 years and the exclusion of concomitant severe disease.

References

1. Bloom B, Fendrick M, Ramsey S (1990) Changes in peptic ulcer and gastritis/duodenitis in Great Britain 1970–1985. J Clin Gastroenterol 12:100–108
2. Fineberg H, Pearlman L (1981) Surgical treatment of peptic ulcer in the United States. Trends before and after the introduction of cimetidine. Lancet I:1305–1307

3. Balfour DC (1922) Factors influencing the life expectancy of patients operated on for gastric ulcer. Ann Surg 76:405–408
4. Freedman M, Berne C (1954) Gastric carcinoma of the gastrojejunal stoma. Gastroenterology 27:210–215
5. Helsingen N, Hillestad L (1956) Cancer development in the gastric stump after partial gastrectomy for ulcer. Ann Surg 143:173–179
6. Peitsch W (1979) Remarks on frequency and pathogenesis of primary gastric stump cancer. In: Herfarth C, Schlag P (eds) Gastric cancer. Springer, New York, pp 137–144
7. Tersmette AC, Giardiello FM, Offerhaus GJA, Tersmette KWF, Ohara K, Vandenbroucke JP, Tytgat GNJ (1991) Geographical variance in the risk of gastric stump cancer: No increased risk in Japan? Jpn J Cancer Res 82:266–272
8. Dockray GJ (1992) Gastric peptides. In: Gustavsson S, Kumar D, Graham D (eds) The stomach. Churchill Livingstone, London, pp 103–127
9. Fischer AB, Graem N, Christiansen L (1983) Causes and clinical significance of gastritis following Billroth II resection for duodenal ulcer. Br J Surg 70:322–325
10. Stael von Holstein C (1992) Gastric stump carcinoma. A clinical study on carcinoma in the gastric remnant after surgery for benign gastroduodenal disease. Thesis, bulletin no 84, Department of Surgery, University of Lund
11. Tatsuta M, Yamamura, Taniguchi H, Tamura H (1982) Gastrin protection against chemically induced gastric adenocarcinomas in Wistar rats: Histopathology of the glandular stomach and incidence of gastric adenocarcinoma. J Natl Cancer Inst 69:59–66
12. Lawson HH (1979) Duodenogastric reflux and epithelial lesions. In: Herfarth C, Schlag P (eds) Gastric cancer. Springer New York, pp 112–119
13. Domellöf L, Janunger KG (1978) Polyps in the gastric remnant after partial gastrectomy. Acta Chir Scand 144:293–298
14. Domellöf L (1979) Gastric carcinoma promoted by alkaline reflux gastritis—with special reference to bile and other surfactants as promoters of postoperative gastric cancer. Med Hypotheses 5:463–476
15. Domellöf L, Reddy BS, Weisburger JH (1980) Microflora and deconjugation of bile acids in alkaline reflux after partial gastrectomy. Am J Surg 140:291–295
16. Salomoni M, Zuccato E, Granelli P, Montorsi W, Doldi SB, Germiniani R, Mussini E (1989) Effect of bile salts on carbonic anhydrase from rat and human gastric mucosa. Scand J Gastroenterol 24:28–32
17. Dewar P, King R, Johnston D (1982) Bile acid and lysolecithin concentrations in the stomach in patients with duodenal ulcer before operation and after treatment by highly selective vagotomy, partial gastrectomy, or truncal vagotomy and drainage. Gut 23:569–577
18. Dahm K, Werner B, Eichen R, et al (1979) Experimental cancer of the gastric stump. In: Herfarth C, Schlag P (eds) Gastric cancer. Springer, New York, pp 44–69
19. Langhans P, Heger R, Hohenstein J, Bunte H (1981) Gastric stump carcinoma—new aspects deduced from experimental results. Scand J Gastroenterol 67 [Suppl]:161–164
20. Kawahara A, Saito T, Kobayashi M (1989) Bile acids promote carcinogenesis in the remnant stomach of rats. J Cancer Res Clin Oncol 115:423–428
21. Mason R, Filipe I (1990) The aetiology of gastric stump carcinoma in the rat. Scand J Gastroenterol 25:961–965
22. Mortensen NJMcC, Houghton PWJ (1988) Bile and enterogastric reflux—a factor in gastric cancer? In: Reeds PI, Hill MJ (eds) Gastric carcinogenesis, Excerpta Medica IV series. Excerpta Medica, Amsterdam

23. Domellöf L, Eriksson S, Janunger KG (1977) Carcinoma and possible precancerous changes of the gastric stump after Billroth II resection. Gastroenterology 73:462–468

24. Correa P, Haenszel W, Cuello C, Tannenbaum S, Archer M (1975) A model for gastric cancer epidemiology. Lancet II:58–59

25. Hill MJ (1988) Gastric carcinogenesis: Luminal factors. In: Reeds PI, Hill MJ (eds) Gastric carcinogenesis, Excerpta Medica IV series. Excerpta Medica, Amsterdam

26. Lundegårdh G (1991) Mortality and cancer incidence following partial gastrectomy for benign ulcer disease. Thesis, Uppsala University

27. Muscroft T, Deane S, Youngs D, Burdon D, Keighley M (1981) The microflora of the postoperative stomach. Br J Surg 68:560–564

28. Marshall BJ, Warren JR (1984) Unidentified curved bacilli in the stomach of patients with gastritis and peptic ulceration. Lancet II:1311–1314

29. Talley NJ, Zinsmeister AR, Weaver A, DiMagno EP, Carpenter HA, Perez-Perez GI, Blaser MJ (1991) Gastric adenocarcinoma and *Helicobacter pylori* infection. J Natl Cancer Inst 83:1734–1739

30. Offerhaus GJA, van der Stadt J, Huibregtse K, Tersmette AC, Tytgat GNJ (1989) The mucosa of the gastric remnant harboring malignancy. Cancer 64:698–703

31. Sipponen P (1989) Atrophic gastritis as a premalignant condition. Ann Med 21: 287–290

32. Konjetzny GE (1928) Die Entzündung des Magens. In: Henke F, Lubarsch O (eds) Handbuch der speziellen pathologischen Anatomie und Histologie, vol 4/2. Springer, Berlin, pp 768–1175

33. Konjetzny GE (1938) Der Magenkrebs. Enke, Stuttgart

34. Konjetzny GE (1943) Die Beziehungen zwischen Gastritis und Magenkrebsentwicklung. Langenbecks Arch Klin Chir 204:4–63

35. Janunger KG, Domellöf L, Eriksson S (1978) The development of mucosal changes after gastric surgery for ulcer disease. Scand J Gastroenterol 13:217–223

36. Siurala M, Lehtola J, Ihamaki T (1968) Atrophic gastritis and its sequelae. Scand J Gastroenterol 3:211–223

37. Eriksson SBS (1983) The operated stomach—A clinical study on late morbidity and mortality rates in patients operated on for benign gastroduodenal diesease, with special reference to the risk of developing gastric cancer. Thesis; bulletin no 36, Department of Surgery, University of Lund

38. Fujita S (1976) Kinetics of cellular proliferation and growth of human cancers. In: Sugimura T, Yamamura Y (eds) Cancer. Iwanami, Tokyo

39. Filipe MI (1988) Intestinal metaplasia in the histogenesis of gastric carcinoma. In: Reeds PI, Hill MJ (eds) Gastric carcinogenesis, Excerpta Medica IV series. Excerpta Medica, Amsterdam

40. Savalgi RS, Corbishley CM, Caygill C, Hill M, Cook MG, Kirkham JS, Northfield TC (1990) Relation between severity and extent of precancerous lesions in the postoperative stomach. Lancet II:413–416

41. Morson BC, Sobin LH, Grundmann E, Johansen Å, Nagayo T, Serck-Hanssen A (1980) Precancerous conditions and epithelial dysplasia in the stomach. J Clin Pathol 33:711–721

42. Graem N, Fischer AB, Beck H (1984) Dysplasia and carcinoma in the Billroth II resected stomach. Acta Pathol Microbiol Immunol Scand [A] 92:185–188

43. Domellöf L, Eriksson S, Helander HF, Janunger KG (1977) Lipid islands in the gastric mucosa after resection for benign ulcer disease. Gastroenterology 72:14–18

44. Laxen F, Sipponen P, Ihamäki T, Hakkilouto A, Dortcheva Z (1982) Gastric polyps; their morphological and endoscopical characteristics and relation to carcinoma. Acta Pathol Microbiol Immunol Scand [A] 90:221–228
45. Norfleet R, Johnson S (1989) Strange bedfellows: Duodenal ulcer and cancer of the stomach. J Clin Gastroenterol 11:382–385
46. Domellöf L (1986) Risk of carcinoma after partial gastrectomy. In: Inokuchi K (ed) Gann monograph on cancer research 31:205–211
47. Tersmette AC, Goodman SN, Offerhaus GJA, Tersmette KWF, Giardiello FM, Vandenbroucke JP, Tytgat GNJ (1991) Multivariate analysis of the risk of stomach cancer after ulcer surgery in an Amsterdam cohort of postgastrectomy patients. Am J Epidemiol 134:14–21
48. Stalsberg H, Taksdal S (1971) Stomach cancer following gastric surgery for benign conditions. Lancet II:1175–1179
49. Stael von Holstein C, Eriksson S, Huldt B, Hammar E (1991) Endoscopic screening during 17 years for gastric stump carcinoma. A prospective clinical trial. Scand J Gastroenterol 26:1020–1026
50. Dilin C, Sarfati E, Chevrel JP (1985) Les cancers dits "du moignon gastrique". J Chir (Paris) 122:193–200
51. Sasako M, Maruyama K, Kinoshita T, Okabayashi K (1991) Surgical treatment of carcinoma of the gastric stump. Br J Surg 78:822–824
52. Krause U (1958) Late prognosis after partial gastrectomy for ulcer. Acta Chir Scand 114:341–354
53. Liavaag K (1962) Cancer development in the gastric stump after partial gastrectomy. Ann Surg 155:103–106
54. McLean Ross AH, Smith MA, Anderson JR, Small WP (1982) Late mortality after surgery for peptic ulcer. N Engl J Med 307:519–522
55. Tokudome S, Kono S, Ikeda M, Karatsune M, Sano C, Inokuchi K, Kodama Y, Ischimiya H, Kanayama F, Faibara N, Koga S, Yamada H, Ikejiri T, Oka N, Tsurumaru H (1984) A prospective study on primary gastric stump cancer following partial gastrectomy for benign gastroduodenal diseases. Cancer Res 44:2208–2212
56. Caygill C, Hill M, Kirkham J, Northfield T (1986) Mortality from gastric cancer following surgery for peptic ulcer. Lancet I:929–931
57. Viste A, Björnestad E, Opholm P, Skarstein A, Thunold J, Hartveit F, Eide GE, Eide TJ, Söreide O (1986) Risk of carcinoma following gastric operations for benign disease: A historical cohort study of 3470 patients. Lancet II:502–505

Part 4
Biology

DNA Ploidy Pattern and Cell Kinetics

Takanori Hattori[1]

Key words. DNA ploidy pattern—Diploid—Aneuploid—Cell kinetics—Cell proliferation—Growth fraction

DNA Ploidy Pattern

Neoplasia is caused by a functional and structural disorder of cellular DNA, and the changes are reflected in the morphology of cells, oncogene expressions, gene amplifications, chromosome numbers, and nuclear DNA content, etc. Recent advances of flow cytometric and cytofluorometric measurements have enabled us to determine the DNA ploidy pattern of cancer cells [1, 2]. In these cytometric studies, the cell nucleus is stained with fluorescent dyes such as pararosaniline, propidium iodine, and diamidino-phenylindole, which specifically bind to DNA, and the DNA content is determined by comparing the fluorescent intensity of the nucleus between cancer cells and normal leukocytes or stromal cells. DNA ploidy patterns of human cancers are classified into diploid and aneuploid modes (Fig. 1). There is also a mosaic type consisting of diploid and aneuploid cell lines, and of different aneuploid cell lines. Each stem cell line is often accompanied with a polyploid cell population(s), the DNA content of which is 2^n-times (n = 1, 2, 3, . . .) the stem DNA content.

DNA Ploidy Patterns of Advanced Gastric Cancers

From a histogenetic point of view, gastric cancers are classified into 2 types, differentiated adenocarcinoma and undifferentiated carcinoma [3]. Table 1 shows the distribution of DNA ploidy patterns of the 63 advanced gastric cancers studied. In the advanced adenocarcinomas, about 46% were diploid, 54% were aneuploid, 26% were mosaics of diploid and aneuploid cell lines, and about 2%

---

[1] Department of Pathology, Shiga University of Medical Science, Seta, Ohtsu, 520-21 Japan

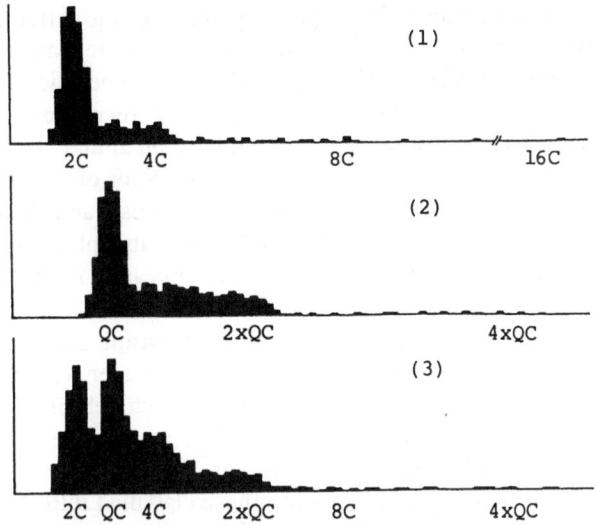

Fig. 1. Modes of DNA ploidy patterns: (**1**) diploid cancer, (**2**) aneuploid cancer, (**3**) mosaic cancer of diploid and aneuploid cell lines. *2C*, diploid; *QC*, aneuploid

Table 1. DNA ploidy patterns of 56 early and 63 advanced cancers.

Type (*n*)		Diploid	Aneuploid (mosaic[a])	Polyploid
Dif. adenocarcinomas				
Early	(26)	8/26	15/26 (8/26)	18/26
Advanced	(35)	16/35	19/35 (10/35)	30/35
Undifferentiated ca.				
Early	(30)	29/30	1/30 (0/30)	11/30
Advanced				
Non-scirrhous	(11)	4/11	7/11 (7/11)	11/11
Scirrhous	(17)	2/17	15/17 (10/17)	17/17

[a] Mosaic of aneuploid and diploid cell lines
Dif., Differentiated, *ca.*, carcinoma

were mosaics of different aneuploid cell lines [4, 5]. The DNA content of aneuploid cancers ranged from 2.4C to 4.3C (2C corresponds to a diploid value of the nuclear DNA), and it was around 3.0C in many cancers. Well-differentiated adenocarcinomas were often uni-modal, consisting of one diploid or aneuploid cell line, whereas moderately and poorly differentiated adenocarcinomas tended to be bi- and multi-modal, composed of diploid and aneuploid cell lines. In most cases, both diploid and aneuploid cells were randomly distributed, and there was no specificity in the distribution of aneuploid cells. In several cases, diploid cells comprised one lesion and aneuploid cells comprised the other one. In such tumors, the histology was more or less different between the diploid and the aneuploid lesions.

In advanced adenocarcinomas, DNA ploidy patterns of the extramucosal lesions (submucosal, muscle layer, subserosal invasive, etc.) were basically similar to those seen in the mucosal lesions. However, there was an occasional difference in the occurrence of mosaicism; for example, there were cancers in which the mucosal lesion consisted of a mosaic of diploid and aneuploid cell lines, but the extramucosal lesion consisted of one of them, or the ratios of the diploid and the aneuploid components were different between the mucosal and the extramucosal lesions. In rare cases (less than 2% of the total), a new aneuploid or polyploid cell line which was not seen in the mucosal lesion appeared in the extramucosal lesion.

DNA ploidy patterns of the metastatic lesions in lymph nodes were basically similar to those of the primary lesions in most advanced adenocarcinomas [6], but there sometimes was a difference in the density of each cell line, and, rarely, a new ploidy appeared in the metastatic lesion. The appearance of a new ploidy class seems to be a kind of progression in the cancer tissue.

Advanced undifferentiated carcinomas are those classified into Borrmann types III (localized ulcerative) and IV (diffusely infiltrative), the latter also being referred to as linitis plastica and scirrhous cancer [3]. About 64% of the Borrmann type III cancers contained aneuploid cells; they were mosaics of aneuploid and diploid lines. About 88% of the Borrmann type IV cancers contained aneuploid cell line(s), of which 59% were mosaic cancers and 29% were uni-modal with an aneuploid cell line. About 12% of the Borrmann type IV cancers consisted of only diploid cell lines [7, 8].

The mucosal and the extramucosal parts of the advanced undifferentiated carcinomas were essentially composed of the same stem cell line(s). However, there was a variation among them in the occurrence of each cell line. In most of the Borrmann type III cancers, diploid and aneuploid cells were distributed both in the mucosal and in the extramucosal layers, but diploid cells were often predominant in the mucosal layer, and groups of aneuploid cells were often

Table 2. DNA ploidy patterns of 57 undifferentiated carcinomas in terms of mucosal sizes, and in the predominance of aneuploidy in the extramucosal lesion. (From [12]).

	Number of cases	Predominance of aneuploidy in the extramucosal part
Early ca.	30	
<0.5 cm	1	1 (100%)
≥0.5 cm	29	0 (0%)
Localized advanced ca.	15	
<2.0 cm	6	5 (83%)
≥2.0 cm	9	2 (22%)
Diffusely infilt. ca.	12	
<3.5 cm	5	5 (100%)
≥3.5 cm	7	2 (29%)

ca., carcinomas; *infilt.*, infiltrative

surrounded by diploid cells. This implies that aneuploid cells are possibly derived from diploid cells. In Table 2, a number of cases of the localized advanced and the diffusely infiltrative undifferentiated carcinomas—the extramucosal parts of which were predominantly composed of aneuploid cells—are comparatively shown in terms of their mucosal sizes. It was characteristic that in 5 (83%) out of 6 localized advanced cancers in which the lesions were smaller than 2 cm in diameter, the predominance of aneuploid cells was noted in the extramucosal parts. These cancers were of an early cancer-mimicking type (macroscopically, they appeared to be early cancers, but microscopically, the invasion was beyond the submucosal layer and the cancers were recognized as being advanced). These findings indicate that aneuploid cells show a strong invasiveness, and that aneuploid cancers are in a state of readiness to become advanced ones.

The metastatic lesions of undifferentiated carcinomas were also mainly composed of the same cell lines seen in the primary lesions. There was no difference in the frequency of metastasis between aneuploid and diploid cancer cells.

DNA Ploidy Pattern of Early Gastric Cancers and Progression of Gastric Cancers

In differentiated adenocarcinomas, the DNA ploidy patterns of the early cancers were similar to those of the advanced cancers; the occurrence of a diploid and an aneuploid cell line was similar between the early and advanced cancers, and even minute intramucosal cancers consisted of similar DNA ploidy patterns [5, 9] (Table 1). Nearly one-half of the adenocarcinomas appeared to be of a diploid origin, and one-fourth may have been of an aneuploid origin, while the others seemed to be of a diploid origin in which an aneuploid cell line could subsequently arise. On the other hand, there was a difference in the occurrence of polyploid cells between the early and advanced cancers. The minute intramucosal and small early cancers consisting of diploid cells often lacked polyploid cells. The appearance of polyploid cells seems to be a time-dependent phenomenon occurring after tumors arise. The change may reflect DNA instability of cancer cells [10, 11].

In undifferentiated carcinomas, there was a marked difference in the DNA ploidy pattern between the early and advanced cancers (Table 1). Most of the early cancers consisted of a diploid cell line. The occurrence of aneuploidy was less than 3% in the early cancers, whereas 64% of the Borrmann type III and 88% of the Borrmann type IV cancers contained aneuploid cell lines [5, 7, 12]. This indicates that DNA ploidy patterns change in the course of tumor progression. However, there was one very small early cancer with submucosal invasion, which consisted of aneuploid cells (Table 2). This was rather an exceptional case, but the finding indicates that aneuploid cells are poised to invade into the extramucosal parts.

The progression of undifferentiated carcinomas can be summarized as follows. Most of them arise having a diploid pattern, and the aneuploid cell lines arise in the course of progression. The occurrence of aneuploid cells also appears to be a time-dependent phenomenon, although this is not the case in differentiated adenocarcinomas. There is no reasonable explanation for this discrepancy between the two cancer types. Undifferentiated carcinomas in earlier stages are mostly comprised of signet-ring cell carcinomas. Signet-ring cell carcinoma may be a less progressive one than adenocarcinoma.

Undifferentiated carcinomas tend to remain in early stages as long as they consist of diploid cell lines. When aneuploid cells arise in the cancer, they seem to attain a greater invasiveness, to eventually become advanced cancers. Small undifferentiated carcinomas consisting of aneuploid cells (this may be of an aneuploid origin or an aneuploidy arises in diploid cancers at earlier stages) progress more rapidly to become advanced cancers [8]. Detection of such small aneuploid carcinomas will contribute to an early diagnosis of scirrhous cancer.

It is also probable that diploid undifferentiated carcinomas become Borrmann types III and IV advanced cancers, but it takes a long time for this to occur.

Prognosis and DNA Ploidy Pattern

It has been reported that DNA ploidy patterns provide a reliable indication of prognosis in many organs [13, 14]. The survival rates of diploid and aneuploid cancers curatively operated at stages III and IV are shown in Fig. 2. The prognosis was poorer in aneuploid than in diploid cancers, thus confirming earlier descriptions [5, 14]. However, it is very difficult to explain why the prognosis is poorer in aneuploid cancers. One possible explanation is that the occurrence of aneuploid cells is a time-dependent phenomenon, as is the case of undifferentiated

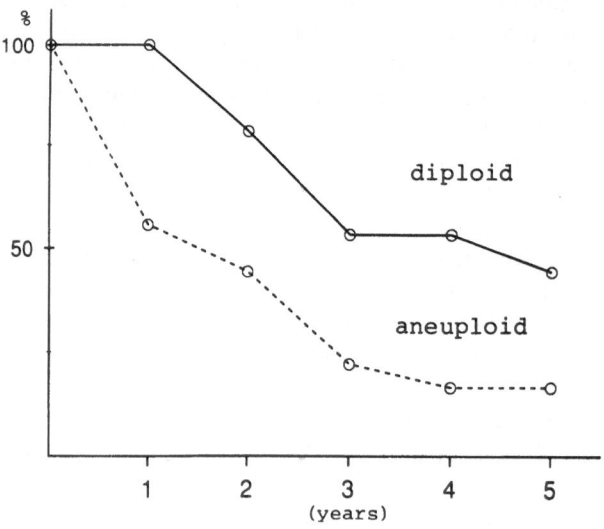

Fig. 2. Survival curves of the patients with *diploid* (15 cases) and *aneuploid* (12 cases) gastric cancers curatively operated at Stage III (T2, 3; N1, 2; M0) and Stage IV (T3, 4; N2, 3; M0, 1)

carcinomas. This implies that a long time is required for the aneuploid cell line to develop; that is, a longer time has elapsed in aneuploid cancers. The neoplastic invasion is widely extended in such cancers, and their prognoses thus become poorer. Another possible explanation may be that aneuploid cells are more aggressive than diploid cells; aneuploid cells may be more mobile, disclosing less adhesiveness.

Cell Kinetics of Gastric Cancers

Cell Cycle Time of Advanced and Early Gastric Cancer Cells

Proliferating cells in the cancer tissue can be determined by flash-labeled autoradiography with ^{3}H-thymidine [15], and, very recently, by immunohistochemical staining with anti-bromodeoxyuridine (BrdU) monoclonal antibody [16]. Generation time (Tg) and DNA synthetic time (Ts) can be determined with ^{3}H-thymidine by either a labeled mitosis chase method or a continuous labeling method [15, 17]. In cell culture, Tg can also be determined by counting the number of cells. Table 3 shows the Tg of ascites cancer cells of undifferentiated gastric carcinoma, and the Tg of metastatic adenocarcinoma cells in the lymph node and skin. It ranges from 1.3 to 3.3 days, and from 2 to 14 days, respectively [17]. In cultured gastric cancer cells, the Tg ranges from 1.4 to 3.3 days [18]. These kinetic parameters are not significantly different from those reported for human cancer cells of other organs proliferating in vivo [19]. Generally speaking, the Tg becomes longer in cancer cells than in normally proliferating cells [15]. In the normal gastrointestinal mucosa, generative cells in the intestinal crypt and at the neck region of gastric glands are known to proliferate with a Tg of 1–1.3 days

Table 3. Labeling indices with ^{3}H-thymidine and generation time of differentiated and undifferentiated carcinomas in early and advanced stages, and of cultured gastric cancer cells.

	LI (%)	Tg (days)
Dif. adenocarcinomas		
Early	14.0–23.8	
Advanced	13.0–38.1	2.0–14.0
Undifferentiated ca.		
Early	2.8– 6.8	
Advanced	5.0–15.9	1.3–3.3
Cultured cells	28.5–38.9	1.4–3.3

LI, labeling indices; *Tg*, generation time; *Dif.*, differentiated; *ca.*, carcinomas

[15]. The elongation of the Tg is caused by the elongation of the Ts. This may reflect a structural abnormality of the nuclear DNA in cancer cells.

There are no analytic data on cellular proliferation in early gastric cancers. Labeling indices of different gastric cancers are shown in Table 3. They range from 13% to 38.1% in advanced adenocarcinomas, from 14% to 23.8% in intramucosal early adenocarcinomas, from 5% to 15.9% in advanced undifferentiated carcinomas, and from 2.8% to 6.8% in early signet-ring cell carcinomas [17]. These values are variable, but it seems that there is no marked difference in the labeling indices between the early and the advanced cancers. It is likely, therefore, that cancer cells in early stages proliferate with the same generation time of 2–4 days as do cells of advanced cancers.

Among previous studies, there was a report that the labeling index with BrdU is higher in aneuploid cancer cells than in diploid cancer cells [5]. Aneuploid cells may disclose a higher proliferative activity. However, this does not mean that the cell cycle time is shorter in the aneuploid cells. There is no study which reveals any relation between the nuclear DNA content and the cell cycle time, whereas the cell cycle parameters in skin cancers were shown not to be different between the diploid and polyploid cells [19].

Growth Fraction of Gastric Cancers

The labeling index with ^{3}H-thymidine is higher in differentiated adenocarcinomas than in undifferentiated carcinomas, and a high labeling index indicates a high proliferation rate.

In tumor biology, there is a problem of growth fraction (GF) [19, 20]. GF is a ratio of proliferative cells to all cancer cells in the tissue. If all cells are proliferative the GF is 1.0. In cell cultures, almost all cells are proliferative (GF = 1.0). However, in human solid tumors, the GF is less than 1.0. In the reported cases, the range is from 0.2 to 0.9 [19]. In previous studies, determination of GF was done by an autoradiographic study with ^{3}H-thymidine [20], but the method was very difficult, and the reported data were not always correct.

Recently, proliferating cell nuclear antigen (PCNA) was used to determine immunohistochemically proliferative cells in cancer tissues [21]. PCNA is a 36 kd, acidic, and non-histone nuclear polypeptide that is associated with cell proliferation. It is expressed not only in the S phase, but also in the G_1 and G_2 phases of a cell cycle, but not in the G_0 phase. Accordingly, with this PCNA method, it is possible to evaluate the GF in human cancers. The percentages of PCNA-positive cells in the early differentiated adenocarcinomas and undifferentiated carcinomas are shown in Fig. 3 (the counting was done in the mucosal lesion). They range from 30.3% to 61.2% in the former, and from 23.2% to 44.6% in the latter (unpublished data), and the mean is significantly higher in the adenocarcinomas. This indicates that the GF is higher in the adenocarcinomas (corresponding to the higher labeling index with ^{3}H-thymidine). Undifferentiated carcinomas have mucin-containing cells, and typical signet-ring cells are no longer proliferative, nor are they labeled with ^{3}H-thymidine or BrdU. They are

Fig. 3. Proliferating cell nuclear antigen (*PCNA*)-positive indices of the differentiated and the undifferentiated carcinomas in early stages (46.7 ± 13.5 vs 36.5 ± 9.3; significantly different, $P < 0.05$)

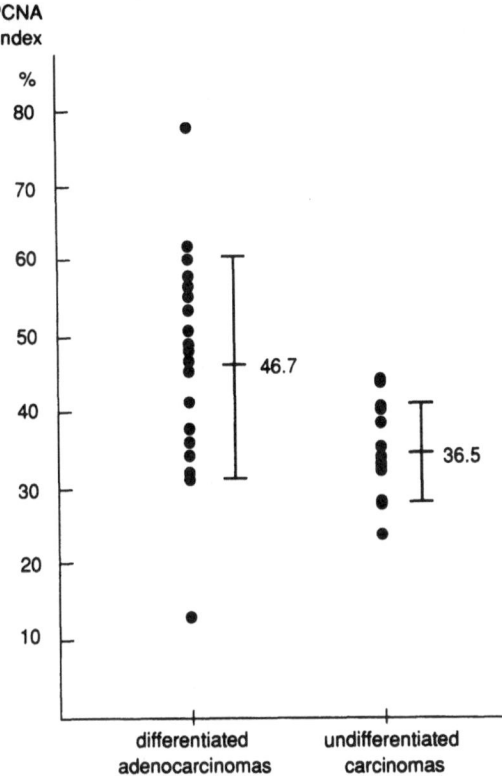

degenerative, or a kind of mature cell, outside the cell cycle. Therefore, the existence of such cells seems to lower the GF in the cancer tissue.

PCNA was expressed in almost all cells in cultured cell lines. However, xenografts of these cell lines which had been transplanted in the nude mouse did not always show high PCNA-positive indices, which, in this case, ranged from 0.5 to 0.9 (unpublished data). This indicates that some proportion of transplanted cells, even if they are essentially proliferative, are excluded from the cell cycle in xenografts. This may be caused by oxygen and nutritional insufficiency in the stroma. Such a phenomenon seems to occur in human cancers, and the GF becomes lower than 1.0, despite the proliferative activity of cancer cells.

Development of Gastric Cancers from Cell Proliferation Kinetics

Recent studies have shown that both differentiated and undifferentiated carcinomas arise at the neck region of gastric glands [22, 23]. In earlier stages, differentiated adenocarcinoma cells seem to proliferate, as do cancer cells of

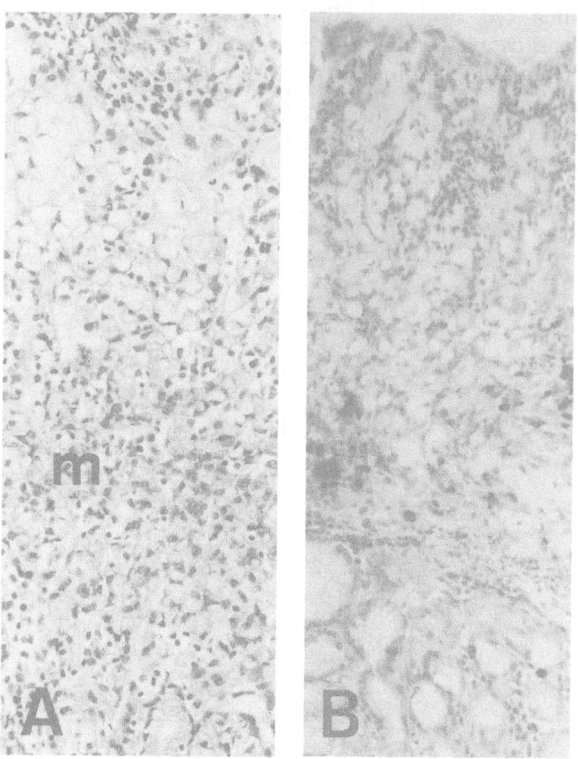

Fig. 4A,B. The layered structure of earlier signet-ring cell carcinoma (**A**) and auto-radiograph with ^{3}H-thymidine (**B**). Cells incorporating ^{3}H-thymidine are small round cells confined to the middle layer (*m*); typical signet-ring cells are not labeled with ^{3}H-thymidine

advanced stages. This was confirmed by PCNA staining, in that proliferative cells were randomly distributed in minute adenocarcinomas (unpublished data). On the other hand, undifferentiated carcinomas in earlier stages disclosed a regional variation in the distribution of proliferative cells [22, 24]. Earlier signet-ring cell carcinomas often disclose a layered structure, the upper and lower layers consisting of signet-ring cells, and the middle layer consisting of small round cells to which cell proliferation is confined (Fig. 4). The signet-ring cells in the outer layers are produced from the cells in the middle layer [22]. This layered structure mimics a mode of cell proliferation and differentiation in the normal gastric mucosa. To the extent that the tumor comprises this layered structure, it expands in the horizontal direction of the mucosa, and the tumor tends to remain a mucosal cancer for a relatively long period.

Growth of Gastric Cancers

The growth rate of human tumors is expressed by the volume-doubling time (Td). The Td of gastric cancers, which was measured on metastatic skin lesions, X-ray, and endoscopic films, is much longer than the Tg of cancer cells. The Td has been reported to be 28 days for metastatic adenocarcinoma in the abdominal skin, 60 days for metastatic adenocarcinoma in lymph nodes, and 17–19 days for metastatic lesions in the abdominal wall of scirrhous cancer [17]. These are values similar to the reported Td (1–3 months) of other human tumors [19]. On the other hand, the Td of early gastric cancers is very long, on the order of 1–3 years. A similarly slow growth rate has been noted in colon and rectal cancers, and in those cancers growing on the surface of the gastrointestinal tract [25–27]. From early to advanced stages, cancer cells must proliferate with a similar Tg without any drastic change in GF. The difference in the growth rate among these tumors may be due to the different places in which the cancers grow. Early mucosal cancers lose a large proportion of cells at the mucosal surface by desquamation, and it takes a long time for them to reach a comparatively large size.

Gastric cancers are thought to grow rather rapidly in an incipient stage. Experimentally, it was shown that microscopic cancers induced in rat stomach by a chemical carcinogen grow with a Td of 14 days. It became a macroscopic lesion of about 5 mm in diameter after 10 months [28]. On the other hand, xenografts of human gastric cancer cell lines in nude mice grew with a Td of 5–14 days; Td is at first short when the tumor is small, and it then becomes elongated as the tumor becomes large [27]. In these models, the Tg of the cancer cells was almost constant, on the order of 1.3–2.5 days (unpublished data) [28, 29]. The difference between the cell proliferation rate and the tumor growth rate in such small lesions is caused by cell loss which inevitably occurs within the cancer tissue. This is also due to stromal insufficiency. Tg and GF do not contribute as much to the growth rate of gastric cancers as does the loss of cells.

In previous studies, there were several reports concerning the difference of labeling indices with ^{3}H-thymidine or BrdU in different sites of cancer growth. Additionally, the grade of malignancy has sometimes been discussed in terms of proliferative activity of the cancer cells [5, 15]. However, it must be kept in mind that neither the proliferation rate nor the cell cycle time of cancer cells are directly related to the growth rate of human cancers.

From the observations described above, the natural history of gastric cancers can be postulated as follows. A gastric cancer arises at the neck region of gastric glands, whether it is differentiated or undifferentiated in type. In an incipient stage, the tumor grows rather rapidly until its size reaches the entire thickness of the gastric mucosa. Theoretically, it takes about 1 or 2 years for the cancer to reach this size. This occurs in a completely subclinical stage. When the tumor grows beyond this size, it appears on the surface of the mucosa. The cancer then comes to be involved in a process of desquamation at the mucosal surface, and the growth rate becomes slower. Many gastric cancers appear to invade into the submucosal layer when they reach a size around 2 cm in diameter, and attaining this condition takes about 2–5 years. The time lapse from the early to the advanced cancers is undoubtedly variable. Many gastric cancers seem to remain early cancers for a long period, since such a large number of gastric cancers are detected while in this stage.

Five to ten years after they arise, the gastric cancers seem to become advanced ones. If untreated, the total duration of the disease may reach 10–20 years in most cases [17]. On the other hand, there are highly infiltrative cancers, in which tumors quickly come to an end stage. Scirrhous cancers of the undifferentiated type and penetrating-type adenocarcinomas [14] are included in such cancers. The DNA ploidy pattern and cell kinetics have been discussed as potential prognostic factors, but there are still many unknown variables related to malignant behaviors of cancer cells, which must be further studied.

References

1. Atkin NB, Kay R (1979) Prognostic significance of modal DNA value and other factors in malignant tumors, based on 1465 cases. Br J Cancer 40:210–220
2. Frankfurt OS, Slocum HK, Rustum YM, et al (1984) Flow cytometric analysis of DNA aneuploidy in primary and metastatic human solid tumors. Cytometry 5:71–80
3. Sugano H, Nakamura K, Kato Y (1982) Pathological studies of human gastric cancer. Acta Pathol Jpn 32:329–347
4. Hattori T, Hosokawa Y, Fukuda M, et al (1984) Analysis of DNA ploidy patterns of gastric carcinomas of Japanese. Cancer 54:1541–1597
5. Yonemura Y, Sugiyama K, Fujimura T, et al (1988) Correlation of DNA ploidy and proliferative activity in human gastric cancer. Cancer 62:1497–1502
6. Rube CH, Valet G, Eder M (1988) Cellular DNA content and metastasis pattern in colorectal carcinomas. Virchows Arch [A] 413:419–424
7. Hattori T, Hosokawa Y, Sugihara H, et al (1985) DNA content of diffusely infiltrative carcinomas in the stomach. Pathol Res Pract 180:615–618
8. Sugihara H, Hattori T, Fukuda M, et al (1993) Progression of signet ring cell carcinomas in the human stomach. Cancer 71:1938–1947
9. Hattori T, Sugihara H, Fukuda M, et al (1986) DNA ploidy patterns of minute carcinomas in the stomach. Jpn J Cancer Res 77:276–281
10. Nowell PC (1976) The clonal evolution of tumor cell populations. Science 194:23–28
11. Wolman SR (1983) Karyotypic progression in human tumors. Cancer Metastasis Rev 2:257–293
12. Sugihara H, Hattori T, Fujita S, et al (1990) Regional ploidy variations in signet ring cell carcinomas of the stomach. Cancer 65:122–129
13. Kouri M, Pyrhonen S, Mecklin JP, et al (1990) The prognostic value of DNA-ploidy in colorectal carcinoma: A prospective study. Br J Cancer 62:976–981
14. Inokuchi K, Kodama Y, Sasaki H, et al (1983) Differentiation of growth patterns of early gastric carcinoma determined by cytophotometric DNA analysis. Cancer 51:1138–1141
15. Lipkin M (1977) Growth kinetics of normal and premalignant gastrointestinal epithelium. In: Drewinko B, Humphrey RM (eds) Growth kinetics and biochemical regulation of normal and malignant cells. Williams and Wilkins, Baltimore, pp 569–589

16. Morstyn E, Hsu SM, Kinsella T, et al (1983) Bromodeoxyuridine in tumors and chromosomes detected with a monoclonal antibody. J Clin Invest 72:155–159
17. Fujita S (1978) Biology of early gastric carcinoma. Pathol Res Pract 163:297–309
18. Motoyama T, Hojo H, Watanabe H (1986) Comparison of seven cell lines derived from human gastric carcinomas. Acta Pathol Jpn 36:65–83
19. Schiffer LM, Braunschweiger PG, Poulakos L (1977) Studies on the cell kinetics of human solid tumors. In: Drewinko B, Humphrey RM (eds) Growth kinetics and biochemical regulation of normal and malignant cells. Williams and Wilkins, Baltimore, pp 663–673
20. Mendelsohn ML (1962) Autoradiographic analysis of cell proliferation in spontaneous breast cancer of C3H mouse. III. The growth fraction. J Natl Cancer Inst 28: 1015–1029
21. Kamel OW, LeBrun DP, Davis RE, et al (1991) Growth fraction estimation of malignant lymphomas in formalin-fixed paraffin-embedded tissue using anti-PCNA/cyclin 19A2. Am J Pathol 138:1471–1477
22. Sugihara H, Hattori T, Imamura Y, et al (1991) Morphology and modes of cell proliferation in earliest signet-ring-cell carcinomas induced in canine stomachs by N-ethyl-N'-nitro-N-nitrosoguanidine. J Cancer Res Clin Oncol 117:197–204
23. Hattori T (1986) Development of adenocarcinomas in the stomach. Cancer 57: 1528–1534
24. Sugihara H, Hattori T, Fujita S, et al (1989) Cell proliferation and differentiation in intramucosal and advanced signet ring cell carcinomas of the stomach. Virchows Arch [A] 411:117–127
25. Kawai K, Miyaoka T, Kohli Y (1974) Evaluation of early gastric cancer from the clinical point of view. In: Grundmann E, Grunze H, Witte S (eds) Early gastric cancer. Current status of diagnosis. Springer, Berlin, pp 63–66
26. Okabe H (1971) Growth of early gastric cancer. Clinical study of growth and invasion patterns of early gastric cancer: Its position in the natural history of gastric cancer. In: Murakami T (ed) Early gastric cancer. Cancer Association GANN Monograph on Cancer Research II. University of Tokyo Press, Tokyo, pp 67–79
27. Welin S, Youker J, Spratt JS (1963) The rates and patterns of growth of 375 tumors of the large intestine and rectum observed serially by double contrast enema study (Malmoe technique). Am J Roentgenol 90:673–687
28. Hattori T, Helpap B, Gedigk P (1984) Cell proliferation and growth of gastric carcinoma induced in inbred Wistar rats by N-methyl-N'-nitro-N-nitrosoguanidine. Cancer Res 44:5266–5272
29. Schmidt M, Deschner EE, Thaler T, et al (1977) Gastrointestinal cancer studies in the human to nude mouse heterotransplant system. Gastroenterology 72:829–837

Oncogenes and Tumor Suppressor Genes

Masaru Katoh and Masaaki Terada[1]

Key words. Oncogene—Tumor suppressor gene—Growth factor—Loss of heterozygosity—Multi-step carcinogenesis—Helicobacter pylori

Introduction

The proliferation of normal cells is regulated by the balance between the growth-promoting signals of proto-oncogenes and the growth-constraining signals of tumor suppressor genes [1, 2]. Multiple steps including initiation, promotion and progression are required for the conversion of normal cells to fully malignant cells with invasive and metastatic capacities. Multiple genetic changes, including activation of proto-oncogenes and inactivation of tumor suppressor genes, occurs during multi-step carcinogenesis which takes 20–30 years [3]. Gastric cancer is still one of the most common malignancies, not only in Japan, but also worldwide. Yet, there has been only limited information available on genetic changes in gastric cancer. In this chapter, all the available information on genetic changes in gastric cancer will be presented, and its perspectives will be discussed.

Proto-Oncogenes

Proto-oncogenes, identified by a variety of approaches, have been shown to function at critical steps in mitogenic signaling. Proto-oncogenes are classified into four groups: growth factor, receptor, signal transducer, and nuclear protein. Proto-oncogenes are activated by amplification, rearrangement, point mutation, or translocation [1]. Receptor tyrosine kinase mediates the mitogenic signal of growth factors through the phosphorylation cascade of signal transducers and

---
[1] Genetics Division, National Cancer Center Research Institute, 5-1-1 Tsukiji, Chuo-ku, Tokyo, 104 Japan

nuclear proteins. Several receptor tyrosine kinases are reported to be amplified in human gastric cancer.

Amplification and Altered Expression

Increased DNA content per cell and aneuploidy are often associated with more malignant phenotypes of tumor cells. Gene amplification has been reported in only a limited number of human gastric cancers. K-*sam* [4–6], c-*erb*B2 [7–9], and c-*met* [10–14] are frequently amplified genes in gastric cancer.

K-*sam*

We have isolated an novel gene, K-*sam* (*KATO*-III cell derived *s*tomach cancer *am*plified gene), from cells of the gastric cancer cell line KATO-III (signet-ring cell carcinoma) by the in-gel DNA renaturation method [4]. K-*sam* is amplified in the gastric cancer cell line KATO-III, in nude mice xenografts NSC4, NSC10, and in surgical specimens (Fig. 1). In some cases, K-*sam* amplification is detected only in the metastatic lesion (Fig. 1C), which suggests the possible involvement of K-*sam* amplification in a late stage of gastric carcinogenesis. K-*sam* amplification is detected in 21% (6/29) of undifferentiated types of gastric cancer, but not in differentiated types of gastric cancer (0/17) [4]. K-*sam* encodes a receptor tyrosine kinase that belongs either to the fibroblast growth factor (FGF) receptor family, or the heparin-binding growth factor (HBGF) receptor family [5].

K-*sam* mRNA is overexpressed in KATO-III cells. Structural multiplicity of K-*sam* transcripts is predicted by northern blot analysis with various K-*sam* probes (Fig. 2). Recently, multiple K-*sam* transcripts, encoding a transmembrane receptor as well as a secreted receptor, have been characterized (Fig. 3). K-*sam* cDNA type I (Brain type) and type II (KATO-III type) encode transmembrane receptors. Type I products mediate mitogenic signals of aFGF and bFGF, while type II products mediate mitogenic signals of aFGF and keratinocyte growth factor (KGF). The altered ligand specificity between K-*sam* type I and type II gene products is due to the difference in the latter half of the third immunoglobulin-like domain that is generated by alternative splicing [6]. K-*sam* cDNA type III (with a tyrosine kinase domain) and type IV (without a tyrosine kinase domain) encode secreted receptors that may act as carrier proteins. Alternatively, the secreted receptor may modulate the response of target cells to ligands by competing with the transmembrane receptor. Although the biological role of the secreted receptor remains to be elucidated, detection of secreted K-*sam* products in serum may be a diagnostic indicator for gastric cancer [6].

Epidermal Growth Factor (EGF) Receptor Gene Family

Avian erythro-blastosis virus induces acute erythroleukemia and sarcoma in vivo and transforms erythroblasts and fibroblasts in vitro [15]. v-*erb*B was isolated from the genome of the ES4 strain of avian erythro-blastosis virus. Three v-*erb*B-related human genes, c-*erb*B1/EGF receptor [16], c-*erb*B2/*neu* [7], and c-*erb*B3

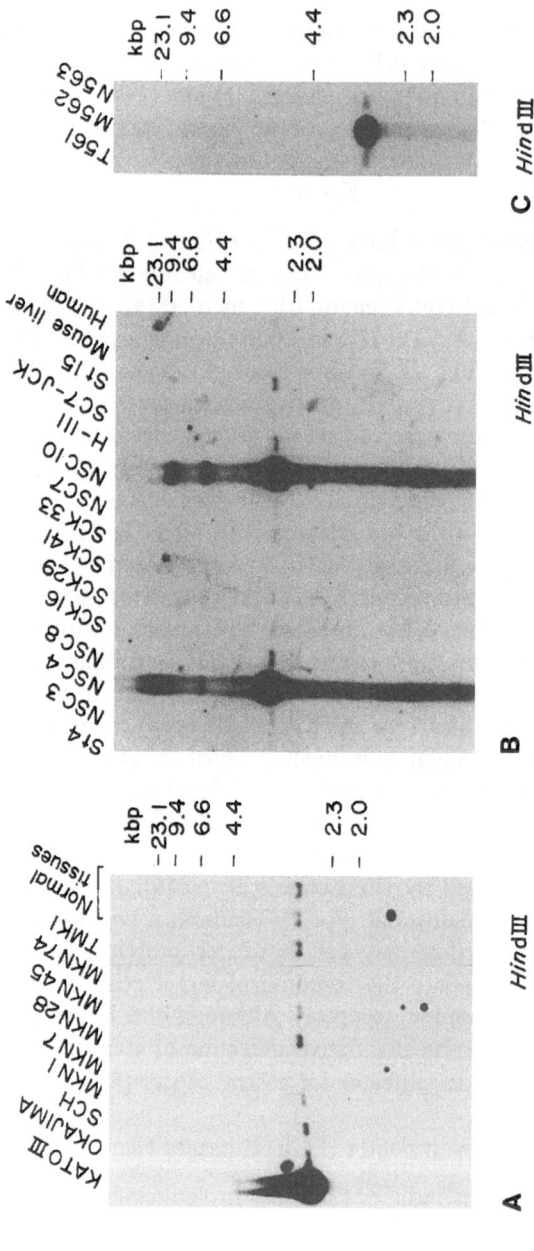

Fig. 1A–C. K-*sam* gene amplification. DNA digested with *Hind*III, were fractionated on agarose gels, transferred to filters, and then probed with ³²P-labelled SAM$_{0.2}$. Amplification of K-*sam* in DNA samples turn figure from gastric cancer cell lines **A**, from human gastric cancers transplanted into nude mice **B**, and from surgical specimens of primary gastric cancer and lymph node metastasis **C**. K-*sam* is amplified in KATO-III cells, in NSC4 and NSC10 xenografts, and in surgical specimens of lymph node metastasis to around 30- to 50-fold

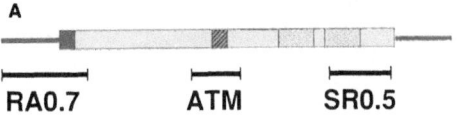

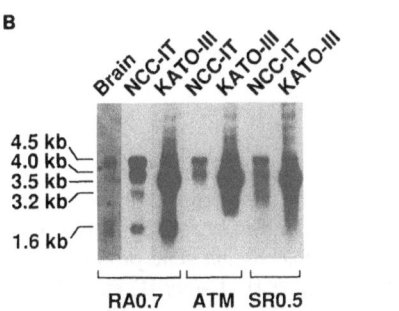

Fig. 2A–B. K-*sam* gene expression. **A** Structure of K-*sam* cDNA type II and location of K-*sam* probes are shown. Noncoding regions are indicated by the *bold bar*. Shown in the schema are hydrophobic signal peptide (*closed box*), transmembrane domain (*hatched box*), and tyrosine kinase domain (*dotted box*). RA0.7 is a specific probe for the K-*sam* gene, corresponding to the 5' noncoding region and a small portion of the coding region. The ATM probe and the SR0.5 probe correspond to the membrane-spanning region and the second part of the tyrosine kinase domain, respectively. **B** Northern blot hybridization with various K-*sam* probes. Two µg of polyadenylated RNA were fractionated on agarose gels, transferred to Nitroplus membranes, and probed with ^{32}P-labeled RA0.7, ATM or SR0.5 probes. K-*sam* transcripts with sizes of 4.5 kb, 4.0 kb and 3.5 kb were hybridized with all the probes. K-*sam* transcripts with sizes of 3.2 kb and 1.6 kb were not hybridized with the ATM probe

[17], make up the EGF receptor gene family. Products of the EGF receptor gene family can transduce growth regulatory signals of the EGF family, such as EGF, transforming growth factor α, and amphiregulin [17]. In adult human gastric mucosa, EGF receptor immunoreactivity was confined to mucus neck cells. c-*erb*B2 immunoreactivity was faintly positive on parietal cells, while c-*erb*B3 immunoreactivity was moderately positive [18].

The EGF receptor was rarely amplified in gastric cancer (3%, 1/37) [19]. EGF receptor mRNA was detected in all gastric cancer cell lines examined. Expression level of EGF receptor mRNA is higher in tumor tissue of gastric cancer than in the adjacent normal tissue [20].

c-*erb*B2 was amplified in 38% (5/13) of differentiated types of gastric cancer, but not in undifferentiated types of gastric cancer (0/27) [8]. 4.6 kb c-*erb*B2 transcript was overexpressed in MKN7 cells with c-*erb*B2 gene amplification [8]. c-*erb*B2 immunoreactivity in the primary lesion of gastric cancer was associated with poor prognosis [9].

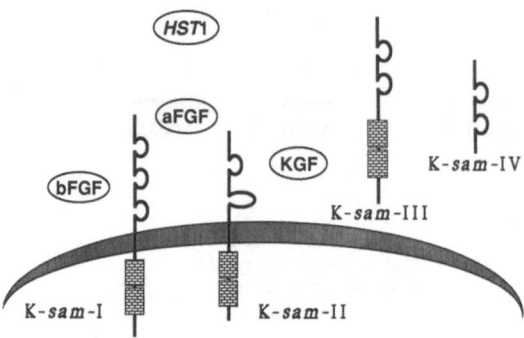

Fig. 3. Structural multiplicity of K-*sam* gene products. K-*sam* encodes a receptor tyrosine kinase that belongs to the FGF receptor family, or the HBGF receptor family. Shown in the schema are the structure of multiple K-*sam* gene products and their possible ligands. K-*sam* cDNA type I (K-*sam*-I) and type II (K-*sam*-II) encode transmembrane receptors. K-*sam*-I products mediate the mitogenic signals of aFGF and bFGF, while K-*sam*-II products mediate aFGF and KGF. The altered ligand specificity between K-*sam*-I and K-*sam*-II is due to the difference in the latter half of the third immunoglobulin-like domain that is generated by alternative splicing. K-*sam* cDNAs type III (K-*sam*-III) and type IV (K-*sam*-IV) encode secreted receptors with or without the tyrosine kinase domain

c-*erb*B3 was not amplified in gastric cancer (0/23). A 6.2 kb c-*erb*B3 transcript, encoding a transmembrane receptor, was detected in all gastric cancer cell lines examined. The 1.4 kb c-*erb*B3 transcript was expressed as strongly as the 6.2 kb c-*erb*B3 transcript in MKN45 cells. *erb*B3-S cDNA, corresponding to the 1.4 kb c-*erb*B3 transcript in MKN45 cells, was isolated by rapid amplification of cDNA ends. Sequence analysis of *erb*B3-S cDNA showed that the 1.4 kb c-*erb*B3 mRNA encoded a secreted receptor. The c-*erb*B3 gene encodes both the secreted as well as the transmembrane receptor tyrosine kinase due to alternative splicing [21].

c-*met*

c-*met* was isolated as a proto-oncogene corresponding to *met* oncogene activated by the rearrangement between the TPR locus and the *met* locus [10]. The c-*met* gene encodes receptor tyrosine kinase, which was identified as a hepatocyte growth factor receptor [11].

The oncogenic TPR-*met* mRNA is expressed in gastric cancer cell lines (MKN1, MKN28, MKN45 and SCH) and was found in biopsy specimens from 12/22 patients [12]. Overexpression of TPR-*met* mRNA in superficial gastritis lesions with hyperplasia of glandular neck cells suggests the possible involvement of TPR-*met* oncogene in an early stage of gastric carcinogenesis [12].

In normal gastric mucosa, a 9.0 kb c-*met* transcript is expressed [13]. In contrast, 9.0, 7.0, and 5.2 kb c-*met* transcripts were overexpressed in the gastric cancer cell line, GTL-16, a subclone derived from MKN45 with c-*met* gene amplification [13]. c-*met* gene was amplified in 26% (10/38) of undifferentiated types of gastric cancer and in 19% (5/26) of differentiated types of gastric cancer [14].

Other Amplified Genes

The *HST1* gene, a transforming gene isolated from a surgical specimen of human gastric cancer, is a member of the FGF or HBGF gene families. It is located on chromosome 11q13, and is frequently amplified in esophageal cancer, head and neck cancer and breast cancer [22–24]. *HST1* is rarely amplified in gastric cancer (2%, 1/43) [24].

c-*myc* is a human equivalent of the v-*myc* oncogene of avian retrovirus MC29. c-*myc* was rarely amplified in gastric cancers transplanted into nude mice (2/11) [25].

The v-*akt* oncogene, which was isolated from the AKT8 murine retrovirus genome, has two human-related genes, *AKT1* and *AKT2* [26]. *AKT1* and *AKT2* encode serine/threonine kinases homologous to adenylate cyclase and protein kinase C [27]. *AKT1* and *AKT2* may be cytoplasmic signaling proteins regulated by receptor tyrosine kinase, because they have a SH2 domain. *AKT1* is rarely amplified in gastric cancer (1/5) [26].

Point Mutational Activation of the *ras* Gene Family

c-Ki-*ras* is a homologous human gene of the v-Ki-*ras* oncogene. The c-Ki-*ras* gene product, p21, can transduce mitogenic signals of receptor tyrosine kinases. c-Ki-*ras* is activated by point mutation. c-Ki-*ras* point mutation was detected in 18% (3/17) of differentiated types of gastric cancer, but not in undifferentiated types of gastric cancer (0/18) [28].

Other Proto-Oncogenes

Seven membrane-spanning receptors coupled to phospholipase C, such as the serotonergic receptor (5-HT1c), muscarinic receptors (M1, M3, M5), and the adrenergic receptor (α1B), were found to transform NIH 3T3 cells [29]. These receptors may be considered as a new class of proto-oncogene that might transform cells by enhancing the phosphoinositide-derived signals of inositol(1,4,5)-triphosphate and diacylglycerol. Gastrin receptors also mediate the mitogenic signal of gastrin through phospholipase C which modulates growth and differentiation of gastric mucosa during normal development [30]. There is controversy whether enterochromaffin-like cell carcinoma is induced by hypergastrinemia, secondary to proton-pump inhibitor treatment. Genetic alterations of gastrin receptors in human gastric cancer remain to be elucidated.

Tumor Suppressor Genes

The existence of tumor suppressor genes was first proposed for the rare childhood eye tumor, retinoblastoma [31]. The gene was isolated later and designated *RB*. Since then, seven additional tumor suppressor genes have been identified, including p53, *DCC*, *APC*, *MCC*, *WT1* and *NF1*. Tumor suppressor genes are inactivated by a deletion or by a point mutation in cancer [2]. Unlike genetic alterations of proto-oncogenes, tumor suppressor genes on both alleles are altered; often the gene on one allele is inactivated by a point mutation or a minor deletion and the other allele by a large deletion including the gene. The large deletion of one segment of chromosome was identified by classical cytogenetics. Restriction fragment length polymorphism (RFLP) analysis made it easier to identify the deleted chromosomal loci which predicted the possible existence of a tumor suppressor gene. The large deletion on one allele could be recognized as loss of heterozygosity (LOH) in RFLP analysis.

p53

p53 was found initially through its association with the SV40 large T oncoprotein in virus-transformed cells. LOH at the locus corresponding to the p53 gene on chromosome 17p which is often detected in diverse types of human cancer. Loss of one allele and a mutation in the remaining allele are typical aberrations of the p53 gene [32]. p53 gene mutations are screened by polymerase chain reaction single-strand conformation polymorphism analysis (PCR-SSCP) (Fig. 4). p53 gene is mutated in four out of eight gastric cancer cell lines (KATO-III, OKAJIMA, TMK1 and MKN1) [33]. p53 gene mutations were detected in 64% (9/14) of aneuploid tumor cells but not in diploid tumor cells (0/10) [34].

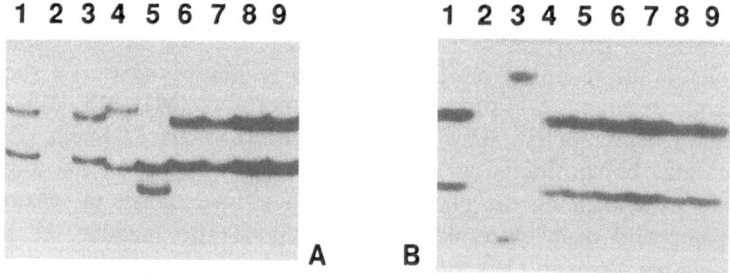

Fig. 4A,B. PCR-SSCP analysis of p53 gene in gastric cancer. PCR products were heat-denatured and run on a 6% neutral polyacrylamide gel. Autoradiogram of PCR-SSCP analysis for the exon 5–6 region **A**, and the exon 10 region **B** of the p53 gene are shown. *Lane 1*, human placenta; *lane 2*, KATO-III; *lane 3*, OKAJIMA; *lane 4*, TMK1; *lane 5*, MKN1; *lane 6*, MKN7; *lane 7*, MKN28; *lane 8*, MKN45; *lane 9*, MKN74. SSCP analysis showed no band in KATO-III, in which both alleles of p53 were deleted. The mobility shift of the bands was detected in TMK1, MKN1 and OKAJIMA

p53 immunoreactivity was detected in 34% (34/99) of advanced gastric cancer, and in 22% (11/50) of early gastric cancer. Histologically, a nuclear accumulation of the p53 protein was frequently detected in papillary adenocarcinoma, well- to moderately-differentiated adenocarcinoma, and poorly-differentiated adenocarcinoma with solid nests or focal tubular structures (43/101, 43%), but it was rarely seen in signet-ring cell carcinoma, mucinous adenocarcinoma, or poorly-differentiated adenocarcinoma growing in a scattered manner (2/48, 4%) [35].

DCC

DCC, a recently identified tumor suppressor gene located on chromosome 18q, is altered during colorectal carcinogenesis. DCC encodes a cell surface, transmembrane protein with considerable homology to neural cell adhesion molecules [36]. LOH at the DCC locus is detected in 61% (14/23) of surgically resected gastric cancers, excluding the diffuse type [37].

APC

APC, a gene responsible for familial polyposis coli, was recently isolated and characterized [37]. The APC gene was located on chromosome 5q, and is frequently mutated out only in familial colorectal cancers but also in sporadic colorectal cancers [38]. LOH at the APC locus was detected in 36% (5/14) of differentiated types of gastric cancer, but not in undifferentiated (0/15) [39] APC gene mutation was detected in 3 out of 44 cases of gastric cancer. The mutation was a miss-sense mutation, a nonsense mutation, or a 5-base pair deletion resulting in a frame shift which causes truncation of the gene product [40].

Other Tumor Suppressor Genes

Genetic alterations of other tumor suppressor genes, such as NF1 or Rb, in gastric cancer remain to be elucidated. There may be other tumor suppressor genes implicated in gastric cancer, because LOH was also detected on chromosome 1q (4/6, 67%) and chromosome 7p (5/15, 33%) in differentiated types of gastric cancer, but not in undifferentiated [39].

Gene Expressed in Fetal Stomach and Gastric Cancer

Several genes preferentially expressed in fetal rat stomach were identified by the newly developed technique of PCR-based cDNA subtraction [40]. As many as six out of eight clones isolated by this method were highly expressed in gastric cancers. Four cDNAs were identified, with partial nucleotide sequence analysis, as profilin, pro-α_1 (1) collagen, nucleolar protein B23.2, and elongation factor 1 α subunit. The remaining two clones were derived from novel genes. These results suggest that many genes expressed preferentially in embryonic stomach are likely to be highly expressed in gastric cancer [41]. Tumor markers expressed in fetal stomach, such as carcinoembryonic antigen and α-fetoprotein, were also expressed in some gastric cancers. Genes expressed in the stomach during fetal development might be expressed in some types of gastric cancer.

Helicobacter pylori (H. pylori)

The incidence of gastric cancer may be largely determined be environmental factors rather than genetic or hereditary factors, because the incidence of gastric cancer can change dramatically from place to place and from one generation to the next [42]. H. pylori is a Gram-negative bacterium with urease, oxidase, and catalase activity, which was recently isolated from gastric mucosa [43]. H. pylori was associated with peptic ulcer and chronic gastritis [44]. Although there are some reports indicating that H. pylori was also associated with gastric cancer [45, 46], the association between H. pylori and gastric cancer remains to be elucidated.

We have developed a PCR method to detect the urease B gene of H. pylori. We have reported that urease B gene of H. pylori was detected in 50% (8/16) of wash-out samples from the biopsy-suction channel of a gastro-fiberscope after manual Hyamine washing, and that bacterial culture revealed viable H. pylori in 19% (3/16). However, H. pylori was not detected by either of the above methods in the biopsy-suction channel of the gastro-fiberscope after mechanical washing. These findings indicated that manual Hyamine washing of gastrofiberscope was insufficient to prevent iatrogenic H. pylori transmission [47]. We also checked the possibility of H. pylori DNA integration by using PCR. The urease B gene of H. pylori was detected in normal gastric mucosa and in the primary lesion of gastric cancer, but not in gastric cancer cell lines nor in the metastatic lesion of gastric cancer (Katoh M, Saito D, Sugimura T, Terada M 1992, unpublished data). Further studies, such as large scale epidemiological studies in the younger generation and intervention study, are required to clarify the roles of H. pylori in gastric carcinogenesis.

Multiple Genetic Alterations in Gastric Cancer

Genetic alterations in gastric cancer so far reported are summarized in Table 1. K-sam and c-met are amplified preferentially in undifferentiated types of gastric cancer [4, 14], whereas c-erbB2 is amplified preferentially in differentiated types of gastric cancer [8]. c-Ki-ras gene is mutated in differentiated types of gastric cancer [28] while p53 gene is mutated in both types of gastric cancer [31]. LOH at chromosomes 5q (APC), 1q, or 7p was detected in differentiated types of gastric cancer [39]. These results indicate that there are two different pathways of genetic alterations in gastric cancer, one (c-Ki-ras, p53, c-erbB2 or c-met) for the differentiated types, and another (p53, K-sam or c-met) for the undifferentiated types.

Table 1. Genetic alterations in gastric cancer.

Gene	differentiated type	undifferentiated type	Ref.
(Amplification)			
K-sam	0% (0/17)	21% (6/29)	[4]
c-erbB2	38% (5/13)	0% (0/27)	[8]
c-met	19% (5/26)	26% (10/38)	[14]
(Point mutation)			
c-Ki-ras	18% (3/17)	0% (0/18)	[28]
p53	42% (5/12)	33% (4/12)	[34]

Perspectives

Genetic alterations in gastric cancer have been studied but there is still limited information available. The elucidation of an increasing number of proto-oncogenes and tumor suppressor genes will lead to a better understanding of multiple genetic changes involved in carcinogenesis of the stomach. Knowledge on genetic changes in gastric cancer could be utilized not only as a diagnostic marker, but also as a prognostic factor. In the future, TNMG classification (Tumor, Node, Metastasis and Gene) for the staging of cancer patients will be widely spread superceding TNM classification. Studies will also lead to the identification of high risk people for gastric cancer by detecting early genetic change. Finally, accumulation of the knowledge on multiple genetic alterations will lead to a better management of gastric cancer.

Acknowledgements. This study was supported by Grants-in-Aid from the Ministry of Health and Welfare of Japan for the comprehensive 10-Year Strategy for Cancer Control; by grants from the Ministry of Education, Science, and Culture of Japan; and from the Bristol-Myers Squibb Foundation.

References

1. Bishop JM (1991) Molecular themes in oncogenesis. Cell 64:235–248
2. Weinberg RA (1992) Tumor suppressor genes. Science 254:1138–1146
3. Sugimura T, Terada M, Yokota J, Hirohashi S, Wakabayashi K (1992) Multiple genetic alterations in human carcinogenesis. Environ Health Perspect 98:5–12
4. Nakatani H, Sakamoto H, Yoshida T, Yokota J, Tahara E, Sugimura T, Terada M (1990) Isolation of an amplified DNA sequences in stomach cancer. Jpn J Cancer Res 81:707–710
5. Hattori Y, Odagiri H, Nakatani H, Miyagawa K, Naito K, Sakamoto H, Katoh O, Yoshida T, Sugimura T, Terada M (1990) K-sam, an amplified gene in stomach cancer, is a member of the heparin-binding growth factor receptor genes. Proc Natl Acad Sci USA 87:5983–5987

6. Katoh, M, Hattori Y, Sasaki H, Tanaka M, Sugano K, Yazaki Y, Sugimura T, Terada M (1992) K-*sam* gene encodes secreted as well as transmembrane receptor tyrosine kinase. Proc Natl Acad Sci USA 89:2960–2964

7. Yamamoto T, Ikawa S, Akiyama T, Semba K, Nomura N, Miyajima N, Saito T, Toyoshima K (1986) Similarity of protein encoded by the human c-*erb-B-2* gene to epidermal growth factor receptor. Nature 319:230–234

8. Yokota J, Yamamoto T, Miyajima N, Toyoshima K, Nomura N, Sakamoto H, Yoshida T, Terada M, Sugimura T (1988) Genetic alterations of the c-*erb*B-2 oncogene occur frequently in tubular adenocarcinoma of the stomach and are often accompanied by amplification of the v-*erb*A homologue. Oncogene 2:283–287

9. Yonemura Y, Ninomiya I, Ohoyama S, Kimura H, Yamaguchi A, Fushida S, Kosaka T, Miwa K, Miyazaki I, Endou Y, Tanaka M, Sasaki T (1991) Expression of c-*erb*B-2 oncoprotein in gastric carcinoma. Immunoreactivity for c-*erb*B-2 protein is an independent indicator of poor short-term prognosis in patients with gastric carcinoma. Cancer 67:2914–2918

10. Park M, Dean M, Kaul K, Braun MJ, Gonda MA, Vande Woude G (1987) Sequence of *MET* protooncogene cDNA has features characteristic of the tyrosine kinase family of growth-factor receptors. Proc Natl Acad Sci USA 84:6379–6383

11. Bottaro DP, Rubin JS, Faletto DL, Chan AML, Kmiecik TE, Vande Woude GF, Aaronson SA (1991) Identification of the hepatocyte growth factor receptor as the c-*met* proto-oncogene product. Science 251:802–804

12. Soman NR, Correa P, Ruiz BA, Wogan GN (1991) The *TPR-MET* oncogenic rearrangement is present and expressed in human gastric carcinoma and precursor lesions. Proc Natl Acad Sci USA 88:4893–4896

13. Di Renzo MF, Narsimhan RP, Olivero M, Bretti S, Giordano S, Medico E, Gaglia P, Zara P, Comoglio PM (1991) Expression of the Met/HGF receptor in normal and neoplastic human tissues. Oncogene 6:1997–2003

14. Kuniyasu H, Yasui W, Kitadai Y, Yokozaki H, Ito H, Tahara E (1992) Frequent amplification of c-*met* gene in scirrhous type stomach cancer. Biochem Biophys Res Commun 189:227–232

15. Graf T, Beug H (1983) Role of the v-*erb*A and v-*erb*B oncogenes of avian erythroblastosis virus in erythroid cell transformation. Cell 34:7–9

16. Ullrich A, Coussens L, Hayflick JS, Dull TJ, Gray A, Tam AW, Lee J, Yarden Y, Libermann TA, Schlessinger J, Downward J, Mayes ELV, Whittle N, Waterfield MD, Seeburg PH (1984) Human epidermal growth factor receptor cDNA sequence and aberrant expression of the amplified gene in A431 epidermoid carcinoma cells. Nature 309:418–425

17. Kraus MH, Issing W, Miki T, Popescu NC, Aaronson S (1989) Isolation and characterization of *ERBB3*, a third member of the *ERBB*/epidermal growth factor receptor family: Evidence for overexpression in a subset of human mammary tumors. Proc Natl Acad Sci USA 86:9193–9197

18. Prigent SA, Lemoine NR, Hughes CM, Plowman GD, Selden C, Gullick WJ (1992) Expression of the c-*erb*B-3 protein in normal human adult and fetal tissues. Oncogene 7:1273–1278

19. Yoshida K, Tsuda T, Matsumura T, Tsujino T, Hattori T, Ito H, Tahara E (1989) Amplification of epidermal growth factor receptor (EGFR) gene and oncogenes in human gastric carcinomas. Virchows Archiv [B] 57:285–290

20. Yoshida K, Kyo E, Tsujino T, Sano T, Niimoto M, Tahara E (1990) Expression of epidermal growth factor, transforming growth factor-α and their receptor genes in human gastric carcinomas: Implication for autocrine growth. Jpn J Cancer Res 81:43–51

21. Katoh M, Yazaki Y, Sugimura T, Terada M (1993) c-*erb*B3 gene encodes secreted as well as transmembrane receptor tyrosine kinase. Biochem Biophys Res Common 192:1189–1197
22. Sakamoto H, Mori M, Taira M, Yoshida T, Matsukawa S, Shimizu K, Sekiguchi M, Terada M, Sugimura T (1986) Transforming gene from stomach cancers and a noncancerous portion of stomach mucosa. Proc Natl Acad Sci USA 83:3997–4001
23. Yoshida T, Miyagawa K, Odagiri H, Sakamoto H, Little PFR, Terada M, Sugimura T (1987) Genomic sequence of *hst*, a transforming gene encoding a protein homologous to fibroblast growth factors and the *int-2*-encoded protein. Proc Natl Acad Sci USA 84:7305–7309
24. Yoshida MC, Wada M, Satoh H, Yoshida T, Sakamoto H, Miyagawa K, Yokata J, Koda T, Kakinuma M, Sugimura T, Terada M (1988) Human *HST1* (*HSTF1*) gene maps to chromosome band 11q13 and coamplifies with the *INT2* gene in human cancer. Proc Natl Acad Sci USA 85:4861–4864
25. Nakasato F, Sakamoto H, Mori M, Hayashi K, Shimosato Y, Nishi M, Takao S, Nakatani K, Terada M, Sugimura T (1984) Amplification of the c-*myc* oncogene in human stomach cancers. Jpn J Cancer Res (Gann) 75:737–742
26. Staal SP (1987) Molecular cloning of the *akt* oncogene and its human homologous of *AKT1* and *AKT2*: Amplification of *AKT1* in a primary human gastric adenocarcinoma. Proc Natl Acad Sci USA 84:5034–5037
27. Cheng JQ, Godwin AK, Bellacosa A, Taguchi T, Franke TF, Hamilton TC, Tsichlis PN, Testa JR (1992) *AKT2*, a putative oncogene encoding a member of a subfamily of protein-serine/threonine kinase, is amplified in human ovarian carcinomas. Proc Natl Acad Sci USA 89:9267–9271
28. Kihana T, Tsuda H, Hirota T, Simosato Y, Sakamoto H, Terada M, Hirohashi S (1991) Point mutation of c-Ki-*ras* oncogene in gastric adenoma and adenocarcinoma with tubular differentiation. Jpn J Cancer Res 82:308–314
29. Berridge MJ (1993) Inositol triphosphate and calcium signaling. Nature 361:315–325
30. Kopin AS, Lee YM, McBride EW, Miller LJ, Lu M, Lin HY, Kolakowski LF, Beinborn M (1992) Expression cloning and characterization of the canine parietal cell gastrin receptor. Proc Natl Acad Sci USA 89:3605–3609
31. Knudson AG (1971) Mutation and cancer: Statistical study of retinoblastoma. Proc Natl Acad Sci USA 68:820–823
32. Baker SJ, Fearon ER, Nigro JM, Hamilton SR, Preisinger AC, Jessup JM, Tuinen P, Ledbetter DH, Barker DF, Nakamura Y, White R, Vogelstein B (1989) Chromosome 17 deletions and p53 gene mutations in colorectal carcinomas. Science 244:217–221
33. Yamada Y, Yoshida T, Hayashi K, Sekiya T, Yokota J, Hirohashi S, Nakatani K, Nagano H, Sugimura T, Terada M (1991) p53 gene mutations in gastric cancer metastases and in gastric cancer cell lines derived from metastases. Cancer Res 51:5800–5805
34. Tamura G, Kihana T, Nomura K, Terada M, Sugimura T, Hirohashi S (1991) Detection of frequent *p53* gene mutations in primary gastric cancer by cell sorting and polymerase chain reaction single-stranded conformation polymorphism analysis. Cancer Res 51:3056–3058
35. Uchino S, Noguchi M, Hirota T, Itabashi M, Saito T, Kobayashi M, Hirohashi S (1992) High incidence of nuclear accumulation of p53 protein in gastric cancer. Jpn J Clin Oncol 22:225–231
36. Fearon ER, Cho KR, Nigro JM, Kern SE, Simons JW, Ruppert JM, Hamilton SR, Preisinger AC, Thomas G, Kinzler KW, Vogelstein B (1990) Identification of a chromosome 18q gene that is altered in colorectal cancers. Science 247:49–56

37. Uchino S, Tsuda H, Noguchi M, Yokota J, Terada M, Saito T, Kobayashi M, Sugimura T, Hirohashi S (1992) Frequent loss of heterozygosity at the *DCC* locus in gastric cancer. Cancer Res 52:3099–3102

38. Nishisho I, Nakamura Y, Miyoshi Y, Miki Y, Ando H, Horii A, Koyama K, Utsunomiya J, Baba S, Hedge P, Markham A, Krush AJ, Petersen G, Hamilton SR, Nilbert MC, Levy DB, Bryan TM, Preisinger AC, Smith KJ, Su LK, Kinzler KW, Vogelstein B (1991) Mutations of chromosome 5q21 genes in FAP and colorectal cancer patients. Science 253:665–669

39. Sano T, Tsujino T, Yoshida K, Nakayama H, Haruma K, Ito H, Nakamura Y, Kajiyama G, Tahara E (1991) Frequent loss of heterozygosity on chromosomes 1q, 5q, and 17p in human gastric carcinomas. Cancer Res 51:2926–2931

40. Horii A, Nakatsuru S, Miyoshi Y, Ichii S, Nagase H, Kato Y, Yanagisawa A, Nakamura Y (1992) The *APC* gene, responsible for familial adenomatous polyposis, is mutated in human gastric cancer. Cancer Res 52:3231–3233

41. Tanaka M, Sasaki H, Kino I, Sugimura T, Terada M (1992) Genes preferentially expressed in embryo stomach are predominantly expressed in gastric cancer. Cancer Res 52:3372–3377

42. Haenszel W, Kurihara M, Segi M, Lee RKC (1972) Stomach cancer among Japanese in Hawaii. J Natl Cancer Inst 49:969–988

43. Warren JR, Marshall B (1983) Unidentified curved bacilli on gastric epithelium in active chronic gastritis. Lancet 1:1273–1275

44. Blaser MJ (1992) Hypothesis on the pathogenesis and natural history of *Helicobacter pylori*-induced inflammation. Gastroenterology 102:720–727

45. Parsonnet J, Friedman GD, Vandersteen DP, Chang Y, Vogelman JH, Orentreich N, Sibley RK (1991) *Helicobacter pylori* infection and the risk of gastric carcinoma. N Engl J Med 325:1127–1131

46. Nomura A, Stemmermann GN, Chyou P-H, Kato I, Perez-Perez GI, Blaser MJ (1991) *Helicobacter pylori* infection and gastric carcinoma among Japanese Americans in Hawaii. N Engl J Med 325:1132–1136

47. Katoh M, Saito D, Noda T, Yoshida S, Oguro Y, Yazaki Y, Sugimura T, Terada M (1993) *Helicobacter pylori* may be transmitted through gastrofiberscope even after manual Hyamine washing. Jpn J Cancer Res 84:117–119

Growth Factors in Gastric Cancer

Eiichi Tahara, Hiroshi Yokozaki, and Wataru Yasui[1]

Key words. Growth factor—Growth factor receptor—Proto-oncogene—Transcription factor—Cytokine—Cancer-stromal interaction—Adhesion molecules

Introduction

Growth factors may play an important role in mammalian embryogenesis, cell proliferation, differentiation, and repair after injury [1]. Normal epithelial cells of the gastrointestinal (GI) tract produce multiple growth factors including epidermal growth factor (EGF), transforming growth factor alpha (TGF alpha), *cripto*, amphiregulin, pS_2, and TGF beta [2–8]. These growth factors positively or negatively function as autocrine, paracrine, and luminal factors in regulating the cell growth, motility, and digestion of the GI tract. EGF may regulate expression of gastrin that stimulates gastric acid secretion and has a trophic effect on the growth of GI epithelial cells [9].

Gastric carcinoma reveals marked heterogeneity of morphology and function, as does lung carcinoma. In addition, gastric carcinoma overexpresses multiple growth factors, gut hormones, and cytokines [10, 11]. Receptors for a number of these ligands are also expressed on the tumor cells, indicating that multiple autocrine loops of growth factors and cytokines may be operative in gastric cancer [11]. Interestingly, the scenario of the gene alterations in proto-oncogenes encoding tyrosine kinase receptors, such as c-*met*, K-*sam*, and c-*erb*B-2, differs depending on the histological types of gastric cancer [11]. Moreover, differences are observed in the expression of growth factors between intestinal type cancer or well-differentiated adenocarcinoma and diffuse type cancer or poorly differentiated adenocarcinoma of the stomach [11].

The following is a description of what a crucial role the alteration and expression of growth factors and their receptor genes play in development and progression of gastric cancers.

[1] The First Department of Pathology, Hiroshima University School of Medicine, 1-2-3 Kasumi, Minami-ku, Hiroshima, 734 Japan

The EGF Family of Growth Factors

Most of the gastric carcinoma tissues and cell lines coexpress TGF alpha and EGF receptor genes [10]. Recent evidence indicates that TGF alpha and EGF precursors produced by tumor cells act as a positive autocrine growth factor for gastric carcinoma. Overexpression of EGF is frequently associated with well-differentiated adenocarcinoma. Synchronous overexpression of EGF or TGF alpha and EGF receptor evidently contributes to biological malignancy [12, 13]. However, no amplification of EGF or TGF alpha genes has been observed. EGF receptor genes also are not frequently amplified in gastric cancer [14]. The EGF receptor and TGF alpha promoters contain guanine cytosine (GC)-rich sequences to which several transcription factors bind. The transcription factor, Sp1, enhances transcription of the EGF receptor gene, whereas the GC-factor (GCF) represses expression of EGF receptor or TGF alpha mRNAs [15, 16]. A transcriptional abnormality including hyperfunction of Sp1 or hypofunction of GCF may bring about overexpression of EGF receptor and TGF alpha without gene amplification in gastric cancer.

In addition to EGF and TGF-alpha, new members of the EGF family such as *cripto* and amphiregulin are expressed in gastric carcinoma [4–6]. The *cripto* gene shares structural homology with EGF, TGF alpha, and amphiregulin. The interaction of *cripto* with EGF receptor, c-*erb*B-2, or c-*erb*B-3 has not yet been investigated. Most of well-differentiated gastric adenocarcinomas as well as colorectal adenocarcinomas express the *cripto* gene at higher levels than those in normal gastric mucosa [4]. The *cripto* protein is overexpressed in 44% of early gastric cancers, even in those under 1 cm in diameter [11]. Overexpression of *cripto* is also correlated with tumor stage and patient prognosis. An exciting observation is that there is a good correlation between *cripto* expression and grade of gastric intestinal metaplasia in which absorptive cells reveal strong immunoreactivity to *cripto* [11]. It is likely that *cripto* overexpression in gastric intestinal metaplasia may have some implication for the pathogenesis of well-differentiated adenocarcinoma of the stomach.

Amphiregulin is a secreted heparin-binding growth factor, of which COOH-terminal 40-amino acid residue has 38% and 32% homology with EGF and TGF alpha, respectively. In contrast to EGF and TGF alpha, amphiregulin has two putative nuclear targeting sequences [15], since amphiregulin is localized to the cytoplasm and/or nucleus of the cells [5, 6, 17]. Amphiregulin as well as EGF or TGF alpha bind to the EGF receptor and act as an autocrine growth factor for colon carcinoma [18]. Overexpression of amphiregulin is often associated with gastric carcinoma regardless of histological types. Most of gastric carcinoma cell lines also express amphiregulin at high levels. There is the possibility that amphiregulin may function as an autocrine growth stimulator for gastric cancer.

TGF Beta/Receptor System and Other Growth Factors

TGF beta 1, a negative growth factor, is also commonly expressed in gastric carcinoma [8]. With regard to the relationship between the incidence of TGF beta 1 overexpression and histological types, overexpression of TGF beta 1 is frequently observed in poorly differentiated adenocarcinoma. Our recent study on a gastric carcinoma cell line, TMK-1, which expresses TGF beta 1, has demonstrated that TGF beta 1 inhibits DNA synthesis by TMK-1 and that the type I receptor for TGF beta 1 is mainly linked to the growth-inhibitory signal by a decrease in retinoblastoma protein phosphorylation by $p34^{cdc2}$ without suppression of c-*myc* expression [19]. Interestingly, over 80% of gastric carcinoma tissues display a reduction in TGF beta type I receptor regardless of histological types [20]. Moreover, the reduction of the type I receptor in the tumor tissue is closely correlated with the depth of tumor invasion. These results suggest that most advanced gastric cancers escape from growth inhibition by TGF beta 1 through reduction in the type I receptor [20].

In addition to TGF beta 1, platelet-derived growth factor (PDGF), insulin-like growth factor II (IGF-II), and basic fibroblast growth factor (FGF) are also often overexpressed in poorly differentiated adenocarcinoma [10, 11, 21]. In particular, the development of scirrhous gastric carcinoma, which corresponds to diffusely infiltrating carcinoma or Borrmann's type IV carcinoma of the stomach, may require synchronous overexpression of TGF beta 1, PDGF, IGF-II, and basic FGF in the same tumor, all of which may function mainly as paracrine growth

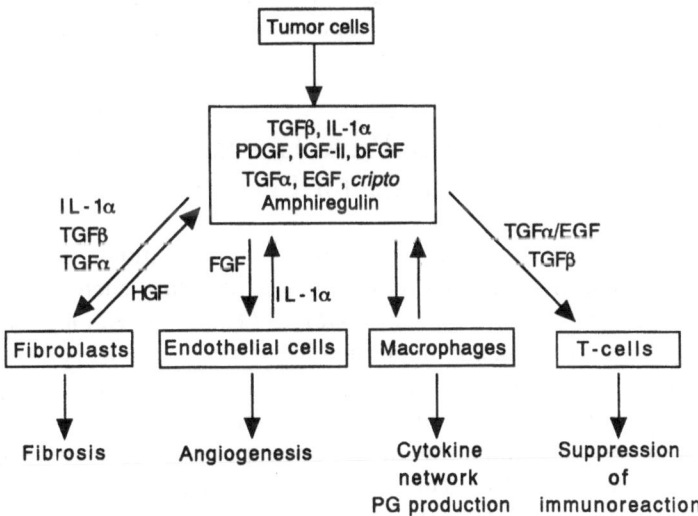

Fig. 1. Interaction of tumor-derived growth factors and cytokines with stromal cells of microenvironment. *TGF*, Transforming growth factor; *EGF*, epidermal growth factor; *PDGF*, platelet-derived growth factor; *IGF*, insulin-like growth factor; *FGF*, fibroblast growth factor; *HGF*, hepatocyte growth factor; *IL-1*, interleukin-1

factors. This reflects the close interaction of tumor cells and stromal cells including fibroblasts, endothelial cells, macrophages, and lymphocytes (Fig. 1).

Cytokines

Gastric carcinoma can produce not only growth factors but also cytokines. Surprisingly, the IL-1 alpha gene is expressed at various levels by most of the gastric carcinoma cell lines, among which MKN-7 secretes a large amount of IL-1 alpha into the condition medium [11]. Over 60% of the gastric carcinoma tissues reveal higher levels of IL-1 alpha mRNA compared to their normal mucosas. More recently, we found that IL-1 alpha enhances the cell growth of gastric carcinoma cell lines and that TGF alpha or EGF induces enhanced secretion of IL-1 alpha by tumor cells. Tumor-derived IL-1 alpha may bring about an increase in proteolytic enzyme activity, cell-adhesion molecules, and interleukin production and decrease production of the extracellular matrix by stromal cells. Therefore, cytokines as well as growth factors produced by tumor cells not only may serve autocrine or paracrine growth and motility of tumor cells themselves, but may also bind to each of the receptors on stromal cells, leading to fibrosis, angiogenesis, activation of cytokine network, and suppression of T cell function (Fig. 1).

On the other hand, fibroblasts, endothelial cells, macrophages, and lymphocytes stimulated by tumor cells may cause the secretion of multiple growth factor and cytokines, resulting in proliferation, enhanced motility, and cell death or necrosis of tumor cells (Fig. 1). In fact, Yasumoto et al. reported the synergistic induction of IL-8 production by TNF alpha and IFN alpha in a gastric carcinoma cell line, MKN-45 [22].

Gene Alterations in Proto-Oncogenes Encoding Growth Factor Receptors

Gastric carcinoma involves gene alterations in multiple tumor suppressor genes and multiple oncogenes encoding tyrosine kinase receptors, such as c-*met*, K-*sam*, c-*erb*B-1 (EGF receptor gene), and c-*erb*B-2 (Table 1). Among these proto-oncogenes, the most frequently implicated in gastric carcinoma is the c-*met* gene. The c-*met* gene encodes hepatocyte growth factor (HGF) receptor composed of a 50-kDa alpha subunit disulfide linked to a 145-kDa beta subunit to form a 190-kDa heterodimer [23]. Amplification and overexpression or abnormal expression of the c-*met* gene frequently occur in gastric carcinoma and closely correlate with tumor progression and metastasis [11]. The c-*met* gene is amplified in approximately 40% of scirrhous gastric carcinomas (Table 1). Interestingly, all of five scirrhous carcinoma cell lines, including HSC-39, KATO-III, NTAS, NKPS, and HSC-43 cells, share the gene amplification. A good correlation is observed between c-*met* amplification and the clinical stage or patient prognosis [24].

Table 1. Genetic alterations in two types of stomach cancer.

Genetic alterations	Frequency of occurrence (%)	
	Poorly differentiated cancer type	Well-differentiated cancer type
Mutation		
K-*ras*		9
p53	66	50
APC	30[a]	40
Deletion		
p53	76	60
Chromosome 5q (*APC* locus)		60
Rb	7	5
bcl-2		43
Chromosome 18q (*DCC* locus)		50
Chromosome 1q		44
Chromosome 1p	38	25
Chromosome 7q (c-*met* locus)		50
Amplification		
c-*met*	39[b]	19
K-*sam*	33[b]	
c-*erb*B2		18
Abnormal expression		
c-*met* 6.0 kb	73[b]	50

[a] Signet ring cell carcinoma; [b] Scirrhous carcinoma

Moreover, a 6.0 kb transcript of the c-*met* gene is expressed only in gastric carcinoma of both cell lines and tumor tissues [11]. In addition, the expression of this abnormal transcript of 6.0 kb is closely linked with the tumor staging, lymph node metastasis, and depth of tumor invasion. Recently, Soman et al. reported that the *tpr-met* rearrangement was expressed in gastric carcinoma as well as in chronic gastritis [25].

In addition to c-*met*, the K-*sam* gene, which encodes a tyrosine kinase receptor belonging to the fibroblast growth factor (FGF) receptor family, is amplified preferentially in poorly differentiated adenocarcinoma or scirrhous carcinoma [11]. It is significant that in cases of scirrhous carcinoma, K-*sam* amplification often occurs independently of c-*met* amplification. Moreover, there is a tendency for the K-*sam* gene to be amplified in tumors of females under 40 years of age, and for the c-*met* gene to be amplified in tumors of males over 50 years of age. In terms of gene expression, various transcripts of the K-*sam* gene have been reported with sizes of 4.5 kb, 4.0 kb or 3.5 kb, 3.2 kb, and 1.6 kb or 1.8 kb [26]. Of these, the 3.5 kb one, which is truncated in the 3' noncoding region, is detected in gastric carcinoma tissues and the gastric carcinoma cell line KATO-III, in which the K-*sam* gene was first identified as amplified DNA.

On the other hand, amplification and overexpression of c-*erb*B-2 is frequently associated with well-differentiated adenocarcinoma. High expression of c-*erb*B-2 in tumor cells without gene amplification may be responsible for transcriptional abnormality, including TATA box-binding protein or Sp1 and GCF [27]. Amplification of the c-*erb*B-2 gene is often detected in distant metastatic tumors rather than in primary ones [14], and c-*erb*B-1 (EGF receptor) gene amplification is a rare event of gastric carcinoma. Co-overexpression of c-*erb*B-2 protein and EGF receptor on tumor cells contributes to a high degree of malignancy which may develop by cross-phosphorylation of both the receptor proteins induced by TGF alpha or EGF. Recently, several ligands for the c-*erb*B-2 receptor, such as gp30 and NAF (*neu* activating factor), have been reported [17]. However, which ligands are expressed by gastric carcinoma is not presently clear.

Hepatocyte Growth Factor/c-*met* System

With regard to the complex interaction between tumor cells and stromal cells, hepatocyte growth factor (HGF), which is a ligand for the c-*met* protein, may play an important role in progression and morphogenesis of gastric cancer [11]. HGF, a heparin-binding polypeptide, is a heterodimeric molecule composed of a 69-kDa alpha subunit and a 34-kDa beta-subunit, and is derived from a single-chain precursor of 728 amino acids [28]. Although HGF was initially identified as a mitogen for hepatocytes, HGF is expressed by stromal fibroblasts, and stimulates proliferation of epithelial cells expressing c-*met* protein [29]. Moreover, HGF is essentially identical with scatter factor which enhances cell motility and stimulates the diversion of epithelial and vascular endothelial cells [30]. In addition, HGF has the property of epithelial morphogenesis [31]. Therefore, HGF is a multifunctional polypeptide that may act as a paracrine mediator of epithelial/mesenchymal interaction in enhancement of cell growth (mitogen), enhancement of cell motility (motogen), and promotion of epithelial tubules (morphogen).

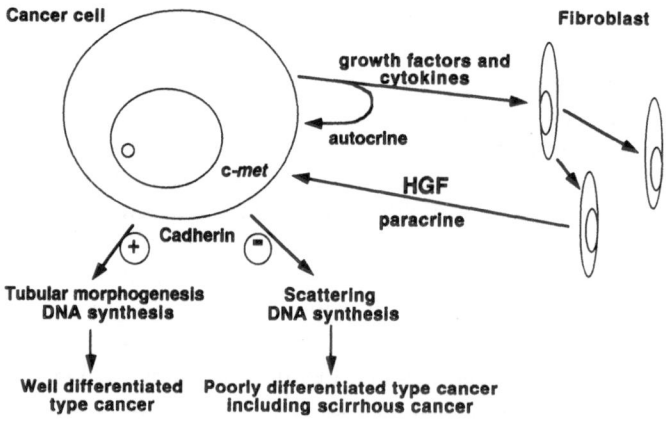

Fig. 2. Interaction between cancer cells and stromal cells implicated in morphogenesis of two types of stomach cancer

The results of our recent study provide a plausible hypothesis that the interaction of HGF in fibroblasts and cell adhesion molecules in c-*met* overexpressing tumor cells is implicated in the morphogenesis of two types of stomach cancer (Fig. 2). Stromal fibroblasts, stimulated by TGF alpha, TGF beta, or IL-1 alpha, may secrete HGF in a paracrine manner which can bind to c-*met* protein on tumor cells. If this happens, in the case of a clone maintaining the expression of E-cadherin, HGF could enhance the growth of tumor cells and promote tubular formation, leading to well-differentiated adenocarcinoma of the stomach. Conversely, in the case of a clone having diminished expression or loss of E-cadherin, HGF may cause scattering and proliferation of tumor cells, resulting in poorly differentiated adenocarcinoma of the stomach [11]. As to the mechanism of E-cadherin involvement in tumor invasion or metastasis, the following should be taken into account: (1) decrease in expression of E-cadherin and (2) disturbance in function of E-cadherin due to tyrosine phosphorylation of the cadherin-catenin complex or loss of catenin [11]. It is of considerable interest to determine whether or not c-*met* receptor kinase may be linked with tyrosine phosphorylation of the cadherin-catenin complex.

Conclusions

The multiple growth factor/receptor system and cytokines are overexpressed in gastric cancer. They act as autocrine and/or paracrine growth factors which induce the complex interaction of tumor cells and stromal cells. The accumulation of their overexpression, associated with reduction of TGF beta type I receptor, are responsible for the development and progression of gastric cancer.

Of the gene alterations in the multiple oncogene encoding tyrosine kinase receptor, the one most frequently implicated in gastric cancer is the activation (abnormal expression and amplification) of the c-*met* gene. Moreover, interaction between cell-adhesion molecules in tumor cells expressing c-*met* and HGF from stromal cells may participate in the morphogenesis of two types of gastric cancer.

References

1. Rappolee DA, Brenner CA, Schultz R, Mark D, Werb Z (1988) Developmental expression of PDGF, TGF-alpha, and TGF-beta genes in preimplantation mouse embryos. Science 241:1823–1825
2. Kajikawa K, Yasui W, Sumiyoshi H, Yoshida K, Nakayama H, Ayhan A, Yokozaki H, Ito H, Tahara E (1991) Expression of epidermal growth factor in human tissues: Immunohistochemical and biochemical analysis. Virchows Arch [A] 418:27–32
3. Yasui W, Ji Z-Q, Kuniyasu H, Ayhan A, Yokozaki H, Ito H, Tahara E (1992) Expression of transforming growth factor alpha in human tissues: Immunohistochemical study and Northern blot analysis. Virchows Arch [A] 421:513–519
4. Kuniyasu H, Yoshida K, Yokozaki H, Yasui W, Ito H, Toge T, Ciardiello F, Persico MG, Saeki T, Salomon DS, Tahara E (1991) Expression of cripto, a novel gene of the

epidermal growth factor family, in human gastrointestinal carcinomas. Jpn J Cancer Res 82:969–973

5. Saeki T, Stromberg K, Qi C-F, Gullick WJ, Tahara E, Normanno N, Ciardiello F, Kenney N, Johnson GR, Salomon DS (1992) Differential immunohistochemical detection of amphiregulin and cripto in human normal colon and colorectal tumors. Cancer Res 52:3467–3473

6. Ciardiello F, Kim N, Saeki T, Dono R, Persico MG, Plowman GD, Garrigues J, Radke S, Todaro GJ, Salomon DS (1991) Differential expression of epidermal growth factor-related proteins in human colorectal tumors. Proc Natl Acad Sci USA 88: 7792–7796

7. Theisinger B, Welter C, Seitz G, Rio M-C, Lathe R, Chambon P, Blin N (1991) Expression of the breast cancer associated gene $p5_2$ and the pancreatic spasmolytic polypeptide gene (hSP) in diffuse type of stomach carcinoma. Eur J Cancer 27: 770–773

8. Yoshida K, Yokozaki H, Niimoto M, Ito H, Ito M, Tahara E (1989) Expression of TGF-beta and procollagen type I and type III in human gastric carcinomas. Int J Cancer 44:394–398

9. Godley JM, Brand SJ (1989) Regulation of the gastrin promoter by epidermal growth factor and neuropeptides. Proc Natl Acad Sci USA 86:3036–3040

10. Tahara E (1990) Growth factors and oncogenes in human gastrointestinal carcinomas. J Cancer Res Clin Oncol 116:121–131

11. Tahara E (1993) Molecular mechanism of stomach carcinogenesis. J Cancer Res Clin Oncol 119:265–272

12. Yasui W, Sumiyoshi H, Hata J, Kameda T, Ochiai A, Ito H, Tahara E (1988) Expression of epidermal growth factor receptor in human gastric and colonic carcinomas. Cancer Res 48:137–141

13. Yasui W, Hata J, Yokozaki H, Nakatani H, Ochiai A, Ito H, Tahara E (1988) Interaction between epidermal growth factor and its receptor in progression of human gastric carcinoma. Int J Cancer 41:211–217

14. Tsujino T, Yoshida K, Nakayama H, Ito H, Shimosato T, Tahara E (1990) Alterations of oncogenes in metastatic tumours of human gastric carcinomas. Br J Cancer 62:226–230

15. Kitadai Y, Yasui W, Yokozaki H, Kuniyasu H, Haruma K, Kajiyama G, Tahara E (1992) The level of a transcription factor Sp1 is correlated with the expression of EGF receptor in human gastric carcinomas. Biochem Biophys Res Commun 189:1342–1348

16. Kitadai Y, Yamazaki H, Yasui W, Kyo E, Yokozaki H, Kajiyama G, Johnson AC, Pastan I, Tahara E (1993) GC factor represses transcription of several growth factor/receptor genes and causes growth inhibition of human gastric carcinoma cell lines. Cell Growth and Differentiation 4:291–296

17. Prigent SA, Lemoine NR (1992) The type 1 (EGFR-related) family of growth factor receptors and their ligands. Prog Growth Factor Res 4:1–24

18. Johnson GR, Saeki T, Gordon AW, Shoyab M, Salomon DS, Stromberg K (1992) Autocrine action of amphiregulin in a colon carcinoma cell line and immunocytochemical localization of amphiregulin in human colon. J Cell Biol 118:741–751

19. Ito M, Yasui W, Kyo E, Yokozaki H, Nakayama H, Ito H, Tahara E (1992) Growth inhibition of transforming growth factor beta on human gastric carcinoma cells: Receptor and postreceptor signaling. Cancer Res 52:295–300

20. Ito M, Yasui W, Nakayama H, Yokozaki H, Ito H, Tahara E (1992) Reduced levels of transforming growth factor-beta type I receptor in human gastric carcinomas. Jpn J Cancer Res 83:86–92

21. Tanimoto H, Yoshida K, Yokozaki H, Yasui W, Nakayama H, Ito H, Ohama K, Tahara E (1991) Expression of basic fibroblast growth factor in human gastric carcinomas. Virchows Arch [B] 61:263–267
22. Yasumoto K, Mai M, Okamoto S, Mukaida N, Matsushima K (1992) Analysis of the synergistic induction of IL-8 production by TNF-alpha and IFN gamma in a human gastric cancer cell line. Proceedings of the Japanese Cancer Association 51st Annual Meeting, p290
23. Bottaro DP, Rubin JS, Faletto DL, Chan AM-L, Kmiecik TE, Vande Woude GF, Aaronson SA (1991) Identification of the hepatocyte growth factor receptor as the c-met proto-oncogene product. Science 251:802–804
24. Kuniyasu H, Yasui W, Kitadai Y, Yokozaki H, Ito H, Tahara E (1992) Frequent amplification of the c-met gene in scirrhous type stomach cancer. Biochem Biophys Res Commun 189:227–232
25. Soman NR, Correa P, Ruiz BA, Wogan GN (1991) The TPR-MET oncogenic rearrangement is present and expressed in human gastric carcinoma and precursor lesions. Proc Natl Acad Sci USA 88:4892–4896
26. Katoh M, Hattori Y, Sasaki H, Tanaka M, Sugano K, Yazaki Y, Sugimura T, Terada M (1992) K-sam gene encodes secreted as well as transmembrane receptor tyrosine kinase. Proc Natl Acad Sci USA 89:2960–2964
27. Kameda T, Yasui W, Yoshida K, Tsujino T, Nakayama H, Ito M, Ito H, Tahara E (1990) Expression of ERBB2 in human gastric carcinomas: Relationship between p185ERBB2 expression and gene amplification. Cancer Res 50:8002–8009
28. Nakamura T, Nishizawa T, Hagiya M, Saeki T, Shimonishi M, Sugimura A, Tashiro K, Shimizu S (1989) Molecular cloning and expression of human hepatocyte growth factor. Nature 342:440–443
29. Prat M, Narsimhan RP, Crepaldi T, Nicotra MR, Natali PG, Comoglio PM (1991) The receptor encoded by the human c-met oncogene is expressed in hepatocytes, epithelial cells and solid tumors. Int J Cancer 49:323–328
30. Bhargava M, Joseph A, Knesel J, Halaban R, Li Y, Pang S, Goldberg I, Setter E, Donovan MA, Zarnegar R, Michalopoulos GA, Nakamura T, Faletto D, Rosen EM (1992) Scatter factor and hepatocyte growth factor: Activities, properties, and mechanism. Cell Growth and Differentiation 3:11–20
31. Montesano R, Matsumoto K, Nakamura T, Orci L (1991) Identification of a fibroblast-derived epithelial morphogen as hepatocyte growth factor. Cell 67:901–908

Tumor Markers

Kohzoh Imai[1] *and Toshiro Sugiyama*[1]

Key words. Tumor marker—Gastric cancer—Monoclonal antibody—Diagnosis—Early detection

Introduction

Many monoclonal antibodies (mAb) have been identified in the 15 years since the advent of hybridoma methodology. Antibodies which detect gastric cancer-associated antigens have made a place for themselves as an essential, non-invasive diagnostic tool for the clinician. The name 'tumor markers' has been coined for these antigens and for cancer-associated proteins, amino acids, and glycolipids. The name has been found to apply further afield, to genes, including oncogenes and suppressor oncogenes, as well as their mRNAs, if they are expressed preferentially in tumor cells or tissues.

Here we describe the newest information concerning gastric cancer-associated tumor markers and briefly discuss the significance of these markers from the viewpoint of tumor biology.

Tumor Markers Detected in the Serum and the Tissue

Many monoclonal antibodies have been established to aid in detecting gastric cancer-associated antigens [1, 2]; some have been shown to be capable of providing precise measurements of circulating antigens in the serum. Table 1 shows the incidence of the antigens in sera from patients with gastric cancer. It is well known that carcinoembryonic antigen (CEA) occurs in 20%–30% of patients with gastric cancer [3]. The CA19-9 antigen, which carries the sialyl Le^a epitope, shows a 32% incidence [4], while sialyl SSEA-1 bearing molecules, recognized by

[1] Department of Internal Medicine (Section 1), Sapporo Medical University, S-1, W-16, Chuo-ku, Sapporo, 060 Japan

Table 1. Incidence of positivity of various tumor markers in the sera of patients with gastric cancer.

Monoclonal antibody	Antigenic structure	Positive ratio (No. positive/no. tested)	Reference
NS19-9	Sailyl Le^a (CA19-9)	32% (30/94)	[4]
FH-6	Sialyl SSEA-1	13%	[5]
B72.3/CC49	Sialosyl-2 6 α-N-acetyl galactosamyl epitope (TAG-72)	43% (40/94)	[4]
NCC-ST-439	High molecular weight glycoprotein (sialosyl type)	19% (48/249)	[10]
YH206	High molecular weight glycoprotein (asialo-type)	32% (22/69)	[8]
MUSE11	MUC-1 gene core protein	32% (9/28)	[16]
c-erbB-2	185 kDa glycoprotein	10% (4/40)	(T. Ishida et al.[a])

[a] Significance of erbB-2 gene product as a target molecule, submitted for publication

the FH6 mAb, have an incidence of only 13% [5]; it seems that gastric cancer cells produce sialyl Le^a-bearing molecules more frequently than sialyl SSEA-1 molecules. The B72.3 mAb, which has recently been found to recognize the sialosyl Tn epitope [6], appears in the sera in 43% of gastric cancer cases [4]. In the case of the YH206 antigen [7, 8], the ratio is 32%, the same as that of CA19-9 [4]. Interestingly, this mAb recognizes high molecular weight asialo-type glycoproteins, which belong to the class of classic mucin molecules [9], while the NCC-ST-439 mAb recognizes the sialosyl-type glycoprotein, showing a 19% incidence [10].

Recently, the cDNA of mucin genes has been extensively cloned; as of the beginning of 1992, four mucin genes have been reported, designated MUC-1, 2, 3, and 4 [11–14]. We do not know at present to which gene our YH206 antigen belongs. It is interesting, however, that at least one of the mucin gene products carries the asialo-type sugar chain; this epitope can be frequently detected in the sera of gastric cancer patients. It is noteworthy that there was no correlation between CA19-9 and YH206 levels in the sera of gastric cancer patients [9].

The MUSE11 mAb, originated in our laboratory [15], was found to recognize the MUC-1 gene core protein [16]. The binding activity of MUSE11 to a synthetic peptide corresponding to the tandem repeat motif of the MUC-1 gene protein was compared with the DF3 mAb (Table 2), which is the antibody used in the CA15-3 assay kit for monitoring breast cancer; the MUSE11 mAb showed a higher binding activity than the DF3 mAb [17]. It is known that the DF3 mAb detects epitope structures containing sialylated carbohydrate chains. The serum levels of the MUSE11 and CA15-3 antigens were simultaneously measured in 35 specimens, including gastric cancers, and the relationship between these serum

Table 2. Binding activity of MUSE11 and DF3 mAbs to a synthetic peptide.

mAb	Binding activity (cpm)[a] to peptide[b]
MUSE11	42 852 ± 794
DF3	14 163 ± 46
YH206	1 074 ± 29
P1-255	2 108 ± 46

[a] Detected with a ^{125}I-labeled anti-mouse IgG-Fc antibody
[b] A peptide consisting of one repeat and four amino acids from the tandem repeat region of mucin core protein. Concentrations of the peptide and mAbs used were 100 µg/ml and 5 µg/ml, respectively. Values are mean ± SD of triplicate determinations

Table 3. Relationship between serum levels of MUSE11 and CA15-3 antigens in patients with gastric cancer.

	CA15-3 (+)	CA15-3 (−)
Antigen MUSE11 (+)	7	11
Antigen MUSE11 (−)	2	15

levels was evaluated (Table 3) (K. Imai, unpublished observation). Seven out of 35 serum specimens tested positive for both the MUSE11 and CA15-3 antigens. Eleven out of 35 were positive for the MUSE11 antigen and negative for CA15-3, whereas only 2 were negative for the MUSE11 antigen and positive for CA15-3. These findings indicated a higher incidence of abnormal levels of the MUSE11 antigen, compared to CA15-3, in the sera of gastric cancer patients ($P < 0.01$). It is noteworthy that no significant correlation was observed between the serum levels of the MUSE11 and CA15-3 antigens. In any case, it is of interest that the MUSE11 mAb can detect 32% of gastric cancer patients (Table 1).

ErbB-2 protein, a 185 kDa glycoprotein encoded by the c-*erbB*-2 gene, was found by Yamamoto, Toyoshima, and colleagues in 1986 [18]. Several mAbs to *erbB*-2 protein have been established, including our own (T. Ishida et al., Significance of *erbB*-2 gene product as a target molecule, submitted for publication). With the simultaneous use of two mAbs, is necessary to unambiguously detect *erbB*-2 protein in the serum. As depicted in Table 1, this method was successful in identifying 10% of gastric cancer patients. Furthermore, all the patients with gastric cancer who showed higher levels of *erbB*-2 protein were found to have well-differentiated adenocarcinoma. Therefore, although it is not very common to find *erbB*-2 protein in the circulation, when it is found, it is a dependable indicator for this histological type of tumor. It is also possible that the *erbB*-2 protein-positive patients form a subgroup of patients with well-differentiated adenocarcinoma.

Studies of suppressor oncogenes have also borne fruit. For example, Matozaki and his coworkers [19] have studied the p53 gene, a suppressor oncogene, in 12 human gastric cancer cell lines. After reverse-transcriptase polymerase chain reaction and direct sequencing, seven cell lines showed point mutations of the p53 gene resulting in amino-acid substitutions. Most of these were rare mutations which had not been observed in other types of cancers. Six out of the seven cell lines with mutations of the p53 gene also lost one allele of chromosome 17p. Immunoblotting of cell lysates with an antibody specific to p53 demonstrated high levels of p53 protein in five cell lines, all of which contained mutations of the p53 gene. These results suggest that human gastric cancer tissue may show certain abnormalities either at the genetic level or at the protein/mRNA level. In fact, preliminary results of experiments performed by Shiku et al. at Nagasaki University School of Medicine showed that 15 out of 30 cases showed point mutations of the p53 gene and that 12 out of 27 cases showed positive nuclear staining with the antibody to p53 protein. Eleven of these 12 cases were found to have structural abnormalities in the p53 gene (Prof. Hiroshi Shiku personal communication, 1992). Other suppressor oncogenes or candidates for suppressor oncogenes, such as DCC, APC, and PTP will be examined in the near future.

Tumor Markers and Early Detection of Gastric Cancer

In many parts of the world, mass endoscopy-based screening for gastric cancer is not feasible because of the relatively low incidence of the disease. Alternative approaches, such as screening with cancer-associated markers, are not, as yet, reliable enough to be used.

To be clinically useful for screening, as distinct from "monitoring" the progress of an established disease, a marker for gastric cancer should also be sensitive enough to allow detection of cancer before it becomes symptomatic or detectable with the usual diagnostic tools. Additional requirements would include that the marker could be assayed with an easily performed test, cause a minimum of tissue damage and discomfort to the patient, have a low cost/effectiveness ratio, and give reproducible results.

Farinati et al. [20] have identified the CA50 mAb, which bears sialosyl fucosyl-lactotetraose, corresponding to the sialylated blood group antigen Lewis[a], in the serum, gastric juice, and urine of patients undergoing upper gastrointestinal tract endoscopy: this study employed 22 control subjects (no macroscopic or microscopic lesions), 29 patients with chronic atrophic gastritis, 20 with epithelial dysplasia, and 16 with gastric cancer. Gastric juices were also tested for pH, protein concentration and specific gravity, and urine samples were tested for protein concentration and osmolarity. Serum and gastric juices were also tested for CEA levels. Comparison of the results obtained with the two markers revealed that in patients with gastric cancer, CA50 gastric juice levels were statistically higher than in controls; a wide overlap was, however, present among groups, and the sensitivity and specificity were, respectively, 38% and 85% for serum and 69% and 82% for gastric juice. Sensitivity and specificity were, respectively, 23% and 89% for CA50 determination in urine. In this case, no statistically significant difference was observed between gastric cancer and control patients. A trend toward higher median values was observed in advanced with respect to early gastric cancer. A correlation was found between gastric juice and serum CA50 levels, as well as between serum and urine levels of the marker. A correlation was also observed between CA50 values and protein concentration in gastric juice and with osmolarity in urines. Overall, CA50 levels were statistically higher in patients with intestinal metaplasia than in those who had no lesions. Increased CA50 gastric juice levels were also observed in patients with chronic atrophic gastritis and epithelial dysplasia. CA50 levels in gastric juice and urine appear to depend, at least in part, on the concentration of the protein in the fluid. Horinouchi et al. [21], using an immunohistochemical method, investigated alterations of carbohydrate chain antigens in relation to histological malignant changes in 62 patients with atypical gastric epithelial lesions (adenomas) which were diagnosed as Group-III (according to *The general rules for gastric cancer study in surgery and pathology, 10th edn.* [Japanese Research Society for Gastric Cancer]) at the first biopsy. These patients were followed up after more than 1 year. Among the seven carbohydrate chain antigens related to the Lewis antigen, the sialyl Le^x-i antigen showed the most impressive findings; the ratio of positive indications from the first biopsy specimens of Group-III was 6%; however, this rose to 33% in the final biopsy specimens of Group-IV, 50% in the resected specimens of border-line lesions, and 67% in the resected specimens of carcinomas. These results indicate that there exists a close correlation between malignant changes in atypical gastric epithelial lesions and alterations in carbohydrate chains in terms of sialylation.

The mAbs to the ras oncogene product p21 have been used to analyze precancerous lesions. Ohuchi et al. [22], using the RAP-5 mAb, showed that dysplastic and noncancerous lesions immediately contiguous to cancerous tissue tested positive for p21. Using the rp-12 mAb, which recognizes both the H- and K-ras p21 products, we have also found a high number of cells expressing p21 in atypical gastric epithelial lesions more than 1 cm in diameter (Imai et al., unpublished observation) (Fig. 1). An in situ hybridization assay in conjunction with an H-ras gene probe in our laboratory confirmed this tendency at the mRNA level. Yoshida et al. [23], who have followed this line of investigation using their RASK-3 mAb, which reacted with all the Ki-, N- and Ha-ras p21s, have proposed an interesting hypothesis. They showed a marked expression of p21 in moderately- to well-differentiated cancer, intestinal metaplasia, and atypical hyperplasia, but not in normal epithelial cells and hyperplastic polyps; this

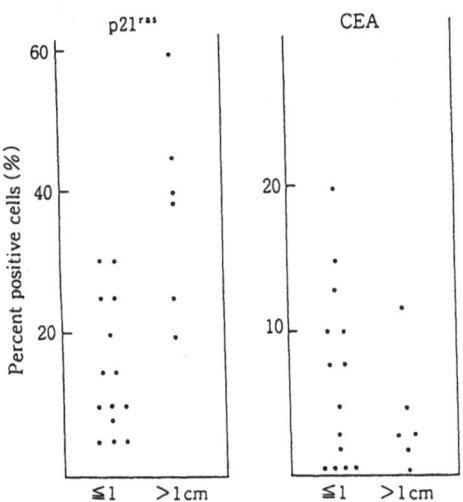

Fig. 1. Percentage of cells positive for ras p21 and carcinoembryonic antigen (*CEA*) in atypical epithelial lesions (determined by immunoperoxidase technique)

indicates that the expression of p21 in the epithelial cells of the stomach had increased as a consequence of cellular changes to premalignant status, manifesting such conditions as intestinal metaplasia and atypical hyperplasia.

Helicobacter pylori (*H. pylori*) infection has recently been implicated in a majority of gastritis cases [24]. Investigations into the epidemiology of *H. pylori* infection have been assisted by a large body of information. Moreover, a number of excellent indirect studies have shown a consistent link between the frequency of *H. pylori* and the prevalence of gastric carcinoma in various populations. Recently, the results of three case-control studies [25–27] have confirmed and extended the indirect association between *H. pylori* and gastric cancer. We have developed several mAbs to *H. pylori* [28]. Since we found that the serum of patients with gastritis reacted strongly with the 25 kDa *H. pylori* antigen, we developed an enzyme-linked immunosorbent assay (ELISA) system for detecting serum antibody against this 25 kDa antigen [29]. The serum titer of anti-25 kDa antibodies (mainly IgG type) was significantly higher in patients with gastritis than in healthy controls. In addition, the titer of IgA type anti-25 kDa antibodies in gastric juice correlated closely with the histological grade of gastritis, suggesting that a local immune response to *H. pylori* in gastric mucosa might also be associated with the development of gastritis [30]. Asaka et al. [31] reported that levels of serum pepsinogen I and II (markers of gastritis and gastric atrophy) were significantly higher in *H. pylori*-infected volunteers than in uninfected volunteers. Graham et al. [24] suggested an interesting epidemiological way of thinking: their prospective study in Japan (Fig. 2) has given us further insight into the changes in the epidemiology of *H. pylori* associated with the westernization of Japanese

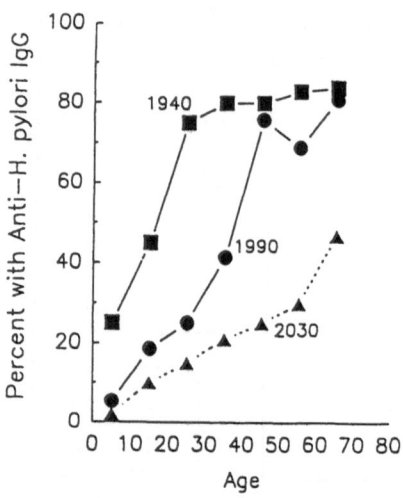

Fig. 2. The effect of westernization on the epidemiology of *Helicobacter pylori* in Japan. The 1940 curve shows the pattern of incidence in a typical underdeveloped country, which would have been expected from a study in that year. The 1990 curve shows the current pattern, and the 2030 curve represents the prevalence of *H. pylori* that may be expected to occur with continued improvements in the standard of living in Japan. *IgG*, immunoglobulin G. (From [24], with permission)

society, and this change is consistent with ongoing changes in the epidemiology of gastric cancer in Japan [31]. Although we need more data, especially regarding the disease-specific features of *H. pylori*, in order to connect *H. pylori* infection and gastric cancer, we must keep in mind that *H. pylori* provides the proper environment, i.e., chronic atrophic gastritis and/or intestinal metaplasia, for the development of gastric cancer.

Tumor Markers and Prognosis of Gastric Cancer

Many tumor markers have already been used to detect malignancies, as well as to assess the efficacy of treatment. Tumor markers also play important roles in predicting prognosis and detecting recurrence. In this section, we survey some recent studies concerning these points.

A recent study [32] using a mAb specific to estrogen receptors showed receptors in 28% of gastric adenocarcinomas, particularly in poorly-differentiated lesions. Harrison et al. [33] showed the correlation of estrogen receptor-related protein status with long-term survival in a group of 188 consecutive patients undergoing surgery for gastric cancer; those who tested negative for the presence of this protein had a significant survival advantage over those who tested positive. Prognostic factor analysis with a Cox proportional hazards model showed tumor stage and estrogen receptor-related protein to be significantly independent factors in gastric cancer.

In 1970, Bourreille et al. [34] reported the first case of α-fetoprotein (AFP)-producing gastric cancer with liver metastasis. In the literature, there have been few reported cases of advanced and early gastric cancer that produced AFP. The incidence of AFP-producing gastric cancer is reported to be from 1.3% to 15%, depending on the writer (about 5% average) in Japan [35]. Chang et al. [35] compared 27 cases of AFP-positive gastric cancer with 478 cases of AFP-negative gastric cancer. Although sex, age distribution, pathologic type, and serum CEA levels were similar in these two groups, Borrmann III-type cancer, lymph node metastasis, and incidence of synchronous and metachronous liver metastasis occurred more often in the AFP-positive group. Liver metastasis occurred in 72% of the AFP-positive patients, all of whom died within 2 years. The long-term survival of the AFP-positive group was clearly worse than that of the others. These investigators also reported three patients with AFP-producing early gastric cancer, in all of whom liver metastasis occurred shortly after curative gastrectomy; all died within 2 years [36] (Fig. 3). These findings suggest that AFP-producing cells are more prone to liver metastasis. Chang discussed the possibility that the liver may offer a suitable environment for AFP-producing tumors to proliferate. It also is possible that AFP-producing cells are associated with early vascular invasion. In any case, AFP-producing gastric cancer seems to have a poor prognosis. Establishment of an AFP-producing gastric cancer cell line [37] may help in elucidating the mechanisms responsible for this disease process.

Using CA19-9 as a marker, Ikeda et al. [38] compared two groups: 57 patients who died of recurrence or metastasis within 2 years (group I) and 58 patients who survived 5 years or more after resection (group II). In undifferentiated type carcinoma, the staining pattern peculiar to stromal type was seen in 65% of group

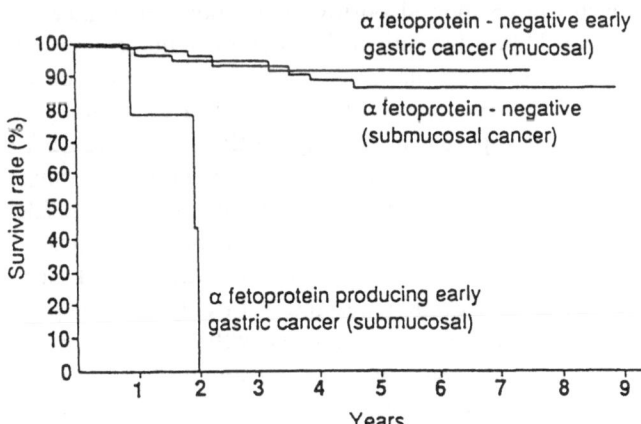

Fig. 3. Survival curves of α fetoprotein-producing and α fetoprotein-negative early gastric cancers calculated by the Kaplan-Meier method. (From [36] with permission)

I and 23% of group II. They therefore proposed that the immunohistochemical localization of CA19-9 in tumorous tissues, particularly in undifferentiated carcinoma, would be useful in predicting the prognosis of patients with advanced gastric carcinoma.

Recent studies have shown that the *erbB*-2 proto-oncogene is amplified in 25%–33% of human mammary carcinomas and that there is a significant association between *erbB*-2 amplification and prognosis, as well as with lymph node metastasis [39]. In gastric carcinoma, however, there have been conflicting results in the literature. Yonemura et al. [40], using a polyclonal antibody, reported that expression of *erbB*-2 protein was associated with serosal invasion, lymph node metastasis, and lymphatic invasion, and that patients with *erbB*-2 protein-positive tumors had a five-fold greater relative risk of death, compared with those with *erbB*-2 protein-negative tumors. Jain et al. [41], on the other hand, described apparently opposite results. They claimed that, overall, patients with tumors expressing this proto-oncogene had a significantly improved prognosis and that within the group of intestinal-type tumors, those that were c-*erbB*-2-positive formed a distinct sub-population which had a better prognosis, suggesting possible differences in etiology. Both Yonemura and Jain used formalin-fixed paraffin-embedded tissue sections and polyclonal anti-c-*erbB*-2 product antisera, although the epitope recognized by each of the antisera seems to be different. We would think that the *in situ* hybridization method or Northern blot analysis might be helpful to elucidate these conflicting results.

Yamaguchi et al. [42] examined the possibility of urinary pepsinogen I being a tumor marker of stomach cancer after total gastrectomy. Because of the high blood and urine concentration of pepsinogen isozymes derived from the gastric mucosa, it is difficult to detect trace amounts of the pepsinogen isozymes produced by gastric cancer cells. However, when the stomach is totally resected, the urinary concentration of "background" pepsinogen isozymes decreases to lower levels. They reported that 22 out of 74 patients who had undergone total gastrectomy for stomach cancer showed positive indications for urinary pepsinogen I, and that 20 of these 22 positive patients had definite clinical signs of recurrence of stomach cancer. This suggests that urinary pepsinogen I could be a usefur tumor marker in detecting the recurrence of stomach cancer after total gastrectomy.

Asao et al. [43] have reported interesting results after using CEA in peritoneal washings. They determined CEA levels in the peritoneal washings of 120 patients with gastric cancer and 9 patients with benign diseases. Elevated values (>100 ng/g of protein) were observed in 20 of 25 patients with gastric cancer with visible dissemination and in 16 of 25 patients with serosal invasion but no dissemination. The same elevation was found in only 9 of 70 patients with no serosal invasion and in none of the patients with benign diseases. The 2-year survival rates after curative operations for the patients with and without elevation of CEA levels were 21% and 100%, respectively ($P < 0.001$). They concluded from this study that the CEA level in peritoneal washings could be a sensitive detector of peritoneal dissemination that is not grossly visible and that this could be a new predictor for the postoperative prognosis of gastric cancer.

Acknowledgments. We acknowledge the secretarial assistance of Ms Y. Himoro. This work was financed by a Grant-in-Aid for Scientific Research on Priority Areas and by Grants-in-Aid for Cancer Research from the Ministry of Education, Science and Culture, Japan.

References

1. Yachi A, Imai K, Ban T, Hinoda Y, Wada T (1987) Serodiagnosis of digestive-tract malignancies employing novel monoclonal antibodies. In: Wada T, Aoki K, Yachi A (eds) Current status of cancer research in Asia, the Middle East, and other countries. The University of Nagoya Press, Nagoya, pp 111–117
2. Imai K, Moriya Y, Fujita H, Tsujisaki M, Kawaharada M, Yachi A (1984) Immunological characterization and molecular profile of carcinoembryonic antigen by monoclonal antibodies. J Immunol 132:2992–2997
3. Koga T, Kano T, Souda K, Oka N, Inokuchi K (1987) The clinical usefulness of preoperative CEA determination in gastric cancer. Jpn J Surg 17:342–347
4. Guadagni F, Roselli M, Amato T, Cosimelli M, Perri P, Casale V, Carlini M, Santoro E, Cavaliere R, Greiner JW, Schlom J (1992) CA 72-4 Measurement of tumor-associated glycoprotein 72 (TAG-72) as a serum marker in the management of gastric carcinoma. Cancer Res 52:1222–1227
5. Kannagi R, Fukushi Y, Tachikawa T, Noda A, Shin S, Shigeta K, Hiraiwa N, Fukuda Y, Inamoto T, Hakomori S, Imura H (1986) Quantitative and qualitative characterization of human cancer-associated serum glycoprotein antigens expressing fucosyl or sialyl-fucosyl type 2 chain polylactosamine. Cancer Res 46:2619–2626
6. Kjeldsen T, Clausen H, Hirohashi S, Ogawa T, Iijima H, Hakomori S (1988) Preparation and characterization of monoclonal antibodies directed to the tumor-associated O-linked sialosyl2-6-N-acetylgalactosaminyl (sialosyl-Tn) epitope. Cancer Res 48:2214–2220
7. Hinoda Y, Imai K, Endo K, et al (1985) Detection of circulating adenocarcinoma-associated antigen in the sera of cancer patients with a monoclonal antibody. Jpn J Cancer Res (Gann) 76:1203–1211
8. Hinoda Y, Imai K, Ban T, et al (1987) A sandwich enzyme immunoassay of an adenocarcinoma-associated antigen, YH206, in cancer sera. Jpn J Cancer Res (Gann) 78:607–613
9. Hinoda Y, Imai K, Ban T, et al (1988) Immunochemical characterization of adeno-carcinoma-associated antigen YH206. Int J Cancer 42(5):653–658
10. Ohkura H, Hattori N, Miyazaki I, Sawabu N, Tobe R, Kawai K, Abe O, Ishii M, Kawai T, Kamano T, Kurihara M, Mizumoto R (1987) Clinical study of the NCC-ST-439 EIA kit using serum from patients with various types of cancer and benign diseases (1). Jpn J Cancer Chemother 14: (Part I) 1901–1906
11. Spicer AP, Parry G, Patton S, Gendler SJ (1991) Molecular cloning and analysis of the mouse homologue of the tumor-associated mucin, MUC1, reveals conservation of potential O-glycosylation sites, transmembrane and cytoplasmic domains, and a loss of minisatellite-like polymorphism. J Biol Chem 266(23):15099–15109
12. Toribara NW, Gum JR Jr, Culhane PJ, Lagace RE, Hicks JW, Petersen GM, Kim YS (1991) MUC-2 human small intestinal mucin gene structure. J Clin Invest 88: 1005–1013

13. Niv Y, Byrd JC, Ho SB, Dahiya R, Kim YS (1992) Mucin synthesis and secretion in relation to spontaneous differentiation of colon cancer cells in vitro. Int J Cancer 50:147–152

14. Porchet N, Van Cong N, Dufosse J, Audie JP, Guyonnet-Duperat V, Gross MS, Denis C, Degand P, Bernheim A, Aubert JP (1991) Molecular cloning and chromosomal localization of a novel human tracheo-bronchial mucin cDNA containing tandemly-repeated sequences of 48 base pairs. Biochem Biophys Res Commun 175(2):414–422

15. Ban T, Imai K, Yachi A (1989) Immunohistological and immunochemical characterization of a novel pancreatic cancer-associated antigen, MUSE11. Cancer Res 49:7141–7146

16. Hinoda Y, Nakagawa N, Ohe Y, Kakiuchi H, Tsujisaki M, Imai K, Yachi Y (1990) Recognition of the polypeptide core of mucin by monoclonal antibody, MUSE11, against an adenocarcinoma-associated antigen. Jpn J Cancer Res 81:1206–1209

17. Hinoda Y, Kakiuchi H, Nakagawa N, Ohe Y, Sugiyama T, Masayuki T, Imai K, Yachi A (1992) Circulating tumor-associated antigens detected by monoclonal antibodies against the polypeptide core of mucin. Comparison of antigen MUSE11 with CA15-3. Gastroenterol Jpn 27:390–395

18. Yamamoto T, Ikawa S, Akiyama T, Semba K, Nomura N, Miyajima N, Saito T, Toyoshima K (1986) Similarity of protein encoded by the human c-erbB-2 gene to epidermal growth factor receptor. Nature 319:230–234

19. Matozaki T, Sakamoto C, Matsuda K, Suzuki T, Konda Y, Nakano O, Wada K, Uchida T, Nishisaki H, Nagao M, et al (1992) Missense mutations and a deletion of the p53 gene in human gastric cancer. Biochem Biophys Res Commun 182(1):215–223

20. Farinati F, Holmgren J, Mario FD, Cardin F, Vallante F, Fanton MC, Libera GD, Nitti D, Plebani M, Crestani B, Naccarato R (1991) CA 50 Determination in body fluids: Can we screen patients at risk for gastric cancer? Int J Cancer 47:7–11

21. Horinouchi H, Sato E, Yonezawa S, Tanaka S (1991) Alterations of Lewis-related sugar antigens in gastric atypical epithelial lesions (adenomas or dysplasia) with relation to their malignant changes—An evaluation by follow-up cases. Jpn J Gastroenterol 88:19–27

22. Ohuchi N, Hand PH, Merlo G, Fujita J, Mariani-Costantini R, Thor A, Nose M, Callahan R, Schlom J (1987) Enhanced expression of c-Ha-ras p21 in human stomach adenocarcinomas defined by immunoassays using monoclonal antibodies and in situ hybridization. Cancer Res 47:1413–1420

23. Yoshida K, Hamatani K, Koide H, Ikeda H, Nakamura N, Akiyama M, Tsuchiyama H, Nakayama E, Shiku H (1988) Preparation of anti-ras M_r21 000 protein monoclonal antibodies and immunohistochemical analyses of expression of ras genes in human stomach and thyroid cancers. Cancer Res 48:5503–5509

24. Graham DY, Klein PD, Evans DG, Fiedorek SC, Evans DJ Jr, Adam E, Malaty HM (1992) Helicobacter pylori: Epidemiology, relationship to gastric cancer, and the role of infants in transmission. Eur J Gastroenterol Hepatol 4:S1–S6

25. Parsonnet J, Vandersteen D, Goates J, Sibley RK, Pritikin J, Chang Y (1991) Helicobacter pylori infection in intestinal and diffuse-type gastric adenocarcinomas. J Natl Cancer Inst 83:640–643

26. Forman D, Newell DG, Fullerton F, Yarnell JWG, Stacey AR, Wald N, et al (1991) Association between infection with Helicobacter pylori and risk of gastric cancer: Evidence from a prospective investigation. BMJ 302:1302–1305

27. Nomura A, Stemmermann GN, Chyou P-H, Kato I, Perez-Perez GI, Blaser MJ (1991) *Helicobacter pylori* infection and gastric carcinoma among Japanese Americans in Hawaii, N Engl J Med 325:1132–1136

28. Yachi A, Sugiyama T, Yoshida H, Imai K, Yabana T, Yokota K, Oguma K (1989) Preparation of anti-*Campylobacter pylori* monoclonal antibodies and clinical implications. In: Takemoto T, Kawai K, Shimoyama T (eds) *Campylobacter pylori* and gastroduodenal diseases. Proceedings of the first Tokyo international symposium on *Campylobacter pylori*. IJI, Tokyo, pp 99–104

29. Sugiyama T, Imai K, Yoshida H, Takayama Y, Yabana T, Yokota K, Oguma K, Yachi A (1991) A novel enzyme immunoassay for serodiagnosis of *Helicobacter pylori* infection. Gastroenterology 101:77–83

30. Imai K, Sugiyama T, Takayama Y, Yoshida H, Yabana T, Yachi A, Yokota K, Oguma K (1990) Immunological investigation of *Helicobacter pylori* infection in gastric mucosal lesions. In: Takemoto T, Kawai K, Shimoyama T (eds) Proceedings of the third Tokyo international symposium on *Helicobacter pylori*. IJI, Tokyo, pp 26–30

31. Asaka M, Kimura T, Kudo M, Takeda H, Mitani S, Miyazaki T, Miki K, Graham DY (1992) Relationship of *Helicobacter pylori* to serum pepsinogens in an asymptomatic Japanese population. Gastroenterology 102:760–766

32. Yozozaki H, Takekura N, Takanashi A, Tabuchi J, Haruta R, Tahara E (1988) Estrogen receptors in gastric adenocarcinoma: A retrospective immunohistochemical analysis. Virchows Arch [A] 413:297–302

33. Harrison JD, Jones JA, Ellis IO, Morris DL (1991) Oestrogen receptor D5 antibody is an independent negative prognostic factor in gastric cancer. Br J Surg 78:334–336

34. Bourreille J, Metayer P, Sauger F, et al (1970) Existence d'alpha-foeto proteine au cours d'un cancer secondaire du foie d'origine gastrique. Presse Med 78:1277–1278

35. Chang Y-C, Nagasue N, Abe S, Taniura H, Kumar DD, Nakamura T (1992) Comparison between the clinicopathologic features of AFP-positive and AFP-negative gastric cancers. Am J Gastroenterol 87(3):321–325

36. Chang Y-C, Nagasue N, Abe S, Kohno H, Kumar DD, Nakamura T (1991) α Fetoprotein-producing early gastric cancer with liver metastasis: Report of three cases. Gut 32:542–545

37. Terashima M, Ikeda K, Maesawa C, Kawamura H, Niitsu Y, Satoh M, Saito K (1991) Establishment of an α-fetoprotein-producing gastric cancer cell line in serum-free media. Jpn J Cancer Res 82:883–885

38. Ikeda Y, Mori M, Kido A, Shimono R, Matsushima T, Sugimachi K, Saku M (1991) Immunohistochemical expression of carbohydrate antigen 19-9 in gastric carcinoma. Am J Gastroenterol 86(9):1163–1166

39. Salmon DJ, Clark GM, Wong SG, Levin WJ, Ullrich A, McGuire WL (1987) Human breast cancer: Correlation of relapse and survival with amplification of the HE-2/neu oncogene. Science 235:177–182

40. Yonemura Y, Ninomiya I, Yamaguchi A, Fushida S, Kimura H, Ohoyama S, Miyazaki I, Endou Y, Tanaka M, Sasaki T (1991) Evaluation of immunoreactivity for *erb*B-2 protein as a marker of poor short-term prognosis in gastric cancer. Cancer Res 51:1034–1038

41. Jain S, Filipe MI, Gullick WJ, Linehan J, Morris RW (1991) c-*erb*B-2 Proto-oncogene expression and its relationship to survival in gastric carcinoma: An immunohistochemical study on archival material. Int J Cancer 48:668–671

42. Yamaguchi T, Takahashi T, Yokota T, Kitamura K, Noguchi A, Kamiguchi M, Doi M, Ahn T, Sawai K, Yamane T (1991) Urinary pepsinogen I as a tumor marker of stomach cancer after total gastrectomy. Cancer 68:906–909
43. Asao T, Fukuda T, Yazawa S, Nagamachi Y (1991) Carcinoembryonic antigen levels in peritoneal washings can predict peritoneal recurrence after curative resection of gastric cancer. Cancer 68:44–47

Part 5
Diagnosis

X-Ray Diagosis of Early Gastric Cancer

Heizaburo Ichikawa[1]

Introduction

It may be said that the recent remarkable progress in the field of gastro-fiberscopic examination is apt to lead the medical profession to believe that X-ray examination is no longer necessary in the diagnosis of gastric diseases. In my opinion, however, X-ray examination, particularly with the double contrast method, still plays a major role in diagnosis in this area.

Regarding the history of research on early gastric cancer, many of my predecessors have described the early features of supposed early stage gastric cancer [1–5]. Their enthusiastic, surprising, and respectable achievements are rather fragmentary, however, from the present standpoint. In other words, though at present, we are aware that macroscopic features of early gastric cancer show many varieties, only a limited number of incidental cases had previously been obtained as a basis for discussion. Considerable research on radiological diagnosis of these early cases has also been reported [1, 3, 4]. Gutmann [1] is one of the most famous contributors in the field of X-ray diagnosis. His main achievement was the successive demonstration of very minute radiological changes caused by small cancer of the stomach. The radiological technique at that time was almost entirely dependent upon the so-called filling method, so that very minute changes of those lesions were not always clearly described. After that, mucosal and compression studies were developed and practiced among specialists, and discussions were conducted in order to detect these kinds of early cases. It was not until the 1920s, however, that there were reports of trials involving insufflation of air into the stomach, together with the contrast meal [6]. The technique of coating the barium meal on the mucosal surface of the stomach was reported to be quite difficult at that time, and it was not accepted among specialists.

It is well known that by the mid 1950s, double contrast radiography of the stomach was developed independently by Shirakabe and his group [7, 8]., Ichikawa, Kumakura, and others. By 1960, it had become, after much trial and

---

[1] National Cancer Center Hospital, 5–1–1 Tsukiju, chou-ku, Tokyo 104, Japan

error, an established examination method. Since we had been using the double contrast method for the examination of the colon, particularly for the diagnosis of colon tuberculosis [9, 10, 11], several years before this technique was applied to the stomach, we had already had a fairly clear understanding of the advantages and disadvantages of this method [12]—namely, that adequate distention of the colon wall with insufflated air and uniform coating of barium on the inner surface of the colon were indispensable, and that very low elevated or very shallow depressed lesions of the colon could easily be demonstrated [10]. When we first tried this method for stomach examination, however, a uniform coating of barium was difficult to achieve, though adequate distention of the stomach wall with air was easily obtainable by insertion a of gastric tube. This problem was finally solved by using a large amount and a fairly high concentration of barium (200–250 ml). The reason why the coating of barium on the mucosal surface of the stomach was not so easy to accomplish, compared to the barium coating of the colon, was found to be that the mucosal surface of the stomach is usually covered with a thick and viscous mucus which prevents the barium from directly touching the mucosal surface. This was not observed in the colon.

During the initial stage of our research work, studies were mainly focused not upon the early detection of cancer, but rather on showing better detail in any lesion. Therefore, the first new discovery was the successful demonst-ration of linear ulcers which are not visible on the film taken with the conventional method [13]. At the time, X-ray pictures of gastric cancer illustrated advanced cases, and we did not have enough information about the macroscopic figure of gastric cancer in the early stage.

Murakami's paper [7, 14] on macroscopic figures of gastric cancer in the early stage was the only one of its kind until Shirakabe [7, 14] followed up with a successful attempt at corroborating these findings with the double contrast method. This was the first case of early gastric cancer to be diagnosed before the operation. Gradually, the number of early cases detected by this method increased [15]. The technique was reported and the cases detected were presented many times at radiological conferences; however, even in Japan, not many people trusted diagnoses obtained from double contrast radiography before 1961. It nonetheless gradually came into more widespread use gradually among the specialists.

In 1962, I moved to the newly constructed National Cancer Center Hospital in Tokyo. As shown in Fig. 1, 11 cases of early gastric cancer were detected during the first six months of 1962; there were 37 cases in 1963, 26 cases in 1964, 59 cases in 1965, and so on. This was the highest detection level in Japan. During this period, I was invited to make hundreds of lectures in many hospitals and universities in order to promote the technique within Japan. In 1969, the International Congress of Radiology was held in Tokyo, and in 1970, the International Cancer Congress took place in Houston. These were the first chances for us to present a paper on Radiological Diagnosis of Early Gastric Cancer in an international forum. I have since been invited abroad 55 times to 34 different countries.

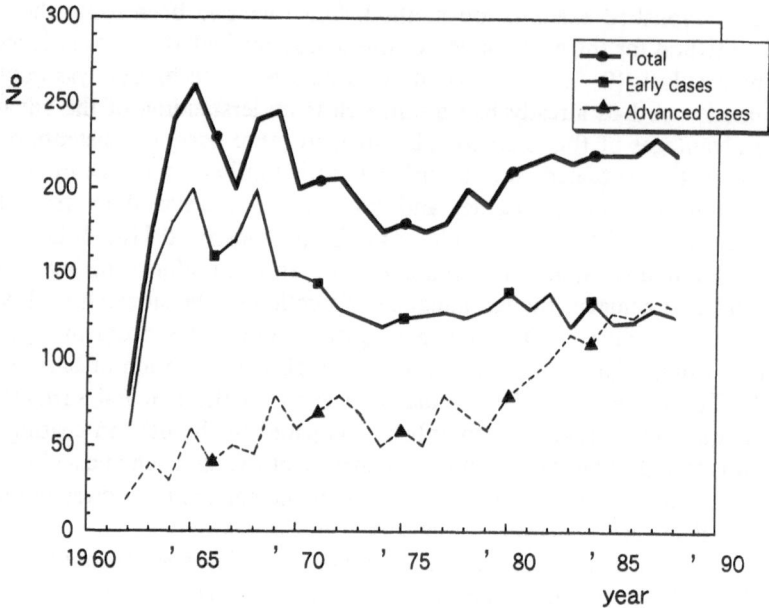

Fig. 1. Number of gastric cancer cases surgically removed at National Cancer Center Hospital

Double Contrast Radiography

The technique of double contrast radiography is described in many reports [14, 16, 17–26], and in order to avoid repetition, I would like to introduce some topics in this paper which were discussed during my lectures abroad and which, I believe, include suggestions that may help convey the idea of this technique.

Main Effects of Insufflation

There were a lot of questions concerning the main purpose of insufflation. The answer was "distention". To illustrate this principle, let us suppose we have written several names on a handkerchief: if we open it, everybody can read them easily, but if it is crumpled up, the names cannot be deciphered. As shown in Fig. 2, there is a small (1.3 × 0.9 cm) cancerous erosion in the middle of the posterior wall of the gastric body, but it is hard to recognize, because the lesion is located among several mucosal folds. However, if you put enough air into the stomach, as shown in Fig. 3, a very small lesion can easily be demonstrated, since the surrounding mucosal folds disappear due to the distention of the gastric wall. The detailed shape of the lesion is clearly shown in Fig. 4.

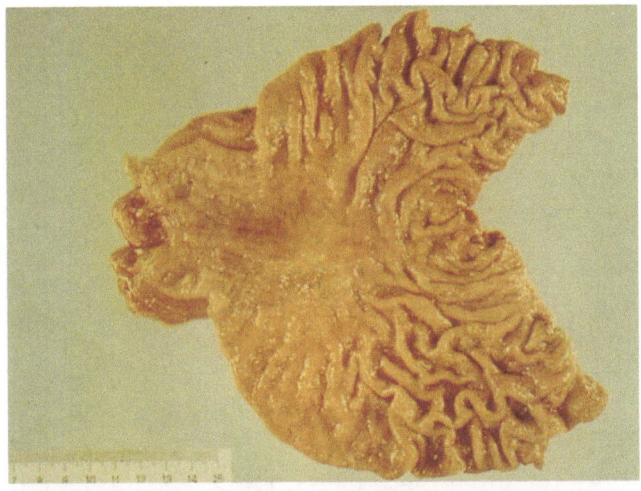

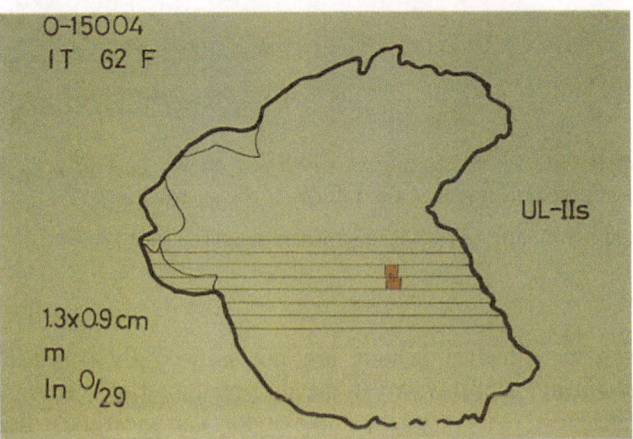

Fig. 2.a,b. a Resected specimen. A small cancerous erosion can be observed in the middle of the posterior wall of the gastric body. The lesion is fairly hard to recognize, because of complicated folds surrounding it. **b** Schematic illustration of Fig. 2 a after histological examination. A cancerous erosion, 1.3 × 0.9 cm, was confirmed. Cancer was limited to the mucosa. There was no lymph node metastasis out of 29 lymph lnodes histologically examined

Quality of Barium Meal

Since the diagnostic accuracy of X-ray double contrast examination has progressed, the number of cases in which lesions are not recognized under palpation of the stomach itself after laparatomy has increased. It is already common knowledge among surgeons that almost all early gastric cancer cases cannot be recognized under palpation during an operation. Furthermore, in

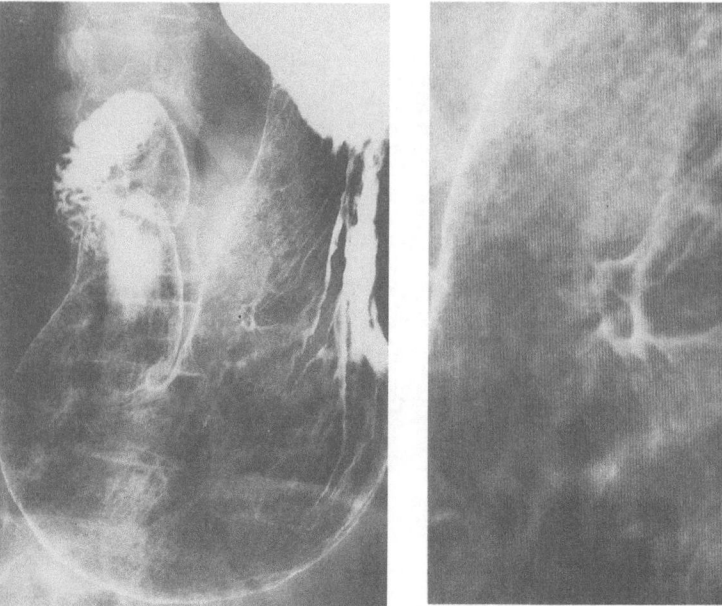

3   4

Fig. 3. Double contrast radiograpy of the lesion shown in Fig. 2. A small cancerous erosion is clearly demonstrated in the middle of the gastric body

Fig. 4. Magnified picture of Fig. 3. The lesion is more clearly shown

several cases, pathological lesions are not noticed by surgeons or even by pathologists during careful observations after opening the stomach cavity, though the appearance and demarcation of the lesion can clearly be demonstrated in double contrast pictures.

The reason is shown in Fig. 5. Here the smallest macroscopic unit of the mucosal surface, the area gastricae, is clearly demonstrated by double contrast examination. If the surface on the resected specimen, is examined, however, it is sometimes quite hard to recognize. This is because the barium meal in double contrast examination is behaving like powder in the case of a fingerprint. From this point of view, the quality of barium must be carefully controlled. Barium with low viscosity is required in order to allow the barium to stick easily to the tiny spaces between the numerous small, elevated area gastricae. The quantity of the barium meal pooling in these spaces is so small that the concentration of barium must be high.

Techniques for Obtaining Good Barium Coating

The quality of coating of the barium meal on the mucosal surface of the stomach is one of the most important keys to effective double contrast examination. While

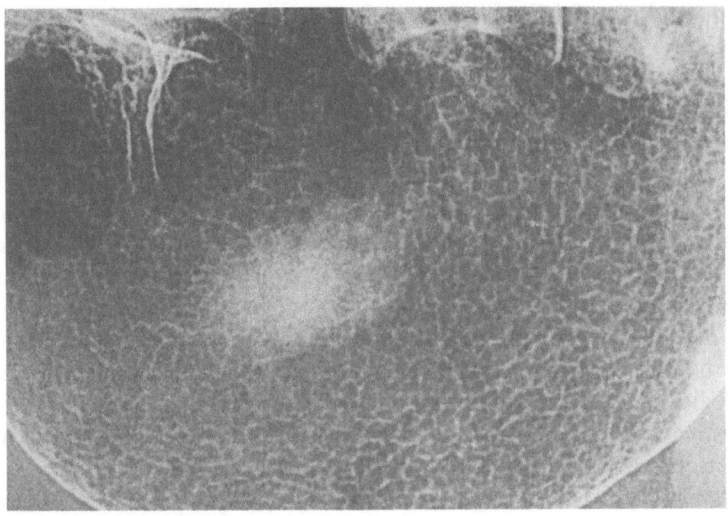

Fig. 5. Double contrast radiograph of a normal area gastricae. Numerous small nodules are clearly demonstrated

in some cases, the barium is good in quality and the amount of air is sufficient, the quality of the picture is nevertheless unsatisfactory. In such cases, the fault lies with the barium "coating". The mucosal surface of the stomach is usually covered with thick or viscous mucus, disrupting the coating of barium. In order to avoid this situation, we have tried to pour several kinds of mucus-dissolving materials into the stomach before starting the examination, but they were not always successful, because these kinds of materials themselves often disrupted the coating as well.

After much trial and error, we reached the conclusion that the washing of the mucosal surface with the barium meal itself was the most efficient way. This method is simple and effective, and for this purpose, the barium meal must be high in concentration with low viscosity. Using this kind of barium, one must change the patient's position fairly quickly, and the barium will flow onto the mucosal surface at a fairly high speed, resulting in a cleaner mucosal surface and therefore more effective coating.

Film Reading and Diagnosis

Figure Recognition

Figure 6 is an example of the characteristic appearance of mucosal cancer demonstrated with the double contrast method. There are many nodules scattering on the mucosal surface of the gastric antrum. When the author presented this picture at several meetings, questions were often raised asking,

"How do you know this is cancer, or what are the characteristic points of cancer in this picture?"

These questions, I believe, bring up a fundamentally important point concerning morphological diagnostic procedures of any kind. Nodules in Fig. 6 are quite different from those seen in Fig. 5. The outline and shapes of each nodules are quite irregular in Fig. 6, the size difference of each nodule is remarkable, the demarcation of the group of nodules can be followed totally, and so on. If science is on the way to describe these phenomena mathematically, any of the above-mentioned wording such as "irregular" or "remarkable" must be regarded as nonscientific. Since in my opinion, morphologic changes represent the final manifestation or integration of numerous molecular changes occuring in or surrounding the lesion, it is as yet impossible to make a complete analysis of morphological changes of living materials for purposes of computerization. We can nevertheless differentiate between the appearance of nodules shown in Fig. 5 and Fig. 6, however.

This capability can be compared to our ability to single out our own son or daughter out of hundreds of similar faces on a picture taken when they graduated from primary school. Though they all look similar, we can still differentiate, not because we can analyze the faces fully, but because we have been so familiar, for such a long period, with the macroscopic characteristics of our sons' and daughters' faces. In other words, the human computer in our brain is still much more elaborate than artificial computers at this time.

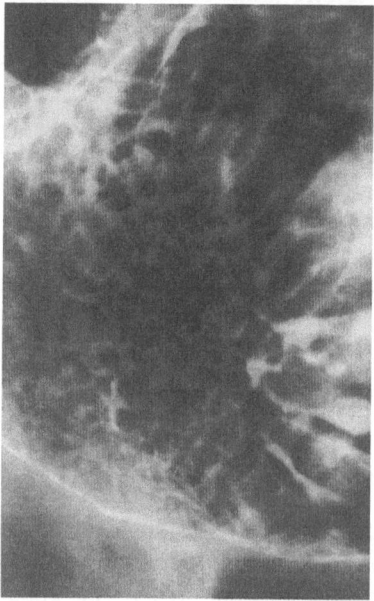

Fig. 6. Double contrast radiograph of the surface of a very superficial type of early gastric cancer. Numerous nodules with irregular shape and size are demonstrated

Diagnosis of Depth of Invasion

In accordance with the progress of diagnostic techniques, papers describing the diagnosis of the depth of invasion of gastric cancer have been appearing with increasing frequency [27]. There have been publications on not only the difference between early cancer and more deeply invaded cases, but also regarding the detailed analysis of differentiation between mucosal cancer and submucosal cancer [27].

Progress in this field is occurring mainly because endoscopic surgery has recently been very much on the rise for mucosal cancer cases. While endeavors with ultrasound equipment have shown fairly good results for the differentiation of depth invasion, ultrasound cannot cover 100% of cases. Diagnosis of depth invasion is therefore still done by X-ray and/or endoscopy in this field.

Nakano et al. [28] mentioned from the radiological standpoint that an irregular and shallow depression with a granular appearance of a floor was mostly mucosal cancer, that an irregular and shallow depression with a flat floor was submucosal cancer, and an irregular and shallow depression surrounded by a petal-like elevation was also to be diagnosed as mucosal cancer.

Mitsunaga et al. [29] mentioned from the endoscopical standpoint that the incidence of submucosal invasion increased when the size of elevated-type lesions was greater than 4 cm. The other findings suggesting submucosal invasion were a wedge-shaped sharp depression, marked erythema, and large nodular elevation. The accuracy of depth diagnosis was 83.6% in the elevated type and 77.4% in the depressed type.

Only in these two examples were there many important key descriptions which are not quite objective. For instance, "shallow", "granular", "flat", "petal-like", "wedge-shaped", "sharp", "marked erythema", and "large nodular elevation" are quite difficult to quantify or to describe objectively. However, where we have become familiar with these delicate findings by careful observations of many similar cases of the disease, we can at least understand what they want to describe. Morphological diagnosis always involves these kinds of linguistic ambiguities, but it is still useful.

Figure 7 is a cancerous erosion (IIc type early gastric cancer) on the posterior wall near the incisula angularis, demonstrated clearly with the double contrast method. The outline of the lesion can clearly be followed, and several characteristic nodules inside the lesion can be observed. In my opinion, these nodules are also one of the indicators for diagnosis of depth invasion. In this particular case, the diagnosis stated that the cancer was almost entirely limited to the mucosal layer, but that, at a very small area in the upper half of the lesion, where there was an accumulation of fairly large, irregular-sized nodules, the cancer had partially invaded the submucosal layer, which was confirmed after the operation.

The lesion shown in Fig. 8 can be described in almost the same way. In this case, a small area where the cancer has partially invaded the submucosal layer is

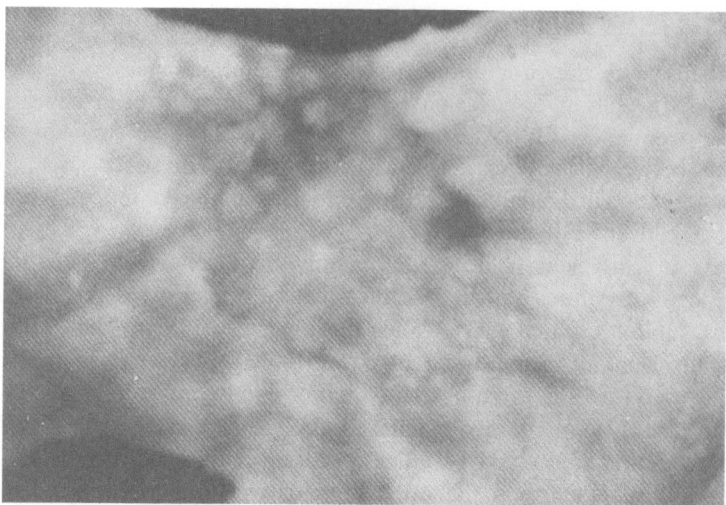

Fig. 7. Double contrast radiograph of a superficial depressed type of early gastric cancer. Size irregularity of the nodules inside the erosion is remarkable on the upper half of the lesion, suggesting that the cancer has invaded somewhat more deeply at this part

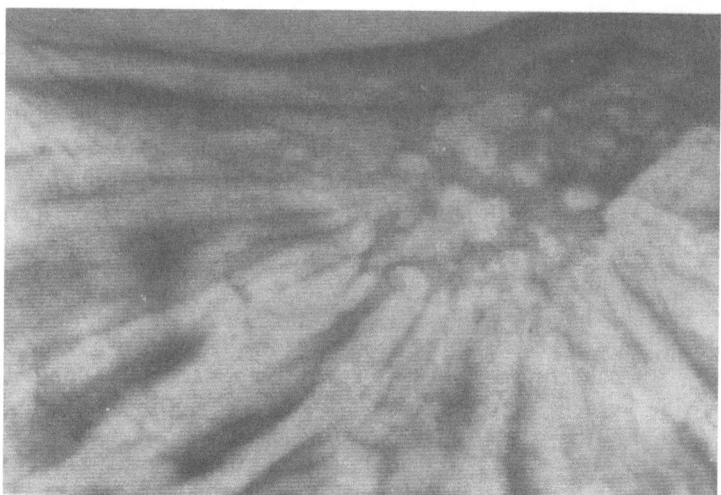

Fig. 8. Double contrast radiograph of another case with superficial depressed type of early gastric cancer. Size irregularity can be noticed on the lower half of the lesion

located at the lower half of the lesion, which was also confirmed after the operation.

In Fig. 9, a very small cancerous erosion is clearly demonstrated on the posterior wall of the antrum, and five small nodules are also demonstrated inside

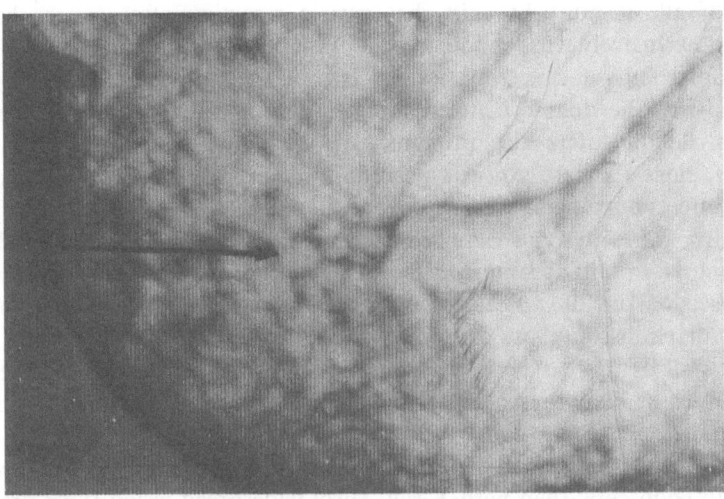

Fig. 9 Double contrast radiograph of a small cancerous erosion. Five small nodules inside the erosion are very similar in their size and outlines compared with the surrounding nodules which are normal area gastricae, suggesting that the cancer is limited to the mucosa in this case

the lesion. However, the size and outlines of these nodules are quite similar to those nodules surrounding it which are normal area gastricae. Thus, the diagnosis in this case was mucosal cancer.

Accuracy of diagnosis of depth invasion is not always 100%, but it has increasingly improved due to more careful monitoring of radiographs and better familiarization with these kinds of morphological features.

Though so-called scientific explanations are quite difficult to provide in some cases, particularly in the field of morphology, almost all of the delicate morphological appearances of cancerous lesions often reflect the deeper molecular change of the human body. One can usually—not 100%, but in a fairly high percentages of cases—differentiate mucosal cancer from submucosal cancer.

Again we can say that diagnoses of this kind with computer technology are still not satisfactory. While Professor Toriwaki of the University of Nagoya is trying to analyze X-ray pictures and make diagnoses with a computer, human eyes are at present still far superior to computers in this field.

Role of X-Ray Examination in Stomach Cancer

Since the recent remarkable progress in endoscopy, there has been something of a tendency among specialists to think that X-ray examination is no longer necessary. It may therefore be appropriate to elaborate upon the advantages and disadvantages of both X-ray and endoscopic examination.

First of all, it must be said that gastric resection after cancer has been diagnosed exclusively with endoscopy can sometimes be quite unreliable, because the proximal end of cancerous lesions is much easier to determine by X-ray diagnosis with the double contrast method than it is by endoscopic diagnosis. Surgeons should know the proximal site of cut immediately prior to the operation, since they are not in a position to determine it by themselves, as the lesion is often nonpalpable during the operation.

Secondly, there are some sections of the stomach for which X-rays produce the best diagnosis; in other sections, conversely, encoscopy is superior. For example, in some sections on the anterior wall of the stomach, small lesions are easier to detect with endoscopy; on the other hand, in certain other sections on the posterior wall of the gastric body, small lesions are much easier to detect with X-ray. In cases like these, a combination of these two methods would be recommended.

Thirdly, while very small lesions, 1–2 mm in size, could be detected more easily with endoscopy than with X-ray, fairly widespread lesion types are harder to demonstrate with endoscopy. In other words, X-ray is more effective in demonstrating the total appearance of the lesion. This is also quite helpful for surgeons considering a plan of operation.

Fourthly, the most important advantage of endoscopy is that it enables observation of the lesion in color and taking biopsies if necessary. Both of these benefits we cannot expect from X-ray examination. It cannot be denied, however, that the color is so beautiful that endoscopists usually have a tendency to believe their own eyes too much, and not to take pictures of other parts of the stomach sereously enough. If they consider the stomach totally, this will be very helpful for the total diagnosis. Reviewing the history of X-ray diagnosis, there was a long period when the leading specialists asked all diagnoses to be decided during fluoroscopy. After the introduction of the double contrast method, however, one series of X-ray pictures was asked to cover every small part of the stomach presenting the mucosal surface, since by then the detection rate of small lesions had become much higher. If endoscopists believe their own eyes too much during fluoroscopy or during endoscopic observation, they tend not to notice their own false negatives.

Recent Results of Mass Screening

According to the data recently published by the *All Japan Statistics of Mass Screening for the Stomach* [30], out of 5 221 116 cases examined in 1988, a total of 6414 cases of gastric cancer was detected, and 4002 cases of early gastric cancer were reported.

Over 95% of early gastric cancer patients have five to ten-year [31, 32] survival rates, and almost half of the other patients are expected to survive as well. Thus, ca. 80% of all patients with gastric cancer are expected to survive five years. This means that about 5000 patients per year could potentially survive longer than 5 years, through the mass screening program in Japan.

It is a fact that the number of early cases detected has been increasing year by year. This is reflected in the high number of cases with 5-year survival rates, and almost all of the associations conducting mass screening in Japan are well-controlled in terms of quality of X-ray pictures, follow-up systems, and the statistical surveys done by many specialists. It must be pointed out, however, that a slight but very important misunderstanding is often presented in many reports. Much of the literature, states the reasons why such a large number of early gastric cancer cases are detected in Japan as being firstly, that the incidence of gastric cancer itself is high in Japan, and secondly, that mass screening is conducted in Japan—with a resulting increase in the chance of detection of such early cases before clinical symptoms appear.

While the former reason—stating that the incidence of stomach cancer is high in Japan—is correct, the latter is not quite right. This is because fairly high numbers of early cases had already been detected from outpatient clinics before the mass screening program began to be implemented widely, and because furthermore, detection rates of early cases from the mass screening field were not as high during the initial period of screening, when double contrast examination was not yet applied widely enough.

In addition, there have been statistics [33] claiming that the number of gastric cancer cases detected and treated at outpatient clinics was ten times those detected through mass screening in some prefectures; in certain other prefectures, five times as many cases were said to have been detected at outpatient clinics. Although there are no exact statistics covering all of Japan, if five times is the average, about 25 000 cases of gastric cancer cases are thought to be surviving longer than five years every year in Japan. This idea is supported by recent data. That is, the number of deaths due to gastric cancer is decreasing, in spite of the increasing incidence of the disease. In other words, mass screening is playing a fairly small part in the decreasing death rate, though it is playing a major role in distributing the technique and in promoting the importance of health checks among people all over Japan.

Conclusion

In this paper, the author has explained the techniques and diagnostic concept of the double contrast method. The role of X-ray examination in comparison with endoscopy, including the recent results of mass screening and its significance in decreasing death rates, has also been discussed.

Lastly, one more point should be mentioned. Magnificent progress in the diagnostic techniques of both X-ray and endoscopy during the last thirty years has produced excellent results in the field of gastric cancer research. Without wholehearted cooperation between surgeon and pathologist, these diagnostic techniques would not have made such remarkable progress. If surgeons never agreed to resect, stomach, specimens would not be in the diagnostician's hand, and detailed comparison between the macroscopic and X-ray or endoscopic findings would be impossible. If pathologists never examined the specimen thoroughly, our diagnosis could not be confirmed. Strong cooperation among at least three kinds of specialists—namely, surgeon, pathologist, and diagnostician- -is indispensable in this kind of research work.

It has often been said that for scientific knowledge to be of practical use, science must come first, and then technology. However, the history of gastric cancer research indicates that detection techniques were the first to open the door to an understanding of the early stages of the disease; moreover, these techniques have played a leading role in subsequent research, and the results they have produced have presented many new aspects, including the natural history of the disease, to the medical profession. In conclusion, then, I would prefer to put it this way: sometimes the converse is true—i.e., techniques must come first, followed by new scientific ideas.

References

1. Gutmann RA, Bertrand DI, Peristiany TJ (1939) Le cancer de l'estomac au début. Doin, Paris
2. Konjetzny GE (1940) Der oberflächliche Schleimhautkrebs des Magens. Chirurg 12:192–202
3. Bucker J (1941) Die Frühdiagnose des Magenkrebses im Röntgenbild. Fortschr Geb Röntgenstr 63:1–28
4. Golden R, Stout AP (1948) Superficial spreading carcinoma of the stomach. Am J Roentgenol Radium Therapy 59:157–167
5. Ayabe S (1949) On mucosal carcinoma. Jpn J Clin Exp Med 26:514–525
6. Hilpert F (1929) Das Pneumo-Relief des Magens. Fortschr Röntgenstr 38:80–87
7. Shirakabe H, Ichikawa H, Kumakura K, Nishizawa M, Higurashi K, Hayakawa H, Murakami T (1966) Atlas of X-ray diagnosis of early gastric cancer. Lippincott, Philadelphia
8. Kuru M, Sakita T, Ichikawa H, Sano R, Miwa K, Yamada Y, Kitaoka H, Takasu S, Omori K, Oguro Y, Ueda I (1967) Atlas of early carcinoma of the stomach. Nakayama-Shoten, Tokyo
9. Fischer AW (1923) Über eine neue röntgenologische Untersuchungsmethode des Dickdarms: Kombination von Kontrasteinlauf und Luftaufblähung. Klin Wochenschr 2:1595–1598
10. Ishikawa N, Shirakabe H, Ichikawa H (1955) Intestinal tuberoulosis. Abdominal X-ray Reading Series No. 6 Kanehara, Tokyo
11. Welin S (1958) Über moderne röntgenologische Dickdarmdiagnostik under besonderer Berücksichtigung der Doppel-Kontrast-methode. Munch Med Wsch 100:1142
12. Shirakabe, H (1963) Advantages and disadvantages of double contrast method in gastro-intestinal X-ray diagnosis. The Jpn J Clin Exp Med 40:768–770
13. Bockus HL (1976) Gastroenterology 2. WB Saunders, Philadelphia
14. Shirakabe H, Kumakura K, Koyama R, Nishizawa M, Horikoshi H, Higurashi K, Yamada T, Doi H, Sawaguchi Y, Okubo H, Yoshida S, Nakajima A., Ichikawa H (1961) X-ray diagnosis of gastro-duodenal ulcer. Jpn J Gastroenterol 58:1187–1191

15. Tasaka S (1962) Statistical study of early gastric cancer collected throughout Japan. Gastrointest Endosc 4:4–14
16. Kumakura K (1960) Roentgenological study on gastric ulcer. Nippon Acta Radiologica 19:2663–2694
17. Fuchigami A, Takagi K (1962) Diagnosis on the mucosal carcinoma of the stomach, particularly on the X-ray diagnosis of 40 cases. Jpn J Gastroenterol, 59:626–627
18. Brown GR (1963) High-density barium-sulfate suspensions: An improved diagnostic medium. Radiology 81:839
19. Ichikawa H, Yamada T, Doi H (1964) Practice of X-ray diagnosis of the stomach: For the diagnosis of early gastric cancer. Bunkodo, Tokyo
20. Shirakabe H, Ichikawa H, Kumakura K, Nishizawa M, Higurashi K, Hayakawa H, Murakami T, Frik W (1969) Frühkarzinom des Magens, Atlas der Röntgendiagnostik. Thieme, Stuttgart
21. Matsue H, Tobayashi K, Yamada T, Horikoshi H, Doi H, Suko H, Ichikawa H (1970) X-ray Diagnosis of lesions in the upper portions of the stomach (in Japanese). Stomach & Intestine 5:1071–1083
22. Shirakabe H (1971) Double contrast studies of the stomach Bunkodo, Tokyo
23. Shirakabe H, Ichikawa H (1973) Early gastric cancer. In Hodes PJ (ed) The esophagus and stomach, an atlas of tumor radiology. Am Coll Radiol, Year Book Med Publ, Chicago, IL pp 277–357
24. Ichikawa H (1976) Differential diagnosis between benign and malignant ulcers of the stomach. Clin Gastroenterol 2:239
25. Shirakabe H , Nishizawa M, Maruyama M, Kobayashi S (1982) Atlas of X-ray diagnosis of early gastric cancer, 2nd edn. Igaku Shoin, Tokyo
26. Laufer I (1979) Double contrast gastrointestinal radiology with endoscopic correlation. WB Saunders, Philadelphia
27. Special Issue (1992) on "Differential diagnosis between mucosal and submucosal early cancer of the stomach" (in Japanese; summary in English). Stomach and Intestine 27(10), Igaku-shoin, Tokyo
28. Nakano H, Kato S, Ogawa H, Nishii M, Ohashi H, Yasuhara R, Takahama K, Watanabe M, Takano E, Kitagawa Y, Miyaji I, Ito M (1992) Radiological diagnosis of the invasivity of small gastric cancers (in Japanese). Stomach and Intestine 27:1139–1148
29. Mitsunaga A, Murata Y, Nagasako H, Suzuki S, Ikeda I, Nakamura S, Haruki K, Chiba M, Yokoyama S, Hashimoto H, Obata H, Suzuki H (1992) Difference between mucosal and submucosal gastric cancer on endoscopic diagnosis (in Japanese). Stomach and Intestine 27:1151–1160
30. All Japan Statistics on Mass Screening for Stomach Cancer (1991) Published yearly by the Japanese Society of Gastro-intestinal Mass Survey (in Japanese). Tokyo
31. Ichikawa H (1978) Mass screening for stomach cancer in Japan. In Miller AB (ed) Screening in Cancer. UICC IC Technical Report Series 40, Int Union Against Cancer, Geneva, pp 279–305
32. Ichikawa H, Yamada T (1985) Double contrast radiography of the stomach. In: Miller AB (ed) Screening for Cancer Academic, Orlando, pp 193–214
33. Arisue T, Tamura K, Yamaguchi Y, Tebayashi A, Yoshida Y, Ikeda S, Ootsuka S, Sasaki M (1990) Quantitative analysis on effect of mass screening for stomach cancer. Comparison between stomach cancer cases detected in mass survey and those detected in out patient clinic. Gastroenterol Mass Survey 88:27–32

Endoscopic Diagnosis: Latest Trends

Shigeaki Yoshida[1], Hajime Yamaguchi, Daizo Saito, and Masaaki Kido[2]

Key words. Early gastric cancer—Gastritis-like early cancer—Chronological trend of early cancer—Endoscopy—Dye spraying endoscopy—Detailed endoscopy—Computed endoscopy

Introduction

Because of the very high risk factor in gastric cancer, its early detection has been a leading project of nationwide cancer control in Japan. As a result, endoscopic diagnosis of early gastric cancer (EGC) has developed remarkably during the past three decades. Currently, EGC is seen regularly in daily clinical practice [1]. In the meantime, endoscopic criteria of EGC have been extended to faint mucosal irregularities which would be undetectable according to the conventional diagnostic criteria [2]. This paper attempts to assess the recent advances of endoscopic diagnosis, mainly by examining the chronological trend in the endoscopic features and surgical results of EGC treated at the National Cancer Center Hospital (NCCH) in Tokyo.

Growth Patterns of Advanced Gastric Cancer and Importance of Detecting Gastritis-Like EGC

As we had shown in a previous paper [3], retrospective observation for rapidly growing advanced cancers, whose malignancy could not be detected by previous endoscopy performed within 3 years before the final examination, revealed the original lesions to have nonulcerative and gastritis-like findings, such as a shallow

Departments of Medicine, [1]National Cancer Center Hospital East, 5-1 Kashiwanoha 6-chome, Kashiwa, Chiba, 277 Japan
[2]National Cancer Center Hospital, 1-1 Tsukiji 5-chome, Chuo-ku, Tokyo, 104 Japan

246

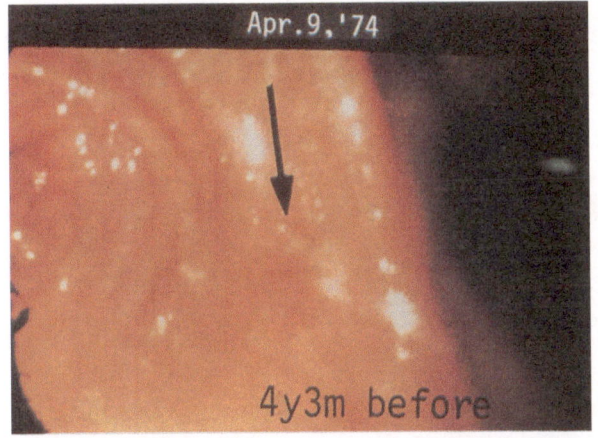

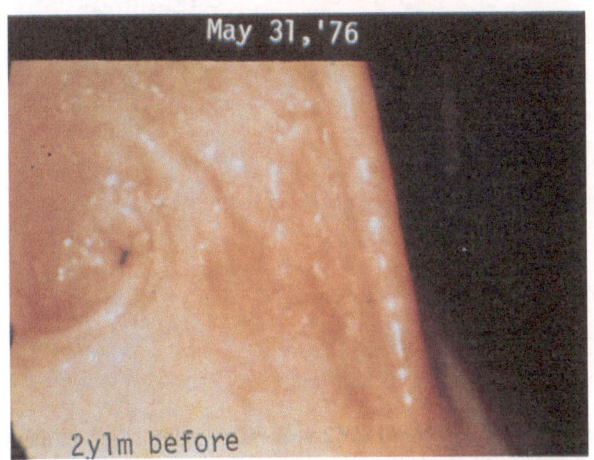

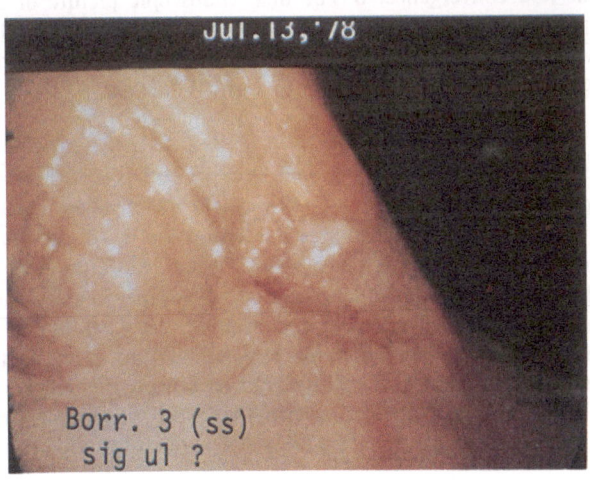

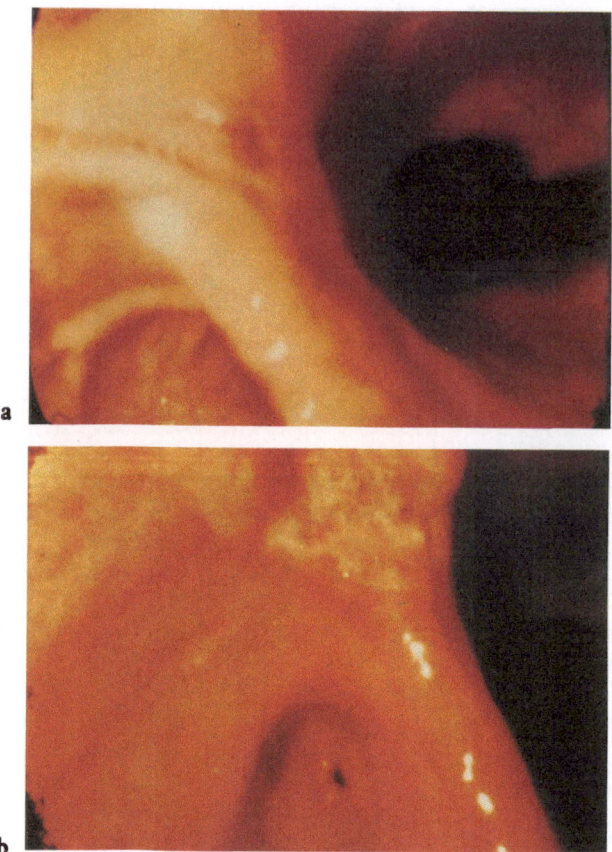

Fig. 2a,b. a An endoscopic picture of case 2 (a 52-year-old female), taken 14 months before the final examination. A tiny reddish shallow depression is seen on the anterior wall of the gastric angulus without fold convergence. **b** The final endoscopic picture of case 2. A shallow depression rapidly grew into an advanced cancer of Borrmann's type II. Histological examination of the resected specimen revealed a mucinous cancer which invaded into the proper muscle layer

←

Fig. 1a–c. a An endoscopic picture of case 1 (a 49-year-old male), taken about 4 years before the final examination. A small reddish area is seen on the lesser curvature of the antrum. **b** An endoscopic picture of case 1, taken about 2 years before the final examination. The small reddish area became large and its color became deeper in association with a slight mucosal depression. **c** The final endoscopic picture of case 1. A tumorous lesion with a deep central excavation with a surrounding elevated wall appeared on the lesser curvature of the antrum, which is compatible with advanced cancer, Borrmann's type III. Histologically the resected specimen revealed a signet-ring cell carcinoma (*sig*) which invaded into the subserosa (*ss*). The presence or absence of peptic ulceration could not be identified (*ul?*)

depression, discoloration, and/or mucosal unevenness without fold convergence in most of the cases.

Two examples (cases 1 and 2) are shown in Figs. 1 and 2, respectively. In case 1, the original lesion, 4 years and 3 months before the final examination, can be seen as a slight redness on the lesser curvature of the antrum (Fig. 1.a). Two years after the initial examination, the surface had become rougher and enlarged without fold convergence (Fig. 1.b); at 2 years after the second examination, the original lesion had rapidly developed into Borrmann's type III advanced cancer (Fig. 1.c). In case 2, the original lesion can be seen retrospectively on the anterior wall of the gastric angulus on the film taken at the initial examination (Fig. 2.a). It developed rapidly into Borrmann's type II of advanced cancer during only 14 months after the initial examination (Fig. 2.b). These cases indicate the importance of the earliest possible detection of gastritis-like malignancy showing nonulcerative and nonpolypoid appearance.

Recent Progress of Early Diagnosis of Gastric Cancer and Surgical Results

During the period between 1962 and 1989, there were 5991 surgical cases of gastric cancers at the National Cancer Center Hospital. Of the 5991, 2046 were solitary EGC, as defined by the Japanese Gastroenterological Endoscopy Society

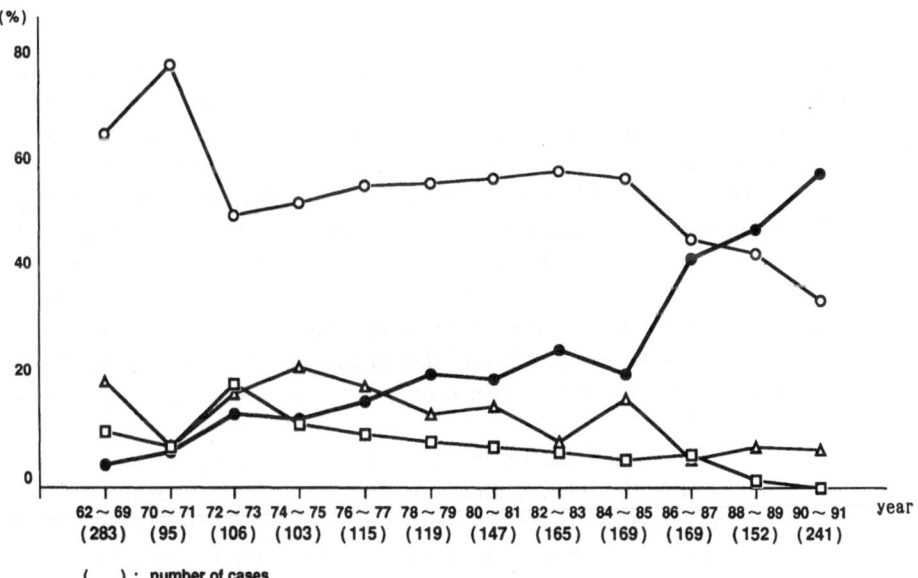

Fig. 3. Chronological trends in endoscopic appearance of early gastric cancer. *Open circles,* Ulcerative; *open triangles,* polypoid; *open squares,* advanced cancer-like; *closed circles,* gastritis-like

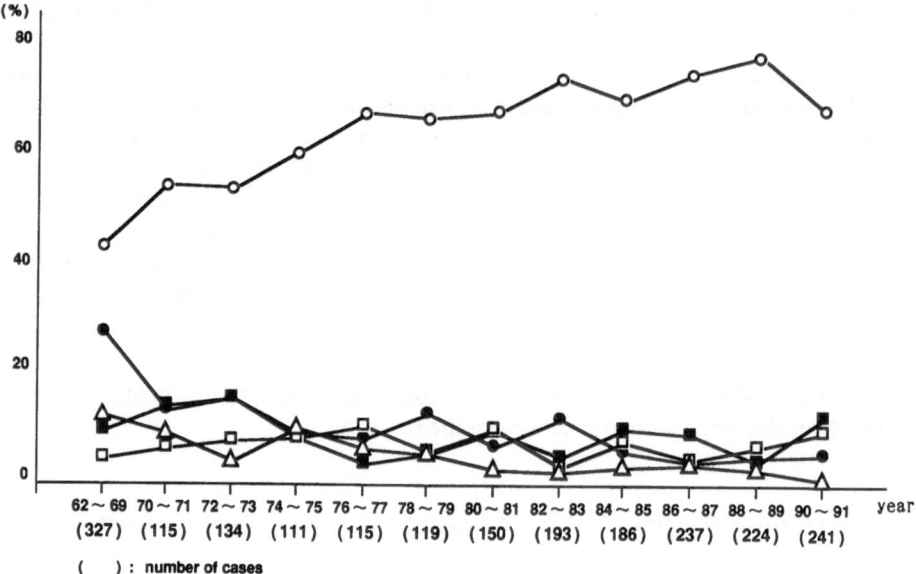

Fig. 4. Chronological trends in macroscopic types of early gastric cancer. *Open circles,* type IIc and IIb; *closed circles,* type III; *open triangles,* type I; *closed squares,* type IIa + IIc; *open squares* type IIa

[4]. Figure 3 shows the chronological trend in the gross endoscopic appearance of the well-documented 1864 EGCs, subclassified into the following four types: polypoid, ulcerative, gastritis-like, and advanced cancer-like. The polypoid type is defined as an EGC showing obvious protrusion, the ulcerative one as that showing ulceration and/or fold convergence, the gastritis-like one as that showing a superficial nonulcerative appearance, and the advanced cancer-like ones that evidently show advanced cancer-like appearances endoscopically. As shown in the figure, the incidence of ulcerative and advanced cancer-like types have been markedly decreasing in recent years (from a maximun of 79% to 35% in the former and 19% to 3% in the latter), and that of the gastritis-like type has been increasing particulary since 1984. As a result, it reached 59% in the past two years (1990 and 1991).

Figure 4 shows the chronological trend in the macroscopic type of EGC which is in accordance with the classification of the Japanese Gastroenterological Endoscopy Society. Types I and III have become rare (less than 5%) in recent years, whereas they had incidences of 10% and 23% in the 1960s, respectively. In the past two decades, the incidence of IIc type ranged between 60%–75%.

Table 1 shows the incidence of EGC and the 5-year survival rate as examined chronologically. The survival rate improved remarkably in recent years proportional to the increase in the incidence of EGC, and during the fifth term

Table 1. Chronological trends in gastric cancer: incidence of early cancer and 5-year survival rate at the National Cancer Center Hospital.

Period	Number of surgical cases	Incidence of early cancer (n)	5-Year survival rate
1962–1969	1628	22% (358)	42%
1970–1974	1020	32% (325)	56%
1975–1979	967	34% (330)	58%
1980–1984	1165	43% (502)	65%
1985–1989	1211	53% (639)	71%

Table 2. Chronological trends in the number of minute (within 5 mm) and small gastric cancers (6–10 mm in maximum diameter). National Cancer Center Hospital.

	Period					
	1962–1969	1970–1974	1975–1979	1980–1984	1985–1989	Total
Minute cancer	1	4	8	17	47	77
	(1)	(5)	(10)	(22)	(61)	(100)
Small cancer	6	13	28	42	83	172
	(3)	(8)	(16)	(24)	(48)	(100)
Total	7	17	36	59	130	249
(%)	(3)	(7)	(14)	(24)	(52)	(100)

Table 3. Chronological trends in 5-year survival rate by stage of gastric cancer. National Cancer Center Hospital.

Stage	Period					
	1962–1969	1970–1974	1975–1979	1980–1984	1985–1989	Total
I	88%	89%	91%	91%	94%	91%
	(429)	(390)	(396)	(536)	(647)	(2398)
II	59%	69%	72%	80%	81%	68%
	(279)	(134)	(94)	(125)	(130)	(762)
III	34%	43%	46%	57%	53%	44%
	(380)	(244)	(235)	(247)	(201)	(1307)
IV	4%	11%	13%	11%	15%	9%
	(534)	(245)	(221)	(234)	(233)	(1467)
Total	42%	56%	58%	65%	71%	56%
	(1622)	(1020)	(967)	(1165)	(1211)	(5991)

Number of cases

(1985–1989), the incidence of EGC reached 53% (639/1211) and the 5-year survival rate was calculated as being 71%.

Table 2 shows the chronological trend in the number of small and minute gastric cancers detected preoperatively. According to the commonly accepted Japanese guidelines, a small cancer is defined as a cancerous lesion ranging from 6 to 10 mm in size, and a minute one as one less than 5 mm in size. Both types increased from year to year, and comparing the fourth to the fifth term, the number of minute cancer cases rapidly increased from 17 to 47 and the small ones from 42 to 83 cases.

The chronological trend of the 5-year survival rate by stage of gastric cancer is shown in Table 3. The 5-year survival rate steadily improved with each year for every stage, except for Stage III in 1985–1989 during which it decreased slightly.

These results apparently show the contribution of recent progress of early detection to the survival of gastric cancer patients, and the importance of early detection based on the differentiation of gastritis-like malignancy.

Diagnostic Findings of Gastritis-Like EGC

Table 4 shows the endoscopic appearance (color patterns and surface structure) of the 132 cases of gastritis-like EGC diagnosed endoscopically as being benign. Their color patterns were devided into discolored, hyperemic, and normocolored ones, and their surface structures into flat well-demarcated, flat poorly demarcated, and uneven groups. In addition, we subclassified the 132 cases endoscopically into flat discolored (27 cases of group A in Table 4), flat hyperemic (63 cases of group B in Table 4) and superficial uneven types (41 cases of group C in Table 4). The endoscopic characteristics of each type could be clarified as follows. In the flat discolored type, well-demarcated lesions are dominant (19/27: 70%), whereas the greater part (45/53: 83%) of the flat hyperemic type shows poorly demarcated lesions. In the superficial uneven type, discolored lesions are rare, and most of them (39/41: 95%) are normocolored or hyperemic.

Table 5 shows the histological and endoscopic types of the 132 gastritis-like EGCs. The histological types were divided into intestinal and diffuse types, according to the Lawrence classification. The incidence of the intestinal type was 30% in the flat discolored type, 62% in the flat hyperemic type, and 93% in the

Table 4. Color and surface patterns in endoscopic appearance of gastritis-like EGCs diagnosed as benign endoscopically. Cases of groups *a*, *b*, and *c* can be subclassified into flat discolored, flat hyperemic, and superficial uneven types, respectively.

Surface pattern	Color pattern			Total
	Discolored	Hyperemic	Normocolored	
Flat				
Well demarcated	19[a]	9[b]		28
Poorly demarcated	8	54	1[A]	63
Uneven	2	20	19[c]	41
	29	83	20	132

[A] One cases of type IIb EGC without any diagnostic findings

Table 5. Size distribution of endoscopic subtype of gastritis-like EGCs diagnosed as benign endoscopically, excluding one case of type IIb showing no diagnostic findings.

Type	Size in maximum diameter (cm)				
	≤1	1< ≤2	2< ≤5	5<	Total
Flat discolored	7	9	8	3	27
	(26)	(33)	(30)	(11)	(100)
Flat hyperemic	16	15	24	8	63
	(25)	(24)	(38)	(13)	(100)
Superficial uneven	19	7	12	3	41
	(47)	(17)	(29)	(7)	(100)
Total	42	31	44	14	131

Table 6. Histological type and endoscopic subtype of gastritis-like EGCs diagnosed as benign endoscopically, excluding one case of type IIb showing no diagnostic findings.

	Histological type		
	Intestinal	Diffuse	Total
Flat discolored	8	19	27
	(30)	(70)	(100)
Flat hyperemic	39	24	63
	(62)	(38)	(100)
Superficial uneven	38	3	41
	(93)	(7)	(100)
Total	85	46	131

superficial uneven type, indicating that this endoscopic subclassification is correlated to the histological characteristics of gastritis-like EGCs.

Table 6 shows the size distribution of the three types. There was a wide range for the flat discolored and the hyperemic types, whereas small lesions less than 10 mm were dominant (19/41: 47%) in the superficial uneven type.

The site distributions are shown in Table 7. In the flat discolored type, most (21/27: 78%) of the lesions were located at the upper (C) and middle third (M) of the stomach. The incidence of location in the lower third (A) of the stomach was more frequent (38%) in the flat hyperemic type than in the flat discolored type (22%), and it was dominant (60%) in the superficial uneven type.

These results may indicate the possibility of screening gastritis-like EGCs as follows: while evaluating the upper two-thirds of the stomach (cardia and gastric body), we should pay attention mainly to the color changes of the mucosa,

Table 7. Site distribution of flat discolored, flat hyperemic and superficial uneven types of gastritis-like EGCs diagnosed as benign endoscopically. C, Upper; M, middle; A, lower one-third of the stomach, respectively.

	C	M	A	Total
Flat discolored type				
Anterior wall		4	2	6 (22)
Lesser curv.		10	1	11 (40)
Posterior wall	2	4	2	8 (30)
Greater curv.		1	1	2 (8)
Total	2 (8)	19 (70)	6 (22)	27 (100)
Flat hyperemic type				
Anterior wall	1	8	4	13 (21)
Lesser curv.	2	20	10	32 (51)
Posterior wall	1	5	4	10 (16)
Greater curv.		2	6	8 (12)
Total	4 (6)	35 (56)	24 (38)	63 (100)
Superficial uneven type				
Anterior wall		2	4	6 (15)
Lesser curv.	1	9	10	20 (49)
Posterior wall		2	6	8 (20)
Greater curv.		2	5	7 (16)
Total	1 (2)	15 (37)	25 (61)	41 (100)

(%)

particularly to the well-demarcated discoloration or the poorly demarcated redness, and for the lower third of the stomach (antrum), be alert to superficial unevenness of the mucosa, such as a tiny depression surrounded with hyperemic or normocolored hyperplastic mucosa. Representative cases of gastritis EGCs are shown in Figs. 5–7.

Value of Dye-Spraying Endoscopy for Detecting EGCs

Even by the most precise observation, it is occasionally difficult to detect the definitive diagnostic findings of gastritis-like malignancy showing faint mucosal irregularities by the conventional endoscopy. The dye-spraying technique, particularly the "contrast method" using 0.1% of Indigocalmin (Tsuda et al. [5]), is indispensable in detecting such fine mucosal irregularities. Table 8 shows the results of a comparative study between conventional and dye-spraying endoscopy on 63 gastritis-like EGCs. The clarity of malignant findings is divided into the

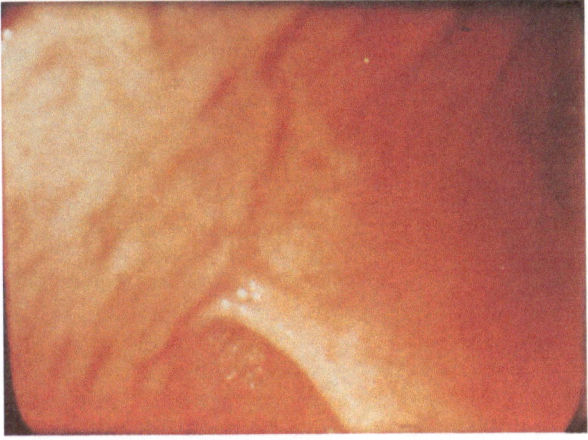

Fig. 5. An endoscopic picture of a case of gastritis-like early gastric cancer, subclassified as a "flat discolored type". A well-demarcated discolored area is seen on the anterior wall of the lower gastric body without fold convergence. The final diagnosis was a mucosal cancer of signet-ring cell carcinoma, whose size waa 12 mm in diameter

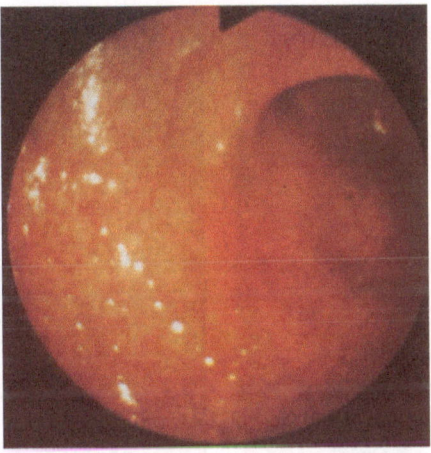

Fig. 6. An endoscopic picture of a case of gastritis-like early gastric cancer (*EGC*), subclassified as a "flat hyperemic type". A poorly demarcated faint reddish area is seen on the anterior wall, near the greater curvature of the lower body. The final diagnosis was an EGC with submucosal invasion and its histological type was well-differentiated tubular adenocarcinoma

following four grades: grade 0 (undetectable malignancy), grade 1 (rather benign), grade 2 (rather malignant), and grade 3 (definitely malignant).

As a result, all the 63 cases was evaluated as grade 0 or 1 by conventional endoscopy. After dye spraying, however, an increase of the grade was seen in

Fig. 7. An endoscopic picture of a case of gastritis-like early gastric cancer, subclassified as a "superficial eneven type". Uneven mucosa is seen on the posterior wall of the antrum. A biopsy taken from the tiny shallow depression surrounded by thickening granular mucosa revealed well-differentiated tubular adenocarcima. The size was less than 5 mm in diameter (minute cancer) on the resected specimen

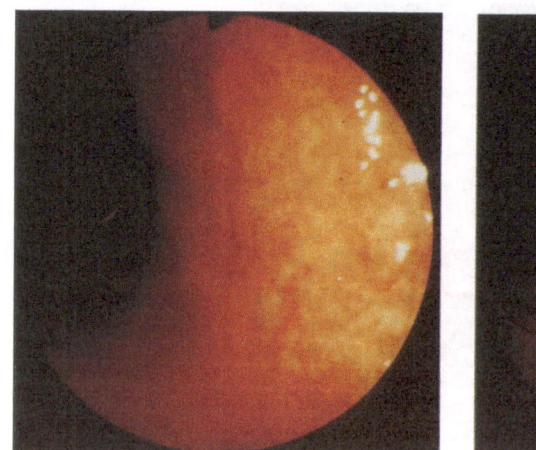
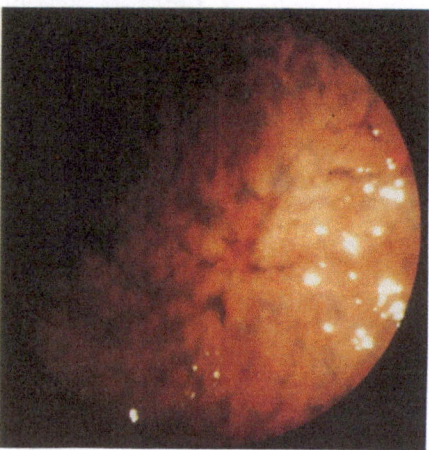

a

b

Fig. 8a,b. Endoscopic pictures of a case of gastritis-like early gastric cancer, taken by conventional (a) and dye-spraying (b) endoscopy. The cancerous lesion with submucosal invasion is located on the lesser curvature of lower gastric body. Although it is difficult to point out the lesion by conventional endoscopy (it is only seen as discoloration with faint redness), the malignant findings such as the moth-eaten appearance on the tip of weakly converging folds or irregular margin of the depressed area are easily detected by dye-spraying endoscopy

Table 8. Grade distribution of findings suggesting malignancy in "gastritis-like" EGCs observed by conventional and dye spraying endoscopy.

Conventional endoscopy	Dye-spraying endoscopy				
	Gr-0[a]	Gr-1[b]	Gr-2[c]	Gr-3[d]	Total
Grade 0[a]	3	4	7	9	23
	(13)	(17)	(31)	(39)	(100)
Grade 1[b]	0	4	17	19	40
		(10)	(42)	(48)	(100)
Total	3	8	24	28	63
	(5)	(13)	(38)	(44)	(100)

(%)
[a] Undetectable of malignancy
[b] Rather benign
[c] Rather malignant
[d] Definitely malignant

87% (20/23) of the cases of grade 0, and in 90% (36/40) of those of grade 1. Particularly, 39% (9/23) of grade 0 and 48% (19/40) of grade 1 were changed into grade 3 after this procedure, clearly indicating the diagnostic usefulness of dye-spraying endoscopy for detecting gastritis-like EGCs. Examples are shown in Fig. 8a,b.

Assessment of Reliability of Biopsy Results

Histological diagonosis by biopsy is indispensable for detecting EGCs with fewer malignant findings such as the gastritis-like type. Figure 9.a,b shows the number of biopsy cases and their incidence in the total number of upper GI endoscopy at NCCH during the period between 1962 and 1989. The number of biopsy cases has been increasing each year, and their incidence in the total number of upper GI examinations has been over 50% since 1980. Table 9 shows the biopsy results of the 5050 gastric lesions which had been diagnosed endoscopically as being benign nonneoplastic ones during the period between 1986 and 1987. The incidence of group IV (highly, suspicious of cancer) or V (cancer) was low (2–6%) in this group, regardless of the gross appearance of the lesion. However, the 136 lesions of group IV and V corresponded to 15% of those detected during the same period, indicating the great efficacy of histological screening by biopsy.

In spite of the above, biopsy is not always a perfect diagnostic tool. As we reported, in 27 of 101 cases of gastric cancer followed-up due to an initial benign diagnosis, biopsy of the original lesions had been performed 56 times within 5 years for endoscopic ruling out of malignancy before the final examination was carried out. The prior biopsy specimens were reviewed histologically with no malignancy being detected, and all were classified as being in either group I (no atypism) or II (benign atypism) [6].

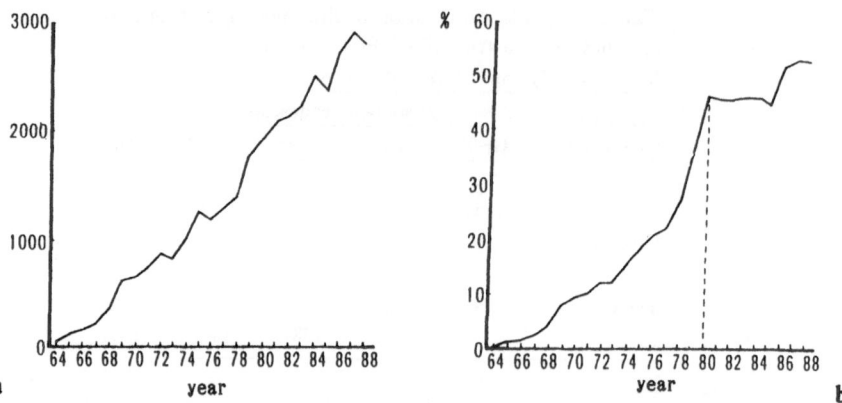

Fig. 9a,b. Chronological trends **a** in the number of gastric biopsy cases and **b** in the incidence of gastric biopsy cases in those examined by upper GI endoscopy

Table 9. Biopsy results of specimens diagnosed as benign non-neoplastic gastric lesions endoscopically. The 136 lesions of groups IV and V correspond to 15% of those detected during the same period. From 1980 to 1987, National Cancer Center Hospital.

Endoscopic diagnosis	Histological diagnosis of biopsy specimens						
	Group classification				RLH	Others	Total
	I or II	III	IV	V			
Hyp. polyp	1072	20	5 (2)	18		7	1122 (100)
Ulcer	501		8 (6)	25			534 (100)
Ulcer scar	1266	4	10 (2)	19	6		1305 (100)
Gastritis	2025	9	11 (2)	40	1	3	2089 (100)
Total	4864	33	34 (3)	102	7	29	5050 (100)

(%)

RLH, Reactive lymphoreticular hyperplasia, *Hyp. polyp*, Hyperplastic polyp

In the lesions diagnosed as group III (gastric adenoma or borderline) by biopsy, the possibility of malignancy is higher, because of the cancer having less cellular or structural atypism [7]. Table 10 shows the final diagnosis of the group III lesions after resection. Of the 243 lesions, 35 (14%) were malignant (25 were cancer and 10 were focal cancer in adenoma), and the malignant potential was significantly higher in the lesions with a depressed component (8/25: 32%) than in those without depression (27/218: 12%) ($P < 0.05$). Table 11 shows the cor-

Table 10. Endoscopic evidence of presence or absence of depressed component and final diagnosis of group III resected lesions.

Endoscopic appearance	Final diagnosis			
	C	F	A	Total
Without depression	19 (12)	8	191	218 (100)
With depression	6 (32)	2	17	25 (100)
Total	25 (14)	10	208	243 (100)

(%)
C, Cancer without adenoma; F, focal cancer with adenoma; A, adenoma

Table 11. Endoscopic appearance and malignant potential of group III lesions; examined on macroscopic type, size, and color of lesion.

	Final diagnosis			
	C	F	A	Total
Macro. type				
Polypoid	7 (16)	3 (7)	35	45 (100)
Flat polypoid	7 (8)	8 (9)	72	87 (100)
Small polypoid	0	1 (2)	41	42 (100)
Fold-like	2 (15)	1 (8)	10	13 (100)
Gastritis-like	3 (12)	7 (28)	15	25 (100)
Depressed	2 (40)	0	3	5 (100)
Total	21 (10)	20 (9)	176	217 (100)
Size				
≤ 1 cm	0	3 (4)	76	79 (100)
1< ≤ 2 cm	9 (11)	6 (7)	67	82 (100)
2 cm<	12 (21)	11 (20)	33	56 (100)
Total	21 (10)	20 (9)	176	217 (100)
Color				
Discolored	5 (5)	2 (2)	90	97 (100)
Normocolored	4 (6)	7 (10)	62	73 (100)
Hyperemic	12 (26)	11 (23)	24	47 (100)
Total	21 (10)	20 (9)	176	217 (100)

(%)
C, Cancer without adenoma; F, focal cancer with adenoma; A, adenoma

Table 12. Partial co-efficient and its statistical significance obtained from multivariate analysis of Hayashi's quantification theory No. 2, examining the correlation between endoscopic and clinicopathological features and malignancy of group III lesions.

Items	Partial coefficient	Statistical significance
Color	0.3562	$P < 0.01$
Size	0.2800	$P < 0.01$
Macroscopic type	0.2448	$P < 0.01$
Depressed component	0.2001	$P < 0.01$
Sex	0.1735	$P < 0.05$
Location	0.1726	$P < 0.05$
Histology (tubular vs papillary)	0.0134	N.S.

N.S., Not significant

relation between other endoscopic appearances and the final diagnoses of the 243 cases. Malignant cases were dominant in the lesions larger than 2 cm, those showing polypoid or gastritis-like appearance, and those which were reddish in color. The multivariate analysis of the 243 lesions, in examining the correlation between endoscopic findings and the malignancy of the lesion according to Hayashi's quantification theory No. 2, revealed that the color of the lesion showed the highest partial coefficient, followed by size, macroscopic appearance, and being in combination with a depressed component (Table 12). These four items have a statistical significance of $P < 0.01$.

These findings clearly indicated a limitation to biopsy and the importance of precisely examining the endoscopic findings of the lesion for succeeding in accurate early detection. When we are confronted with a lesion suggesting the presence of a malignancy endoscopically but not histologically by biopsy, close follow-up examination including repeated biopsy should be required.

Discussion

It is no exaggeration to say that early detection of gastric cancer in Japan started with the proposal of the definition and endoscopic classification of EGC by the Japanese Gastroenterological Endoscopy Society in 1962 [4]. In those days, most EGC was identified from the differential diagnosis of deep ulcerated (type III) or polypoid (type I) lesions, which are easily detected. In the 1970s, early diagnosis progressed, and it became possible to detect EGC lesions with the appearance of an ulcer scar (type IIc) and plateau-like elevation (type IIa). With this advance, early detection of gastric cancer seemed to be almost complete. In the 1980s, however, retrospective studies of advanced cancer revealed that gastritis-like lesions which could not be diagnosed as being malignant by conventional endoscopic criteria rapidly grew into tumorous advanced cancers, indicating the importance of differential diagnosis of superficial nonulcerative malignancy (IIb-like type), seen endoscopically as faint redness, discoloration, and/or unevenness of the gastric mucosa. Consequently, nonulcerative and nonpolypoid EGC, namely, the gastritis-like type, has increased in incidence during the last decade, and it corresponds now to over 50% of all EGC diagnosed at the NCCH each year.

For diagnosing gastritis-like malignancy, precise endoscopic observation with a dye-spraying technique and adequate biopsy is required. The differentiations of faint mucosal irregularities, however, tend to become more subjective and empirical than those of ulcerative or polypoid lesions. Videoimage endoscopy, in which an optical image is changed into quantitative electronic signals corresponding to color values for R (red), G (green), and B (blue) by a charged coupled device (CCD), is expected to be available to make endoscopic diagnosis more objective, as shown in preliminary reports of image analysis obtained from the trials by our study group [8–10]. Computer analysis of faint mucosal irregularity (computed endoscopy) is being developed, and it will be used for screening superficial malignancy which can now be detected only by subjective and empirical endoscopy.

The limitation of biopsy is mostly caused by the very small sizes of the specimens and the heterogeneity of atypism within cancerous invasion. Hence, blind acceptance of biopsy results compromise the clinical management of the patients. When we have a questionable diagnosis by biopsy, we should pay attention to the endoscopic appearance of the lesion in detail and repeat the biopsy without hesitation.

Recently, many oncogenes and antioncogenes have been disclosed as being related to the progression of gastric cancer. Gene analysis of the biopsy specimens for early diagnosis is now ongoing, particularly by examining the mutation on the p53 antioncogene in cases of tubular adenocarcinoma [11]. These new approaches will undoubtedly develop the methodology of endoscopic early diagnosis.

Acknowledgment. This work was supported, in part, by a Grant-in Aid for Cancer Research (No. 3–5) from the Ministry of Health and Welfare of Japan.

References

1. Sakita T (1983) Gastric cancer in Japan: Data from a nationwide questionnaire (in Japanese). Gastroenterol Endosc 25:317–343
2. Yoshida S, Yamaguchi H, Tajiri H, Saito D, Hijikata A, Yoshimori M, Oguro Y, Hirota T (1984) Diagnosis of early gastric cancer seen as less malignant endoscopically. Jpn J Clin Oncol 14:225–241
3. Yoshida S, Yoshimori M, Hirashima T, Yamaguchi H, Tajiri H, Nakamura K, Oguro Y, Hirota T (1981) Nonulcerative lesion detected by endoscopy as an early expression of gastric malignancy. Jpn J Clin Oncol 11:495–506
4. Tasaka T (1962) National questionaire of early gastric cancer in Japan (in Japanese). Gastroenterol Endosc 4:4–19

5. Tsuda Y (1967) Endoscopic observation of gastric lesions with a dye spraying technique (in Japanese). Gastroenterol Endosc 9:189–195
6. Yoshida S, Tsuji Y, Saito D, Yamaguchi H, Boku N, Oguro Y, Hirota T (1990) Clinical and histological issues of endoscopic biopsy in diagnosing gastric cancer (in Japanese with English summary). Stomach and Intestine 25:959–969
7. Fujii T, Yoshida S, Saito D, Yamaguchi H, Tajiri H, Miyamoto K, Ohtsu A, Yoshino M, Watanabe S, Numata K, Yoshihara M, Mizuno Y, Yoshimori M, Oguro Y, Maruyama K, Shirao K, Itabashi M, Hirota T (1989) Endoscopic and clinicopathological features of tubular adenocarcinoma with less atypism (in Japanese with English summary). Prog Dig Endosc 35:151–1556
8. Kawai M, Yamaguchi H, Yoshida S, Saito D, Hijikata A, Miyamoto K, Mukai T, Fujii T, Yamaguchi N, Okazaki H, Tsugiki M, Ishii K, Yoshimori M, Oguro Y (1988) Application of electronic endoscope to colorimeter: An evaluation of clinical utilities (in Japanese with English summary). Prog Dig Endosc 32:69–72
9. Badique E, Ohyama N (1988) Use of color image correlation in the retrieval of gastric surface topography by endoscopic stereopair matching. Appl Opt 27:941–948
10. Yachida M, Ohyama N (1989) Color image restoration using synthetic method. Opt Commun 72:[1, 2]22–26
11. Fukuda H, Saito D, Yoshida S, Uchino S, Ochiai A, Hirohashi S p53 abnormal expression in human gastric tumors by endoscopic biopsy specimens. Jpn J Cancer Res (in press)

A Retrospective Study on Advanced Gastric Cancer Detected by Mass Screening

Taiken Okamura and Masakazu Maruyama[1]

Key words. Advanced gastric cancer—mass screening—retrospective study—photofluorographic technique

Introduction

Mass screening for gastric cancers has helped reduce the gastric cancer mortality rate by detecting early cancers, thus saving the lives of many patients. Its primary objective is to detect lesions with a favorable prognosis (i.e., early gastric cancer). The absolute number of early gastric cancers detected by mass screening and the frequency of detection have certainly been growing as mass screening has come into increasingly widespread use and diagnostic techniques for endoscopic examinations continue to be improved. However, it is also a fact that gastric cancers with a poor prognosis (i.e., advanced gastric cancers) have been detected with high frequency in people undergoing mass screening despite annual examinations. Considering that this problem seriously detracts from the social contribution of mass screening, it is imperative to find the cause of the problem and take corrective action.

Patients and Methods

The results (Table 1) of 10 years (1980–1989) of mass screening at the Mass Survey Center of the Cancer Institute Hospital and the characteristics of gastric cancers detected by this mass screening program are summarized below. Gastric cancer was detected by mass screening in a total of 291 patients, in 198 of whom (or 68.0%) early gastric cancer was diagnosed, and 93 of whom (or 32.0%) suffered from advanced gastric cancer. The rate of detection was 0.21 (0.28 for males and 0.12 for females).

[1] Mass Survey Center, Cancer Institute Hospital, 1-37-1 Kami-Ikebukuro, Toshima-ku, Tokyo 170, Japan

Table 1. Results of gastric mass screening at the Mass Survey Center of the Cancer Institute Hospital (1980–1989).

Total number of gastric mass screenings (A)	137,869
Necessary number of detailed examinations (B)	26,173
Examined number of detailed examinations (C)	24,692
Rate of examined number of detailed examinations (C/B)	94.3%
Detected number of gastric cancers (D)	291
Number of early gastric cancers (E)	198
Rate of detection of gastric cancers (D/A)	0.21%
Rate of early gastric cancers (E/D)	68.0%

The 93 patients with advanced gastric cancer had a mean age of 56.1 years and consisted of 73 males (78.5%) with a mean age of 57.5 years and 20 females (21.5%) with a mean age of 50.8 years.

Of the 93 patients, 82 (88.2%) underwent curative resection, 2 (2.2%) underwent non-curative resection, 1 had complications consisting of liver cirrhosis and hepatocellular carcinoma, and 1 refused operation (after having been diagnosed with advanced gastric cancer by imaging diagnosis). Those 93 patients included 11 cases of advanced gastric cancer (11.8%) detected at other institutions.

Of the 93 patients, 25 (26.9%) were screened for the first time and 68 (73.1%) had a history of prior screening. Of the 68 patients, 55 could have been screened by photofluorography. In the present study, we reviewed 39 patients, whose history of photofluorographic examination could be traced for less than 2 years. These patients' photofluorographic, fluoroscopic, and endoscopic films were reviewed, and clinical and pathological records obtained when the gastric cancer had been detected were reexamined.

The diagnoses based on photofluorographic films were classified into three groups: (1) the diagnostic group whose photofluorographic films permitted various interpretations, (2) the existent group whose photofluorographic films allowed detection of gastric cancers, and (3) the missed group whose photofluorographic films did not permit detection of gastric cancers.

The gross appearance, histological type, depth, and location of gastric cancers were reported as defined in *The General Rules for the Gastric Cancer Study in Surgery and Pathology*, published by the Japanese Research Society for Gastric Cancer [1].

Results

The latest photofluorographic films (traced for periods of up to 23 months) taken before the detection of gastric cancers were reviewed.

Initially, according to the last photofluorographic films (Table 2), there were no patients in the diagnostic group, 8 (20.5%) in the existent group, and 31 (79.5%) in the missed group. The 8 patients in the existent group were given detailed examination, but gastric cancer could not be detected in any of them. A review of

Table 2. Diagnostic results for prior photofluorographic films (39 patients with advanced gastric cancer).

Diagnostic group	Initial diagnosis	Reviewed diagnosis
Diagnostic group	0 patients (0%)	2 patients (5.2%)
Exsistent group	8 patients (20.5%)	19 patients (48.7%)
Missed group	31 patients (79.5%)	18 patients (46.2%)

Table 3. Visualization of abnormal findings in prior photofluorographic films.

| | Traced for period (months) | | | |
Degree of visualization	10–12	13–23	24-	Total
Clear	4 (14.7%)	0 (0%)	0 (0%)	4 (7.3%)
Unclear	13 (46.4%)	5 (45.5%)	2 (12.5%)	20 (36.4%)
Nothing	11 (39.3%)	6 (54.5%)	14 (87.5%)	31 (56.4%)
Total	28 (100%)	11 (100%)	16 (100%)	55 (100%)

Table 4. Demonstration ability of prior photofluorography.

Method	Rate of demonstration	Demonstrated only by this method
Double contrast study	48.7% (19/39)	8 patients
Filling study	30.8% (12/39)	2 patients
Compression study	33.3% (2/6)	1 patient

their photofluorographic films showed that there were 2 patients (5.1%) in the diagnostic group, 19 (48.7%) in the existent group, and 18 (46.2%) in the missed group.

The last photofluorographic films were traced for two periods, 10–12 months and 13–24 months, to evaluate the degree of visualization of lesions in the photofluorographic films (Table 3). For purposes of comparison, photofluorographic films that had been taken 25 months or more before the detection of gastric cancer were also shown. There were 28 patients whose photofluorographic films could be traced for 10–12 months. The visualization of lesions in this group was classified as clear in 4 patients (14.3%), hazy or unclear in 13 (33.3%), and normal in 11 (28.2%). There were 11 patients whose photofluorographic films could be traced for 13–24 months. The visualization of lesions in this group was classified as clear in none of the patients, hazy or unclear in 5 (45.5%), and normal in 6 (54.5%).

Lesions were demonstrated in 19 of 39 patients (48.7%) in the double contrast study, 12 of 39 patients (30.8%) in the filling study, and 2 of 6 patients (33.3%) in the compression study (Table 4). There were 8 patients whose lesions were demonstrated only in the double contrast study. In contrast, there were 2 patients

Table 5. Abnormal findings revealed in prior photo-fluorographic films.

Abnormal findings	Double contrast study	Filling study
Irregular margin	12 patients	9 patients
Converging folds	8 patients	1 patients
Barium fleck	8 patients	0 patients
Linear barium pooling	2 patients	2 patients
Radiolucent shadow	5 patients	0 patients
Abnormal folds	2 patients	0 patients
Niche	0 patients	0 patients

whose lesions were demonstrated only in the filling study. The lesions in these cases were located in the anterior wall of the cardia and the middle lesser curvature of the stomach.

When photofluorographic films were reviewed, abnormal findings reflecting lesions were found in 22 cases. The abnormalities revealed in the double contrast study consisted of conversing mucosal folds in 8 patients, a radiolucent shadow in 5 patients, a barium fleck in 11 patients, a linear barium shadow in 2 patients, an abnormal margin in 12 patients, and abnormal folds in 2 patients. No patients had a niche. The abnormalities revealed in the filling study consisted of conversing folds in 1 patient, a linear barium shadow in 2 patients, and an abnormal margin in 9 patients. The abnormalities seen in the compression study consisted of a radiolucent shadow in 1 patient and a barium fleck in another patient (Table 5).

The photofluorographic films were studied for factors impeding visualization. The impeding factors were, in order of decreasing impediment, (1) coating state of barium (in 23 patients, or 59.0%), (2) overlapping of barium in the intestine (in 18 patients, or 46.2%), (3) insufficient resolution of the X-ray equipment (in 16 patients, or 41.2%), (4) inappropriate position of projection (in 9 patients, or 23.1%), (5) inappropriate condition of exposure (in 7 patients, or 17.9%), (6) compression and overlapping with gas in the large intestine (in 3 patients, or 7.7%), (7) shading by breath or by heartbeats (in 1 patient, or 2.6%), (8) figure of the stomach (in 1 patient, or 2.6%), and (9) excessive gastric juice (in 1 patient, or 2.6%).

Case Studies

A few cases of advanced gastric cancer where retrospective inspection of photofluorographic films revealed abnormalities are discussed in this section.

Case 1: A 52-Year-Old Male

In the double contrast fluoroscopic study in the supine left posterior oblique position (Fig. 1a), the lower greater curvature of the stomach has a niche along

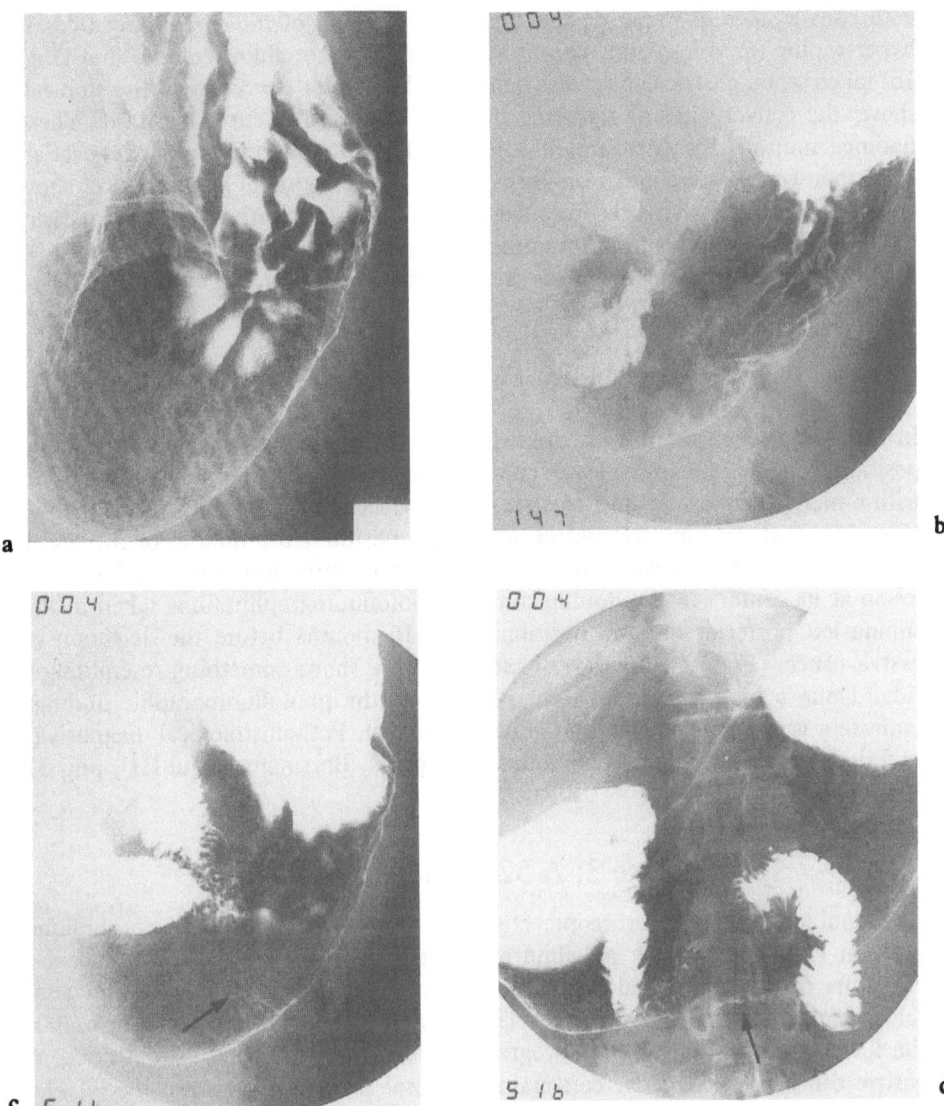

Fig. 1a–c. a Double contrast fluoroscopic study. The lower greater curvature of the stomach has a niche along with convergence of radiating mucosal folds. The tip of the converging folds is hypertrophic and discontinuous. **b** Photofluorographic film taken at detection of gastric cancer. The greater curvature of the stomach shows the convergence of radiating mucosal folds and is curved inward. **c–d** Photofluorographic films taken about 13 months before the detection of gastric cancer. A light shadow and a slightly irregular margin consistent with a lesion indicate a very slight change that is hard to detect

with convergence of radiating mucosal folds. The tip of the converging folds is hypertrophic (or thick) and discontinuous. In the photofluorographic film (Fig. 1b) taken when gastric cancer was detected, the greater curvature of the stomach shows the convergence of radiating mucosal folds and is curved inward. These findings indicate the presence of a lesion. The photofluorographic films (Fig. 1c,d) that were taken about 13 months before the detection of gastric cancer show a light shadow and a slightly irregular margin consistent with a lesion. However, the photofluorographic findings indicate a very slight change that is hard to detect. Pathohistological diagnosis is as follows: adenocarcinoma mucocellulare (sig.), Borrmann III (ul-II), se, 15 × 22 mm.

Case 2: A 59-Year-Old Male

In the double contrast fluoroscopic study in the supine right posterior oblique position (Fig. 2a), the lower lesser curvature of the stomach has an elevated lesion with a niche at its center and erosion of its surface. In the double contrast study (Fig. 2b) in the supine left posterior oblique position, the middle of the lesser curvature above the angle of the stomach has an elevated lesion with a depressed lesion at its center. In the double contrast photofluorographic films taken in the supine left posterior oblique position about 16 months before the detection of gastric cancer (Fig. 2c), the lower lesser curvature shows something resembling a ridge along a high mound of tissue. However, the photofluorographic findings indicate a very slight change that is hard to detect. Pathohistological diagnosis is as follows: adenocarcinoma papillotubulare (pap.), Borrmann II (ul-III), pm, 37 × 35 mm.

Case 3: A 52-Year-Old Male

The double contrast fluoroscopic study in the supine right posterior oblique position (Fig. 3a) reveals an abnormal rugal pattern centering on the lesser curvature of the stomach along with extensive convergence of radiating mucosal folds. A mucosal spread is seen as a clear marginal shadow in the posterior wall of the lower corpus. The photofluorographic film (Fig. 3b), taken at detection of gastric cancer, reveals clear conversing mucosal folds and a barium fleck. The photofluorographic film (Fig. 3c), taken about a year before the detection of gastric cancer, shows a barium fleck with conversing mucosal folds, though the affected region is narrower than seen at detection of gastric cancer. In this case, careful interpretation of the radiological findings led to the detection of the lesion. Pathohistological diagnosis is as follows: adenocarcinoma tubulare (tub. 1), IIc adv. (ul-III), ss, 120 × 102 mm, v(+), ly(3+).

Case 4: A 40-Year-Old Male

In the double contrast fluoroscopic study (Fig. 4a) in the supine right posterior oblique position, the antrum of the greater curvature is sharply curved inward

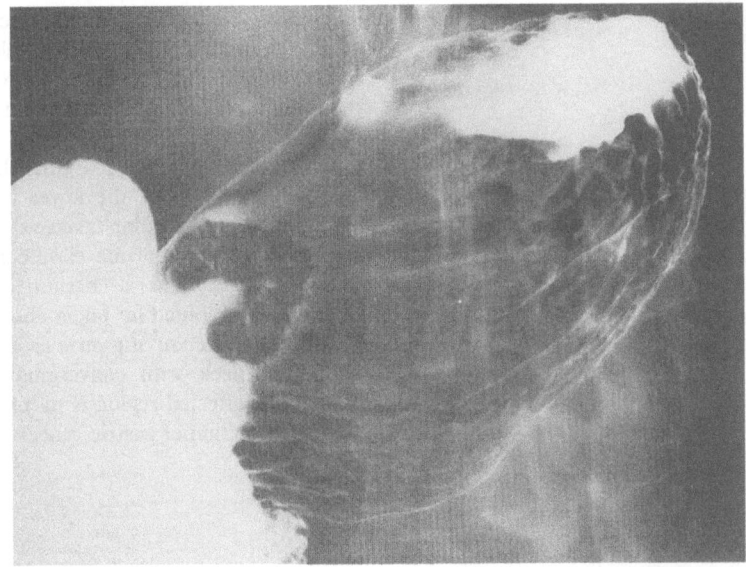

a

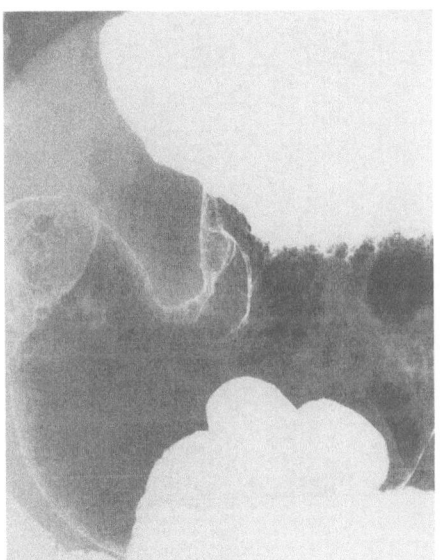

b

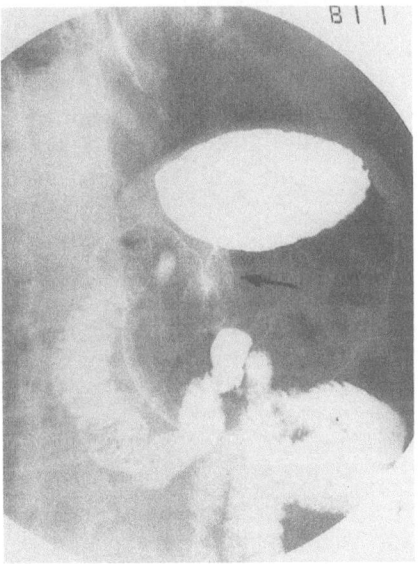

c

Fig. 2a–c. a Double contrast fluoroscopic study. The lower lesser curvature of the stomach has an elevated lesion with a niche at its center and erosion of its surface. **b** Double contrast fluoroscopic study. The middle of the lesser curvature above the angle of the stomach has an elevated lesion with a depressed lesion at its center. **c** Double contrast photofluorographic films taken about 16 months before the detection of gastric cancer. The lower lesser curvature shows something resembling a ridge along a high mound of tissue. The photofluorographic findings indicate a very slight change that is hard to detect

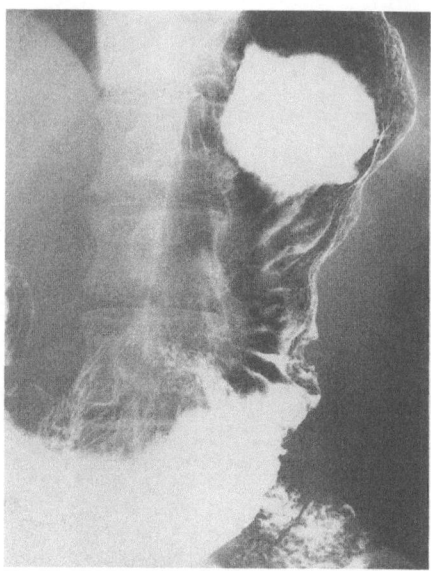

a

Fig. 3a–c. a Double contrast fluoroscopic study showing an abnormal rugal pattern centering on the lesser curvature of the stomach along with extensive convergence of radiating mucosal folds. A mucosal spread is seen as a clear marginal shadow in the posterior wall of the lower corpus. b Photofluorographic film taken at detection of gastric cancer showing clear converging mucosal folds and a barium fleck. c Photofluorographic film taken about 1 year before the detection of gastric cancer shows a barium fleck with converging mucosal folds. The affected region is narrower than seen at detection of gastric cancer

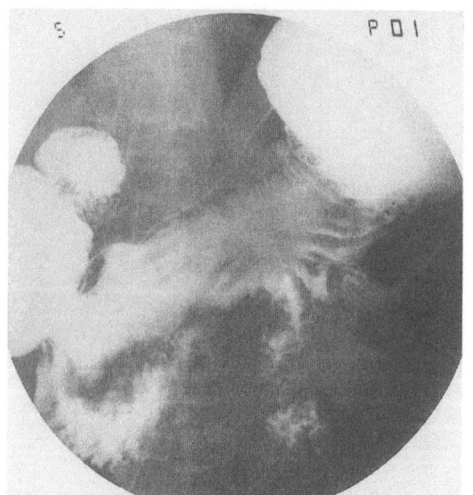

b

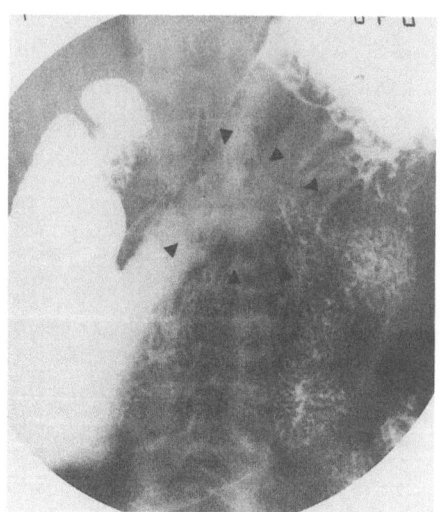

c

and shows the convergence of mucosal folds toward it. In the compression study (Fig. 4b), the same site shows an irregular ulcer and a high mound of tissue around the ulcer. The double contrast photofluorographic film (Fig. 4c) taken in the supine right posterior oblique position about 16 months before the detection of gastric cancer shows convergence of mucosal folds toward the antrum of the

Fig. 4a–c. a Double contrast fluoroscopic study. The antrum of the greater curvature is sharply curved inward and shows the convergence of mucosal folds toward it. **b** In the compression study, the same site shows an irregular ulcer and a high mound of tissue around the ulcer. **c** Double contrast photofluorographic film taken about 16 months before the detection of gastric cancer shows convergence of mucosal folds toward the antrum of the greater curvature. Since artifacts are liable to occur at this site, it may be difficult to interpret this finding as an abnormality

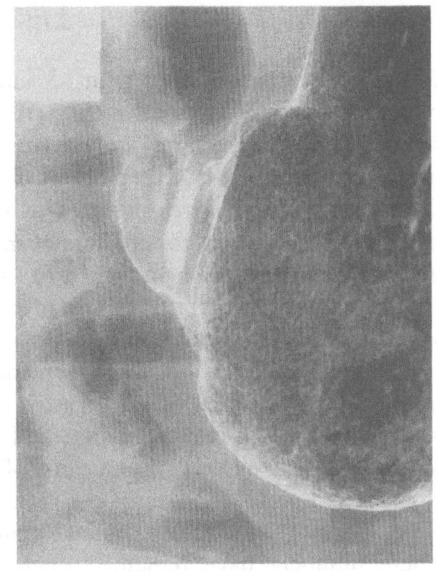

a

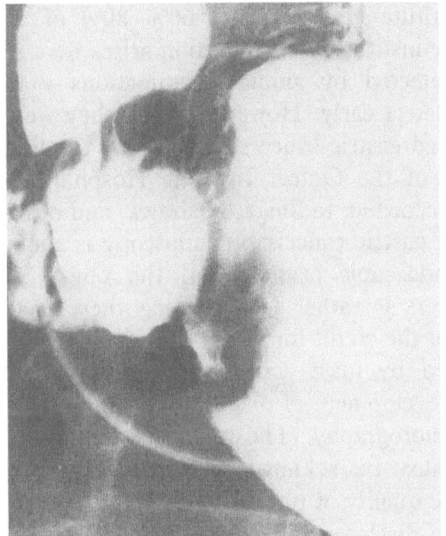

b

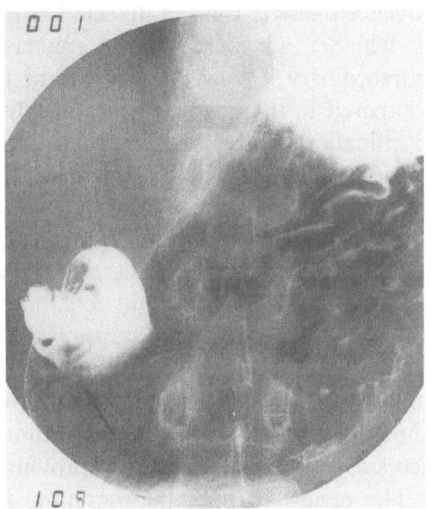

c

greater curvature. Since artifacts are liable to occur at this site, it may be difficult to interpret this finding as an abnormality. Pathohistological diagnosis is as follows: double cancer of the stomach. (1) adenocarcinoma muconodullare (muc.), Borrmann III, pm, 32 × 30 mm, ly(+), (2) poorly differentiated adenocarcinoma (por.), IIc c(ul-II s), m, 20 × 20 mm.

Discussion

Considering that more than 5 million people are now screened by photofluorography in Japan each year, studies on the efficiency, cost, effect, and safety of mass screening are of particular importance. It may therefore be unavoidable that mass screening by photofluorography has limitations regarding the number of exposures, amount of labor, and contrast medium consumption per examinee. In the present state of mass screening for gastric disorders, undue importance appears to be attached to social restrictions (i.e., cost, efficiency, and effect), to the detriment of efforts to improve the accuracy of photofluorography as a means of detecting lesions.

National statistics on mass screening for gastric cancers show that the frequency of detection of early gastric cancers has been increasing from year to year. According to our experience and the literature, the frequency of detection of early gastric cancers by means of photofluorographic examination of the stomach is low [2], and early gastric cancers have been accidentally detected in about 25%–35% of cases while examining other sites by photofluorography. These numbers have remained unchanged for 10 years. Annual examination accounts for 73% of all advanced gastric cancers detected by mass screening at the Mass Survey Center of the Cancer Institute Hospital, and 60%–80% of all advanced gastric cancers detected at other institutions. A question arises here as to whether advanced gastric cancers detected by annual examinations were extraordinary lesions that were hard to detect early. However, when they were compared to the characteristics of advanced gastric cancers detected by the first examination at the Mass Survey Center of the Cancer Institute Hospital, no appreciable difference was revealed [3]. According to Shiga, Nisizawa, and other investigations [4], the rate of detection of gastric cancers by endoscopy is about 1.43%. Compared to the results of endoscopic examination, the power of photofluorography to detect gastric cancers is rather low. Putting these facts together, we cannot help but conclude that the credit for recent improvements in the prognosis of gastric cancers detected by mass screening belongs to the increasingly widespread application and development of diagnostic techniques of endoscopy, not to the impact of photofluorography. The social restrictions of photofluorography in mass screening must be acknowledged, but it seems necessary to study means of improving the quality of photofluorography.

The review of photofluorographic films disclosed 13 cases (33.3%) of barely detectable cancer. In other words, these cases escaped detection by photofluorography in mass screening.

The results of the present study turned out to be the same as the results of previous reviews of photofluorographic films taken for the purpose of early detection of gastric cancer [3, 5]. The main problems of photofluorography were the coating state of barium, the overlapping of barium in the intestine, insufficient resolution of the X-ray equipment, and inappropriate projection positioning in the examination for both early and advanced gastric cancers.

The first problem led to the effort to improve the adhesion of contrast media. The quality and concentration of contrast media should also be given further consideration, however.

As for the second problem, an anatomical knowledge of the gastrointestinal tract, including the stomach and duodenum, should be taken into account in radiological studies of the stomach aiming to reduce the emptying of barium into the duodenum. Roughly speaking, the gastrointestinal tract reaching from the stomach to the duodenum is a cubic structure called a "lumen" that extends, as if drawing a dextrogyratory spiral, from the oral to the anal side. Generally speaking, if a dextrogyratory spiral lumen, containing a little fluid, makes a levogyratory movement in a horizontal position, then the fluid is forced toward the anal side. To improve the adhesion of a contrast medium in photo-fluorographic studies, the basic procedure is dextrogyratory.

As for the third problem of insufficient resolution of X-ray equipment, recent reports should be noted stating that X-ray films of high resolution as produced by sophisticated X-ray equipment can be obtained by the use of contrast media of high concentration and low viscosity.

Regarding the fourth problem, it should be borne in mind that films taken in appropriate positions of projection cannot serve any purpose if the adhesion of a contrast medium is poor. The position of projection deserves consideration only when excellent adhesion of a contrast medium is achieved. Considering the fact that the space occupied by gastric cancer does not differ appreciably from the anterior to the posterior wall, the demonstration of the anterior wall should be given particular consideration.

In 1984, the Japan Society of Gastric Mass Screening published the criteria for gastric photofluorography for the purpose of improving the rate of detection of lesions in the anterior wall or C-region [6]. These criteria have basic defects, however. That is to say, the criteria set the concentration of a contrast medium at about 100 w/v% and make no mention of the coating state of barium suspension. When a 100% concentration of contrast medium is used, the effort to improve its adhesion is often futile. The adhesion of a contrast medium may be improved to some extent by increasing its quantity to, say, 250 ml. However, when large quantities of a contrast medium are used, it becomes difficult to secure a double contrast view of the anterior wall. To cope with this problem, thin-layer or mucous-membrane methods have been adapted to photofluorographic studies of the anterior wall, but these methods do not visualize great details, in view of the time they consume. Since better methods exist, efforts should be made to improve the quality of photofluorography.

Taking into particular consideration the problems of the coating state of barium, overlapping of barium in the small intestine, and inapproriate positions of projection, we have implemented the following measures and obtained excellent photofluorographic films [7, 8]. The effects of these measures in the detection of gastric cancer have yet to be evaluated, but we have the feeling that our improved photofluorographic technique provides for reliable detection of lesions.

Improved Photofluorography: The 8-Projection Method

(1) The patient swallows 4.5 g of effervescent granules and washes them down with 20 ml of water.

(2) While the esophagus is being examined under fluoroscopic control with the patient in the left posterior oblique position on standing, he or she is given 180 ml of 180 w/v% barium suspension containing an antifoaming agent.

(3) With the patient in the supine left posterior oblique position, the tilt table is set into the horizontal position, and the patient is rotated to the right through 360° three times.

(4) The patient is returned to the prone position after rotation, whereupon the barium pooling in the antrum is moved into the corpus by turning the patient onto his or her left side. After the tilt table has been tilted downward (about 45° below the horizontal), the patient is returned to the prone position. A spot film of the anterior wall is obtained in this position with the double contrast.

(5) After setting the tilt table into the horizontal position, the patient is turned to the supine position after one and a half rotations to the right. With the tilt table tilted downward (about 15°), the patient is then turned to the supine right posterior oblique position. A spot film of the posterior wall is obtained in this position with the double contrast.

(6) After setting the tilt table into the horizontal position, the patient is turned to the supine position after one rotation to the right. With the tilt table tilted downward (about 15°), a spot film of the posterior wall is obtained in a frontal projection with the double contrast.

(7) The tilt table is turned to the horizontal position. After being rotated once to the right, the patient is returned to the prone position. With the tilt table tilted downward (about 15°), a spot film of the distal half of the posterior wall and the greater curvature of the stomach is then obtained in the left posterior oblique position with double contrast.

(8) The tilt table is turned into the horizontal position. After undergoing one and a half rotations to the right, the patient is brought into the right lateral position. With the tilt table turned semi-upright (about 30° above the horizontal), a spot film of the lesser curvature of the upper part of the stomach is obtained with the double contrast.

(9) The tilt table is turned into the horizontal position, with the patient in the right lateral position, and the extent of barium flow is adjusted by varying the angle of incline of the tilt table so that a double contrast view of the region from the posterior flexure of the upper part of the stomach to the upper cardia may be obtained. A spot film of the posterior wall of the proximal half of the stomach is obtained in this position with the double contrast.

(10) The tilt table is turned to the horizontal position. After undergoing one rotation to the right, the patient is returned to the prone position and then turned onto his or her right side. With the tilt table turned semi-upright (about 30°), a spot film of the anterior wall of the upper part of the stomach is obtained with the double contrast in the semi-upright right posterior oblique position.

(11) The tilt table is turned to the horizontal position. After undergoing a one-half rotation to the right, the patient is brought into the left lateral position, and barium is made to flow down the greater curvature by bringing the tilt table upright. With the tilt table turned upright to semi-upright, a spot film of the greater curvature of the upper part of the stomach is obtained with the double contrast in the left lateral position.

A disadvantage of this 8-projection method consists in the poor adhesion of barium to the pyloric region of the stomach. To make good this defect, the entire antrum must be well demonstrated by double contrast visualization of the anterior wall before barium is emptied into the duodenum.

Summary

The fact that advanced gastric cancers are detected by annual examinations with high frequency in people who undergo mass screening is a serious problem. Resolving this problem will help save the lives of these people, thus doing much to lower the national gastric cancer mortality rate. In order to identify the problems involved in mass screening and to improve the detection rate of early gastric cancers, we reviewed the last photofluorographic films of 39 cases of advanced gastric cancers detected by mass screening that had been traced for periods of up to 23 months. The impeding factors were found to be, in order of decreasing impediment: (1) the coating state of barium (in 23 patients, or 59.0%), (2) overlapping of barium in the intestine (in 18 patients, or 46.2%), (3) insufficient resolution of the X-ray equipment (in 16 patients, or 41.2%), (4) inappropriate position of projection (in 9 patients, or 23.1%).

As a result of this review, the number of cancers detected increased by 13 to a total of 21, or 53.8%. In the review of photofluorographic films the visualization of lesions was clear in 4 and unclear in 18 cases. These cases might have been detected in the early course of the cancer if photofluorographic films had been inspected more carefully or if photofluorographic films of higher quality had been obtained.

In the last photofluorographic studies, abnormalities were pointed out in 8 cases, but gastric cancer was not ultimately detected. The workup (fluoroscopic and endoscopic studies) appeared to have been defective.

The rate of visualization of lesions was 48.7% (19/39) in the double contrast study and 30.8% (12/39) in the filling study. In the filling study alone, a lesion was demonstrated in 1 case (2.6%), and in the double contrast study alone, a lesion was demonstrated in 8 cases (20.5%). To detect early gastric cancers it seems important that double contrast photofluorographic studies be conducted in mass screening.

The abnormalities demonstrated in the double contrast study consisted of converging mucosal folds in 8 cases, a radiolucent shadow in 5 cases, a barium fleck in 8 cases, a linear barium pooling in 2 cases, an abnormal irregular margin in 12 cases, and an abnormal rugal pattern in 2 cases. No case demonstrated a niche. In the filling study converging mucosal folds were demonstrated in 1 case, a linear barium pooling in 2 cases, and an abnormal irregular margin in 9 cases.

The impeding factors were, in order of decreasing impediment: (1) the coating state of barium (in 23 patients, or 59.0%), (2) overlapping of barium in the intestine (in 18 patients, or 46.2%), (3) insufficient resolution of the X-ray equipment (in 16 patients, or 41.2%), and (4) inapproriate position of projection (in 9 patients, or 23.1%). Problems (1), (2), and (4) can be solved by improving the radiological technique and modifying the use of contrast media.

Conclusion

The present study has shown that the problems of (1) inferior quality of photofluorographic films, (2) inadequate interpretation of photofluorographic films, and (3) overlooking lesions in secondary examinations (fluoroscopic and endoscopic studies) must be resolved to increase the rate of detection of early gastric cancers in mass screening.

Remedies that can simply and readily be implemented include the improvement of techniques of photofluorographic studies and procedures of projection, review of insufflation and contrast media, and improvement of secondary examinations. A modified procedure for photofluorographic studies has been proposed.

However, the improvements in the technique for photofluorographic studies cannot be achieved without the efforts of doctors who concern themselves with mass screening. It is hoped that doctors will bear this problem in mind when engaged in mass screening.

References

1. Japanese Research Society for Gastric Cancer (1985) The general rules for the gastric cancer study in surgery and pathology (11th edn) (in Japanese). Kanehara, Tokyo
2. Mai M, Takahashi Y, Minamoto T (1991) Quantitative evaluation of mass screening program for stomach cancer, diagnostic accuracy of indirect X-ray examination and its problems (in Japanese). J Gastroenterolo Mass Survey 91:23–31
3. Okamura T, Fujii A (1990) A study on indirect X-ray examination for the progress of gastric mass screening. J Gastroenterolo Mass Survey 87:29–38
4. Shiga T, Nishizawa Y, Hosoi K (1991) Evaluation of gastric mass survey from the point of the prevalence of gastric cancer among seemingly healthy individuals (in Japanese). Stomach Intestine 26:1371–1385
5. Togasi S, Yamagisi Z, Yamana T (1993) A study on the problems of indirect X-ray examination in gastric mass screening. J Gastroenterolo Mass Survey (in press)
6. Itikawa H, Yamada T, Arisue T (1984) Standard examination of gastric photofluorography in mass screening (in Japanese). J Gastroenterolo Mass Survey 62:3–5

7. Kumakura K, Baba Y, Sugino Y (1992) Diagnostic radiology of the stomach (in Japanese). Igaku Syoin, Tokyo
8. Igor L (1975) A simple method of routine double-contrast study of the upper gastro-intestinal tract. Diagn Radiol 117:513–518

Part VI
Treatment

Principles of Surgical Treatment

Kunio Okajima and Hiroshi Isozaki[1]

Key words. Gastric cancer—Surgical treatment for gastric cancer—Curative resection—Lymph node dissection—Gastrectomy—Endoscopic mucosectomy—Vagus-preserving gastrectomy

Introduction

Curative treatment of gastric cancer requires complete elimination of all cancer cells. Surgery is the only treatment method that can fully and demonstrably achieve this goal. However, in the clinical setting, the most appropriate procedure for each case must be selected, based on a full grasp and understanding of various local and systemic conditions.

Surgical Indications

Surgical indications must be considered in terms of both systemic and local conditions.

Systemic Conditions

The heart, lung, liver, kidney, and pancreas must be examined preoperatively to determine whether or not they are functioning normally. However, even if there is some organ dysfunction, the possibility of operating on a gastric cancer should not be abandoned. One should aim towards performing surgery after improving the condition of the patient until a stage is reached wherein surgery is permissible by improving organ function as much as possible. In performing surgery in such cases, close collaboration with anesthesiologists is essential.

---

[1] Department of Surgery, Osaka Medical College, 2-7 Daigaku-machi, Takatsuki, Osaka, 569 Japan

Any dehydration or electrolyte imbalances must be corrected, and adjustments in treatment should be made to achieve a hemoglobin level of ≥ 10 g/dl, total protein ≥ 6.0 g/dl, albumin ≥ 3.0 g/dl, white blood cell count $\geq 3000/mm^3$, red blood cell count $\geq 3\,500\,000/mm^3$, and platelet count $\geq 80\,000\,mm^3$. In addition, cardiovascular, hepatic, and renal functions must be checked to determine the systemic condition of the patient.

Local Conditions

Curative Surgical Indications

Curative operation cannot be undertaken in cases preoperatively showing the following condition(s): (1) Virchow's metastasis, (2) Schnitzler's metastasis, (3) cancerous peritonitis, and (4) metastasis to the liver or lung. In addition, curative resection is impossible when laparotomy findings reveal (1) liver metastasis of $>H_2$, (2) carcinomatous dissemination of P_2 or more, (3) invasion to other organs in which the lesion cannot be dissected by combined resection (including direct invasion from lymph node metastasis), or (4) multiple distant lymph node metastases ($\geq N_4$).

Palliative Operations

Palliative operations include (1) palliative dissection of the stomach, (2) by-pass operation (gastrojejunostomy, esophagojejunostomy), and (3) gastric or intestinal fistula. The purpose of a palliative operation is only to dissect the main lesion; therefore, it is mainly a treatment method for cases accompanied by bleeding, stenosis, and perforation. The purpose of bypass surgery is to enable per oral food intake, and that of gastric or intestinal fistula is enteral tube-feeding.

The three main considerations to bear in mind when undertaking a palliative operation are: (1) extension of survival can be expected, (2) immediate death (operative death) can be avoided, and (3) the procedure includes no course of action which can possibly promote the development of advancement of the tumor. In addition, the following conditions should be fulfilled: (1) when possible, enable oral food intake, (2) reduce pain, and (3) resect as much of the lesion as possible. Although these conditions may actually be contradictory at times, the most important policy is to tailor the treatment for the maximum benefit of the patient. It is important to understand that a palliative operation is different from a curative one, and that it should not exacerbate the condition. Although some palliative operations are aimed at reduction surgery for immunological reasons, unless the residual tumor can be made extremely small, immunotherapy and chemotherapy will have little effect.

Since combined resection and multidisciplinary treatment have recently been aggressively undertaken in cases with peritoneal dissemination only in the immediate vicinity of the stomach (P_1) and in cases with metastasis to only one lobe of the liver (H_1), the number of cases in which only exploratory laparotomy is performed has decreased even among cases which do not meet the above conditions for curative surgery. In fact, postoperative results have been improved by combinations of palliative dissection and supplementary treatment. For example, in cases of liver metastasis (H_1 and some H_2 cases), gastrectomy with extensive hepatic resection, lymph node dissection, and continuous intra-arterial infusion chemotherapy via the hepatic artery yields better postoperative results than cases without resection of primary or metastatic lesions.

Furthermore, although cases with peritoneal metastasis used to be considered completely untreatable, chemo-hyperthermia by laparotomy and chemotherapy using new forms of drugs (activated carbon particle adsorbent Mitomicin C, intra-abdominal administration, etc.) have recently been reported to be effective, showing some hope in treatment of such currently inoperable cases in the future.

Fundamental Rules in Selecting Operative Methods

When selecting the operative method, the first fundamental points to think of are (1) whether the procedure can obtain a cure, (2) whether it is a safe method, and (3) preservation of postoperative function (digestive function). The ideal operation method should be appropriate to the degree of development of the lesion without decreasing the curability. Therefore, it is essential to accurately grasp the extent of invasion through preoperative examinations (size, degree of invasion to the wall, the presence and extent of lymph node metastasis, histologic type, etc.) and consider the systemic condition of the patient (function of the heart, lung, liver, and kidneys) when choosing the operative method. In order to accurately comprehend the preoperative condition of invasion of the tumor, diagnostic imaging examinations such as roentogenograms of the stomach and intestine, endoscopy, ultrasound, CT, MRI, and angiography should be fully employed and the findings should be examined systematically.

Deciding the Extent of Resection

Since a curative operation requires complete resection, leaving no remaining malignant cells in residual stomach or other organs, the principles for deciding on the lines of resection for gastrectomy are as follows.

Resection Line on the Oral Side

A review of many clinical cases revealed that the minimum macroscopically recognizable distances from the margin of the tumor to be observed in order to ensure that no remaining tumor is left on the oral side are: (1) ≥ 2 cm for superficial carcinoma (early stage carcinoma), (2) ≥ 3 cm for localized type carcinoma (Borrmann I and II (according to Borrmann's classification [1]), and (3) ≥ 5 cm for infiltrative carcinoma (Borrmann III and IV).

These safety margins were established based on accumulated experience concerning noncontinuous invasion as revealed by histological examination of tumor invasion in the gastric wall. In cases in which the macroscopic distance from the esophagogastric junction (EGJ) to the tumor margin is less than the distance described above, total gastrectomy or gastrectomy on the oral side is required.

In cases of cancer of the upper third of the stomach in which it invades into the esophagus beyond the EGJ, invasion in the esophageal wall shows characteristics according to the macroscopic type of tumor development (the localized, inter-mediate, or infiltrative types of Kajitani's classification [2]). In all three types, the layer of deepest invasion in the esophagus tends to be submucosal, but it was also found that the localized type frequently invades the mucosal epithelium, the intermediate type all layers, and the infiltrative type the lamina propria. The intermediate type also displays a high rate of intralymphatic invasion in the submucosal layer, with a stepping-stone manner of invasion. These data indicate that it is difficult to macroscopically estimate the deepest extent of invasion based only on mucosal features.

The distance between the margin of invasion seen macroscopically and the histological margin on resected specimens were 1.5 cm for the localized type, 2.0 for the intermediate, 3.0 cm for the infiltrative, and 0.5 cm for the superficial. Histological specimens are prepared after being fixed following resection, but are said to be reduced to 65% of the actual size. Therefore, it is calculated that the above-mentioned distances in the body are actually 2.3 cm for the localized type, 3.1 for the intermediate, 4.6 cm for the infiltrative, and 0.8 cm for the superficial. These distances can be considered to represent safety margins for the borderlines on the oral side from the tumor margins in order to avoid leaving any residual tumor cells.

Surgical Margin on the Duodenal Side

The author examined how much the duodenum should be dissected in cases when the intramural invasion reaches the pyloric ring. Most invasion of gastric cancer into the duodenum remains limited to within 2 cm from the pyloric ring. Therefore, in cases of invasion to the duodenum, leaving residual tumor can be avoided if a dissection is made 4–5 cm away from the pyloric ring. More resection is required if the invasion is more extensive, and pancreaticoduodenectomy is necessary in these cases.

Other Factors

Lymph node metastasis must be taken into consideration as another factor when determining the extent of resection. When apparent lymph node metastasis can be observed in the right or left cardiac lymph nodes in cases of lower gastric cancer, total gastrectomy is necessary. When there is metastasis to the lymph node of the spleen or splenic artery, as in cases of cancer of the middle or lower third of the stomach, combined resection of the body and tail of the pancreas and spleen must be performed in addition to gastrectomy.

Concerning the applications of guidelines for determining the extent of re-section mentioned above, subtotal gastrectomy on the pyloric side is performed in many cases of cancer of the lower or middle third of the stomach. Although subtotal gastrectomy is classified as a procedure which resects 4/5 of the stomach, according to "the General Rules for Gastric Cancer Study" [3] prepared by the Japanese Research Society for Gastric Cancer, the author employs subtotal gastrectomy on the pyloric side if the borderline on the lesser curvature is adjacent to the EGJ or if the borderline exists within 2 cm on the lesser curvature from the EGJ.

Lymph Node Dissection

Early Gastric Cancer

The percentages of lymph node metastasis of 564 early gastric cancer treated in the author's department, of which 304 were mucosal carcinoma (m carcinoma) and 260 were submucosal carcinoma (sm carcinoma), are 3.0% for the former and 16.6% for the latter. In terms of extension of metastasis, 2.1% of m carcinoma cases were n_1 (+), 0.6% n_2 (+), and 1.1% n_3 (+), while 13.9% of sm carcinoma were n_1 (+), 2.3% n_2 (+), and 0.6% n_3 (+).

Site of Lesion and Lymph Node Metastasis Occurrence Rate

In early gastric cancer (m, sm carcinoma), 4.2% are upper gastric cancer, 8.3% middle gastric, and 13.2% lower gastric, revealing a high percentage of lymph node metastasis in cases of early lower gastric cancer.

Histologic Types and Lymph Node Metastasis Occurrence Rate

The occurrence rate of lymph node metastasis of poorly differentiated carcinoma (por, sig) is 17.6%, higher than that of highly differentiated carcinoma (pap, tub_1, tub_2) (10.6%). Therefore, even in early gastric cancer, attention must be paid to poorly differentiated carcinomas with a por or sig histologic type because of their having high occurrence rates of lymph node metastasis.

Site of Lesion, Histologic Types, and Lymph Node Metastasis Occurrence Rate

Poorly differentiated carcinomas show lymph node metastasis in 23.5% of cases in the lower third of the stomach, 16.4% in the middle third of the stomach, and 9.1% in the upper third of the stomach. In highly differentiated carcinoma cases, metastasis is observed in 10% of lower gastric cancer cases, 7.3% middle, and 0% upper. Lymph node dissection must be performed out of consideration to the fact that poorly differentiated carcinomas (especially lower gastric cancer) show a high rate of lymph node metastasis even in the early stage.

Sites of Lymph Node Metastasis in Early Gastric Cancer

According to the General Rules for Gastric Cancer Study in Surgery and Pathology [3], lymph nodes are classified into four groups: the first group includes the proximal lymph nodes in the perigastric region, the second includes the intermediate lymph nodes along the celiac axis, and left gastric and splenic arteries, the third includes the distant lymph nodes along the hepatoduodenal ligament and at the root of the mesentery, and the fourth group includes the far-distant lymph nodes in the para-aortic region.

The lymph nodes of the second group or more distant in which metastasis frequently occurs are Nos. 1, 7, 9, 11, and 14V lymph nodes in cases of lower gastric m carcinoma. In middle gastric cancer cases, Nos. 7, 8a, and 14V show frequent metastasis, while in sm carcinomas, Nos. 7, 8a, 11, and 12 in lower gastric cancer and Nos. 7, 8a, 9, 11, and 12 in the middle region. Metastasis in upper early gastric cancer only extends to the first group of lymph nodes.

Largest Dimension of Lesions of Early Gastric Cancer, Macroscopic Types, and Rates of Lymph Node Metastasis

Early gastric carcinomas are macroscopically classified into elevated (I, IIa), depressed (IIc, III), flat (IIb), and elevated + depressed types (IIa + IIc, IIc + IIa). The following data describe the occurrence rate of lymph node metastasis in relation to the maximum dimensions of lesions. (1) No lymph node metastasis is observed in elevated type m and sm carcinomas smaller than 20 mm. When the lesion is 20 mm or more, 7.7% of m carcinoma and 41.2% of sm carcinoma show metastasis. (2) In the elevated + depressed type, no metastasis is observed in m or sm carcinomas smaller than 10 mm. When the lesion is 10–19 mm, 0% of m carcinoma and 8.3% sm carcinoma show metastasis, and when 20 mm or more, the values are 7.7% and 20%, respectively. These include n_3 (+) cases. (3) The depressed type shows no lymph node metastasis when smaller than 10 mm. Lesions between 10 and 19 mm in size show 5.7% metastasis in m cancer and 13.0% in sm cancer, while in those between 20 and 39 mm, metastasis is observed in 1.8% of m cancers and in 11.1% of sm cancers. In m cancers of over 40 mm, metastasis is seen in 13.8% of the cases and sm cancers in 23.1%, including n_3 (+) cases. (4) No metastasis was observed in flat-type cases.

Cases in which no metastasis was observed are m cancers smaller than 20 mm in the elevated type, m cancers smaller than 20 mm, and sm cancers smaller than 10 mm in the elevated + depressed type, as well as both m and sm cancers smaller than 10 mm in the depressed type.

Relative to the above findings, the candidates for reduced surgery are those with depressed m cancers smaller than 20 mm and all patients with m and sm cancers smaller than 10 mm.

Advanced Gastric Cancer

For advanced gastric cancer, the principle of employing surgery applies to cases over R_2. The author has histologically examined resected lymph nodes and summarized the correlation between the site of lesion and lymph node extension (Table 1). The metastasis occurrence rates were 55.6% for upper gastric cancer, 33.8% for middle gastric, 51.9% for lower, and 85.1% for cancer of the entire stomach. Metastases to the 3rd or more distant group were observed most

Table 1. Site of advanced gastric cancer and extension of lymph node metastasis.

Site / Extension	n (−) %	n_1 (+) %	n_2 (+) %	n_3 (+) %	n_4 (+) %	Total (n cases)
Upper third	44.4	23.8	18.5	3.3	9.9	55.6% (151)
Middle third	66.2	18.0	8.3	3.5	4.0	33.8% (373)
Lower third	48.1	23.2	14.5	10.7	3.6	51.9% (393)
Entire stomach	14.9	23.0	33.8	21.6	6.8	85.1% (74)
Total	51.9	21.3	14.2	7.7	4.9	48.1% (991)

frequently in cancers of the entire stomach, followed in descending order by lower, upper, and middle gastric cancers.

The characteristics of sites of metastatic lymph nodes in advanced gastric cancer, according to sites of lesion, are as follows. (1) In upper gastric cancer, there is a high percentage of metastasis to the group 4 lymph nodes, especially the lymph nodes around the abdominal aorta. This is due to its easy access to abdominal para-aortic lymph nodes via the subphrenic lymphatics. On the other hand, no metastasis to the lymph nodes of the head of the pancreas was observed in cases of carcinoma of the upper stomach. (2) In middle gastric cancer, resection of the lymph nodes behind the head of the pancreas is not important, but the lymph nodes of the hepatoduodenal ligament must be completely dissected. (3) In cases of lower gastric cancer, hepatoduodenal ligament lymph nodes must be considered as group 2 lymph nodes and completely dissected. However, metastasis to the splenic hilus lymph nodes is extremely rare.

Indications of Operative Method in Terms of Site and Extent of Resection

Gastrectomy on the Pyloric Side

Since gastric cancers are more frequently located in the lower or middle third of the stomach than in the upper third, gastrectomy on the pyloric side—subtotal gastrectomy in particular—is frequently performed. The previously mentioned basic principles concerning the oral surgical margin must be applied in such cases. Daughter lesions of multiple intramural gastric carcinomas are more frequently located in the middle and lower stomach than in the upper stomach. Therefore, with gastrectomy on the pyloric side, there is less probability of daughter lesions remaining in the residual stomach, although the possibility of multiple lesions must be fully examined.

Gastrectomy on the Oral Side

The *indications* of gastrectomy on the cardiac side were studied in terms of (1) extension in the gastric wall and (2) lymph node metastasis. The following are indications for curative gastrectomy on the cardiac side. (1) The lesion must be limited to the upper stomach with no invasion to the serosa, with the size of the primary lesions being no greater than 4 cm in greatest dimension (with a surgical margin of 2 cm in an anal direction for superficial lesions, 3 cm for the localized type, and 5 cm in infiltrative lesions). (2) Other indications for curative cardiac side gastrectomy are cases in which there is no metastasis to the superior or inferior pyloric lymph nodes or to the lymph nodes on the right side of the greater curvature. These conditions for resection were established as a result of studies showing that, when the greatest dimension was more than 4 cm or in cases where the lesion is located in the upper stomach with invasion to the serosa, metastasis to the lymph nodes of the lesser curvature is extremely frequent, as are metastases to the superior and inferior pyloric lymph nodes and right lymph nodes of the greater curvature.

Furthermore, in some cases, palliative gastrectomy on the cardiac side for the purpose of resecting only the tumor is sometimes performed instead of curative gastrectomy on the cardiac side, due to the overall condition of the patient.

Reconstruction after Gastrectomy on the Oral Side

There are three main approaches to reconstruction after gastrectomy on the oral side (Fig. 1): (1) esophagogastrostomy, (2) interposition between the esophagus and the residual stomach, and (3) esophagojejunostomy. The important points to remember when performing reconstruction of the gastric tract are to ensure the passage of food through the duodenum and to prevent reflux esophagitis. Most procedures for esophagogastrostomy and interposition between the esophagus and the residual stomach allow the passage of food through the duodenum, but a weak aspect of esophagogastrostomy is that it has a high frequency of reflux esophagitis. In esophagojejunostomy, if there is a distance of at least 40 cm between the anastomosis of the esophagus and the jejunum and the jejunojejunostomy site, reflex esophagitis can be prevented, but unless a double tract technique is used with this method, food would not be able to pass the duodenum.

Apart from the esophagogastrostomy and the double tract methods, esophagojejunostomy has the benefit of requiring little operating time and involving less invasiveness, but it does have the above-mentioned drawbacks. From a physiological point of view, the interposition method allows the most natural digestive tract absorption, and, if the interposed intestine is 30 cm or more in length, reflex esophagitis can be prevented. However this method requires a longer operating time, which is its main drawback.

Selection of the operative method must be made in terms of the safest method in consideration of the overall condition of the patient, but one must always strive to achieve the most physiological method with the least likelihood of post-operative complications.

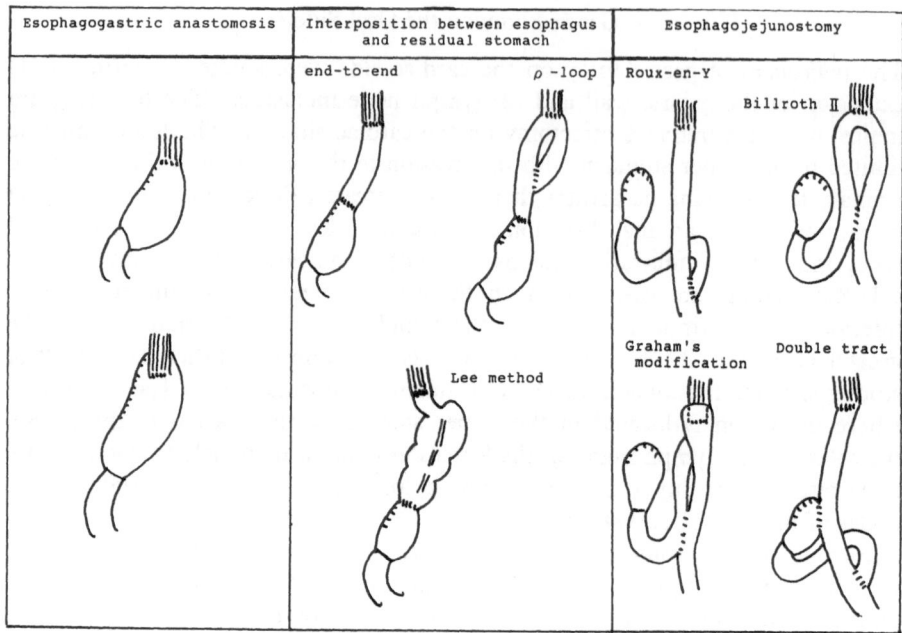

Fig. 1. Gastric resection and reconstruction on the oral side

Total Gastrectomy

Indications

Based on the previously described principles for deciding on the surgical resection line in gastric cancer, total gastrectomy is generally performed in cases in which the lesion extends extensively to the stomach or in which multiple lesions are located extensively within the stomach. Total gastrectomy is also usually performed in cases of cancer of the lower stomach in which there is a distinct metastasis to the left or right cardiac lymph nodes or in cases of cancer of the upper stomach in which there is a distinct metastasis to the superior or inferior pyloric lymph nodes. Furthermore, gastrectomy is performed as a matter of a course in cases in which there is combined resection of the body or of the tail of the pancreas or the spleen due to direct invasion of the body of the pancreas or metastasis to the splenic hilus or the splenic artery lymph nodes in cases of middle or lower stomach.

Reconstruction After Total Gastrectomy

There are 3 main methods: (1) interposition between the esophagus and duodenum, (2) esophagojejunostomy (Roux-en-Y method, Billroth II method), and (3) double tract method (see the previous description of reconstruction after gastrectomy on the oral side). Here, as in gastrectomy on the oral side, it is essential to choose a method which is as physiological as possible and which would have the least likelihood of causing reflex esophagitis; but, again, the safest method must be selected considering the condition of the patient and extent of invasiveness of the operation. The author selects the reconstruction method based on curability as follows. If a cure can be obtained, i.e., in the cases of an absolutely curative resection, the interposition method is chosen. When a cure cannot be obtained, such as in cases of absolutely non-curative resection, then either the Roux-en-Y or the Billroth II method is chosen, whereas in cases of relatively curative resection or cases of relatively non-curative resection, the double tract method is selected. These criteria are based mainly on curability, as well as on the extent of invasiveness of the procedure and the surgical risk.

Reduced Operation for Gastric Cancer

In the past, extended operations in gastric cancer used to be employed in order to give priority to curability of the operative method. However, early gastric cancer is recently being detected with increasing frequency. In light of this, the concept has developed that an extended operation may be too excessive for such cases of early cancer. As a result, the concept that the extent of a surgical procedure should be apposite to the extent of the lesion has gained increasing acceptance. However, the problem is to reach a happy medium that satisfies the opposing points of view that, on the one hand, because the pathology is early gastric cancer in which a cure can be hoped for, it is necessary to perform an operation that would fully ensure curability, and the opposing view, which claims that it is not mandatory to add unnecessary invasiveness and operating fields wider than are required for lesions at such an early stage.

In order to reach a solution to this problem, it is necessary for a surgeon to have extensive knowledge of the clinical pathology of the patterns of development and extension of gastric cancer and, based on that knowledge, to select the most appropriate operative procedure for each individual case. Against this background, the reduced version of the operation for early gastric cancer has received increasing attention. This method involves (1) a limited range of lymph node dissection or no lymph node dissection at all, (2) a reduced resection of the stomach, including wedge resection or gastrectomy of limited extent, and (3) reduced or no resection of perigastric tissue, including reduced or no resection of the greater or lesser omentum or of the lesser peritoneal sac.

In cases of elevated-type lesions with the greatest dimension being less than 20 mm, depressed lesions less than 10 mm, and elevated and depressed lesions less than 10 mm, the author performs reduced gastrectomy, including the site of the lesion and prophylactic dissection of lymph nodes in the vicinity of the lesion, based on studies showing that there is no lymph node metastasis in lesions of these types and dimensions. These procedures can include partial gastrectomy, involving wedge resection, segmental gastrectomy, or gastrectomy preserving the pyloric ring. As to lymph node dissection, apart from the cases described above, in early gastric cancer this involves dissection of the second group of lymph nodes described earlier. In other words, in addition to the group 1 lymph nodes, in early cancer of the lower stomach the numbers 1, 7, 8a, 9, 11, and 12 lymph nodes are dissected, and in cancer of the middle stomach, numbers 7, 8a, 9, 11, 12, and 14V lymph nodes are the main ones that are dissected.

There are points of caution concerning the selection of a reduced operation. The most important problems for reduced operations including endoscopic treatment (see below) are concerned with the accurate pretreatment determination of the presence or absence of lymph node metastasis and the accurate evaluation of multiple lesions. In cases in which the extent of gastrectomy is limited and in which lesions remain in the residual stomach due to multiple cancer, it can be said that the basic principle of cancer treatment has been transgressed. Multiple cancer is more commonly seen to be associated with early stage lesions than with advanced gastric cancer. Even within early gastric cancers it is actually higher in cases of ultra-small gastric lesions (greatest dimension up to 5 mm). Our investigations have indicated the presence of multiple lesions in early gastric cancer in 8.3% as opposed to 5.6% for advanced gastric cancer. Other investigators have reported multiple lesions being 31.8% [4] and 50.7% [5] of ultra-small lesions. Furthermore, while the presence of multiple lesions is often detected only on histological examination of the resected specimen, suggesting that a more extended gastrectomy is safer, there is of course a limit to the possible extent of a resection. Therefore, it is essential that the follow-up of the residual stomach be performed on a regular postoperative basis.

Procedures to Preserve the Vagus Nerve

In early gastric cancer, when the extent of lymph node dissection can be limited in cases of gastrectomy on the pyloric side and gastrectomy with preservation of the pyloric ring, attempts should be made to preserve the hepatic and abdominal branches of the vagus nerve. In addition, in cases of gastrectomy on the oral side, if possible, the hepatic branch, abdominal branch, and Latarget's branch should be preserved in order to preserve the biliary and pyloric function postoperatively.

Endoscopic Treatment of Early Gastric Cancer

The endoscopic treatment of gastric cancer includes (1) treatment of bleeding or stenosis in advanced cases, and (2) treatment aimed at a cure in early gastric cancer. The latter procedure was initially performed only in cases of poor risk in early gastric cancer or in patients that absolutely refused to undergo an operation. However, in recent years, endoscopic treatment has been aggressively pursued in certain types of early gastric cancer. This has come about partly because of increased accuracy in the preoperative diagnosis of early gastric cancer, recognition of the indications and limitations of endoscopic treatment, and also as a result of increased emphasis on the quality of life of the patient after the operation.

Indications for Endoscopic Treatment

In endoscopic treatment, one of the points of greatest interest is in developing a method to accurately determine the presence or absence of lymph node metastasis before embarking on any procedure, but such a methodology has not yet been perfected. Therefore, to solve this problem, although it is a retrospective method, studies were carried out to find out what types of gastric cancer have no lymph node metastasis. The criteria mentioned previously were developed from the results of these studies: i.e., protruding lesions less than 20 mm in greatest dimension and all gastric cancers macroscopically less than 10 mm in greatest dimension. However, in terms of selecting the endoscopic procedure, lesions seen to be accompanied by ulcer scar, such as IIc cases, even if less than 10 mm in greatest dimension, are difficult to treat endoscopically and should not be included in the indications for endoscopic treatment. Other reasons to exclude lesions as being indications for endoscopic treatment include those in which it is difficult to clearly decide on the extent of the lesion and those lesions which are anatomically located in a site that is difficult to treat endoscopically.

Points of Caution Concerning Endoscopic Treatment

Informed Consent

Before treatment, the patient must be made fully aware of advantages, disadvantages, complications, anticipated curability, and type of supplementary treatment that must be applied in cases in which cancer remains. Only if the patient agrees, on the basis of having this information, can the procedure be performed.

Post-Treatment Regular Follow Up

It is essential to perform regular posttreatment endoscopic examinations of both the treated site and the related lymph nodes.

Other

Extended lymph node dissection and combined resection of other organs is treated elsewhere in this volume.

Conclusion

The surgical treatment of gastric cancer is based on a logical surgical approach and the appropriate amount of resection, based on an accurate clinicopathological accumulation of knowledge. The author sincerely hopes that the time will come when surgeons will select the most appropriate method for each individual case, freeing themselves from the habits of the old era when the extended end procedure was usually selected in every case.

References

1. Borrmann R (1926) Geschwülste des Magens. In: Henke F, Lubarsch O (eds) Handbuch der Speziellen pathologischen Anatatomie und Histologie IVth. Julius Springer, Berlin, pp 864–871
2. Kajitani T (1950) Clinical classification of gastric cancer and its significance (in Japanese). Gann 41:76–78
3. Japanese Research Society for Gastric Cancer (1981) The general rules for Gastric Cancer Study in Surgery and Pathology. Jpn J Surg 11:127–145
4. Oohara T, Johjima Y, Tohma H, et al (1980) Comparison between minute gastric cancer and small gastric cancer (in Japanese). Jpn J Cancer Clin 26:1220–1225
5. Hirota T, Itabashi M, Suzuki K, et al (1979) Clinico-Pathological study of 63 cases of micro and small early gastric cancer-histogenesis of gastric cancer (in Japanese). Stomach and Intestine 14:1027–1036

Effectiveness of Systematic Lymph Node Dissection in Gastric Cancer Surgery

Keiichi Maruyama, Mitsuru Sasako, Taira Kinoshita, and Kazuo Okajima[1]

Key words. Gastric cancer—Surgical treatment—Lymph node dissection

Introduction

The National Cancer Center Hospital was established in 1962 and has played a major role in improving diagnostic and treatment methods of gastirc cancer in Japan. In the 30-year period from 1962 to 1991, 6865 patients with primary gastric cancer were treated in the institution, and the overall 5-year survival rate (5YSR) was 55.4%, 55% in resected cases (n = 6540), and 69.5% in curatively resected cases (n = 5416). The 30 years were divided into three equal periods for an analysis of trend. The proportion of Stage I cancer was 30.5% in the first 10-year period (Fig. 1.a), and increased to 53.7% in the last 10-year period. The proportion of Stage IV had decreased from 28.8% to 17.9%. The increase of early stage cancer and decrease of advanced cancer were produced by progress in diagnostic methods and the establishment of a mass screening program. Treatment results were also improved in the 30-year period, with the 5YSR rising from 44.5% to 70.8% in all resected cases. The 5YSR also rose in each stage: from 89% to 94% in Stage Ia, from 79% to 90% in Stage Ib, from 61% to 76% in Stage II, from 39% to 63% in Stage IIIa, from 28% to 39% in Stage IIIb, and from 2.4% to 10.1% in Stage IV (Fig. 1.b). Progress in surgical treatment, particularly systematic lymph node (LN) dissection, played a major role in this improvement. The resection rate rose from 84% to 95%, and the frequency of systematic LN dissection also increased, from 63% to 84% (Fig. 1.c). However, the postoperative mortality rate decreased from 2.3% to 0.4%. Using these data, the effectiveness of LN dissection was evaluated in this study.

---

[1] Department of Surgical Oncology, National Cancer Center Hospital, 5-1-1 Tsukiji, Chuo-ku, Tokyo, 104 Japan

294 K. Maruyama et al.

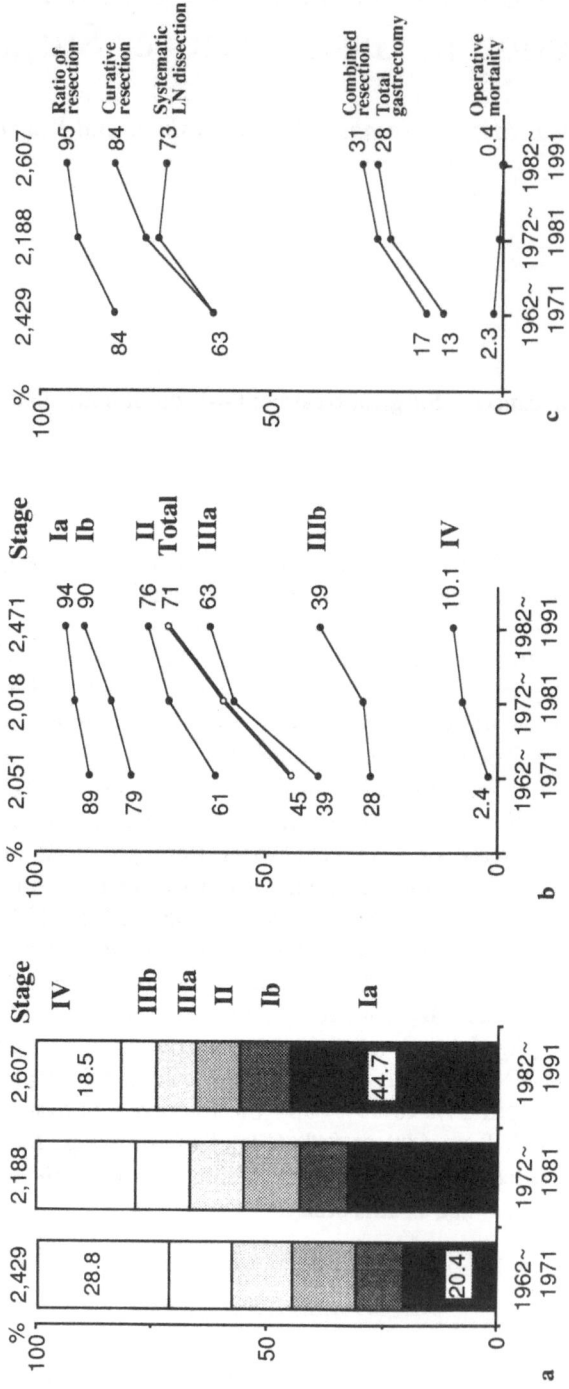

Fig. 1. Trends of stage, 5-year survival rate, and surgical treatment in a 30-year period in the National Cancer Center (Tokyo). **a** Increase of early stage cancer; **b** elevation of 5-year survival rate at every stage; **c** trend of surgical treatment and decrease of operative mortality

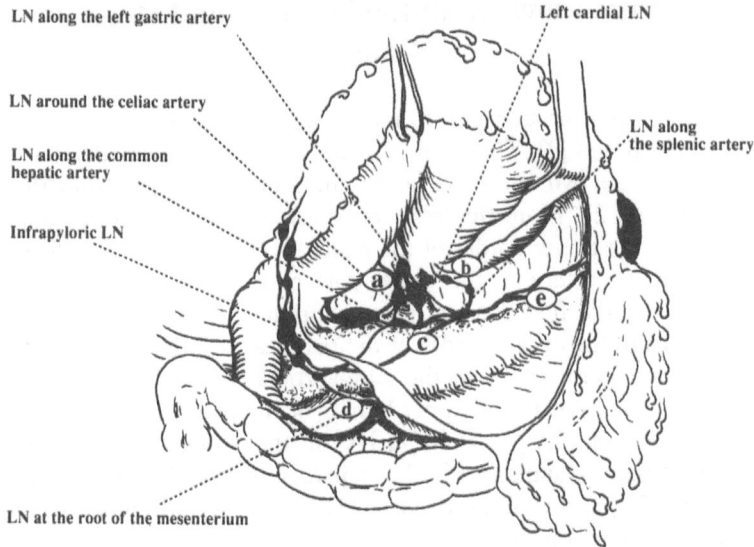

Fig. 2. Schema of five major lymphatic flows (**a–e**) from the Stomach. *LN*, Lymph node. (From [8] with permission)

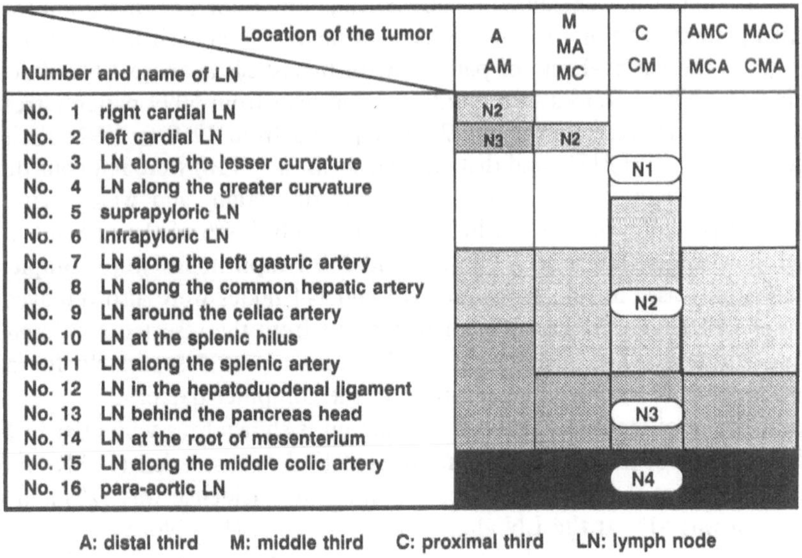

Location of the tumor Number and name of LN	A AM	M MA MC	C CM	AMC MAC MCA CMA
No. 1 right cardial LN	N2			
No. 2 left cardial LN	N3	N2		
No. 3 LN along the lesser curvature			N1	
No. 4 LN along the greater curvature				
No. 5 suprapyloric LN				
No. 6 Infrapyloric LN				
No. 7 LN along the left gastric artery				
No. 8 LN along the common hepatic artery			N2	
No. 9 LN around the celiac artery				
No. 10 LN at the splenic hilus				
No. 11 LN along the splenic artery				
No. 12 LN in the hepatoduodenal ligament				
No. 13 LN behind the pancreas head			N3	
No. 14 LN at the root of mesenterium				
No. 15 LN along the middle colic artery			N4	
No. 16 para-aortic LN				

A: distal third   M: middle third   C: proximal third   LN: lymph node

Fig. 3. Regional lymph nodes of the stomach and the N Classification of the Japanese Research Society for Gastric Cancer

Lymphatic Flows from the Stomach and 16 Regional LN Stations

The lympatic system around the stomach was clarified by anatomical [1] and lymphographic studies [2]. The major streams from the stomach demonstrated by lymphography were two from the lesser curvature and three from the greater curvature [3] (Fig. 2). From the lesser curvature, a stream flowed along the left gastric artery to the upper border of the pancreas (**a**), and the other flowed along the left subphrenic artery to the upper part of para-aortic LN (**b**). From the greater curvature, the first channel passed through the subpyloric LN and the pancreas surface to the upper border of the pancreas (**c**), the second passed along the superior mesenteric artery to the para-aortic LN (**d**), and the third wound through the splenic hilus to the upper border of the pancreas (**e**).

Based on these studies, regional LNs of the stomach were anatomically classified into sixteen stations by the Japanese Research Society for Gastric Cancer in 1963 [3], and were grouped as N1, N2, N3, and N4 according to the location of the tumor (Fig. 3).

Complete removal of the N1 and N2 groups was called "R_2 dissection" or "systematic LN dissection", and was considered as being the minimum requirement for effective gastric cancer surgery and the standard surgical operation.

Rationale of Lymph Node Dissection Planning

Two factors should be considered when devising a plan for LN dissection for an individual patient. The first is the incidence of metastasis at each LN station, and the second is the survival rate of patients with metastasis at these LNs after the dissection [4]. These factors were studied using data from 5099 patients treated by means of gastric resection in the 23-year period from 1969 to 1991. Patients with early cancer ($n = 2171$) and distant metastasis ($n = 716$) were not considered as being appropriate for the evaluation of LN dissection, and were excluded, leaving 2212 patients for analysis in this study. Only 3.4% of the patients were lost to follow-up in this series. The N1 and N2 lymph nodes were completely dissected in all cases in this series and N3 and N4 nodes were also removed in most cases. All LNs were carefully dissected out from the resected specimen by attending surgeons. The histological results were reported separately for each LN station, and the results were recorded in the computer database.

The incidence of metastasis at each LN station is shown by a white bar in Fig. 4, and the 5YSR of metastatic patients treated by LN dissection (5YSR+meta) by the black bar at the same site. For example, the incidence was 12% and the 5YSR+meta was 41% at the LN along the celiac artery (LN No. 9) in cancer of the middle third of the stomach. Dissection of these nodes was indicated because of the high incidence of LN metastasis and apparent effectiveness of LN dissection. The figure shows also the effectiveness of LN dissection in the para-

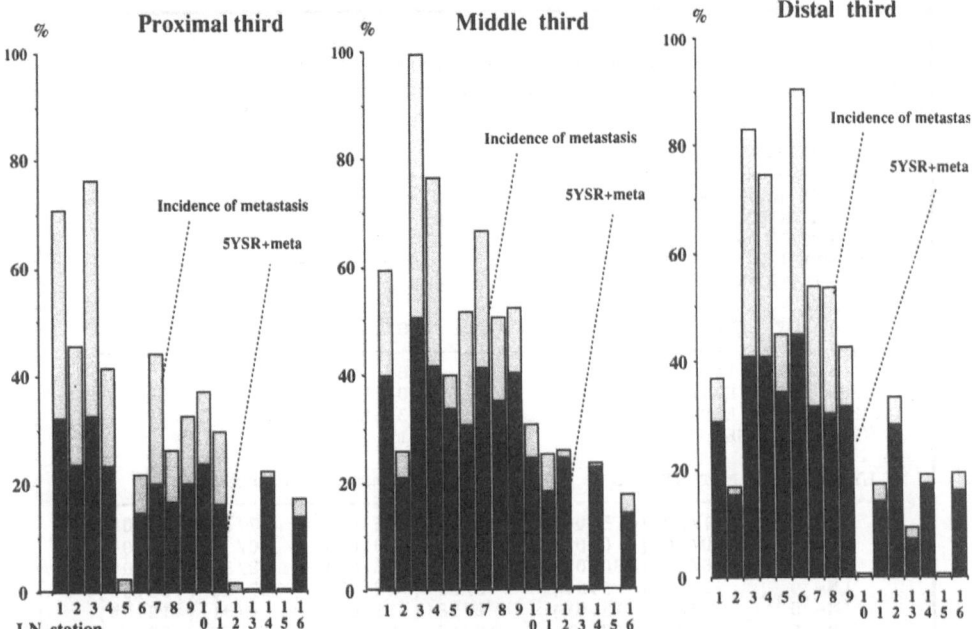

Fig. 4. Incidence of metastasis and 5-year survival rate (*5YSR*) of patients with metastasis (*meta*) at each lymph node (*LN*) station. There were 2212 patients treated by gastric resection in 1969–1991, excluding early cancer and distant metastasis

aortic area (LN No. 16): the 5YSR+meta was 14%, 14%, and 16% for proximal, middle, and distal cancer, respectively.

It is not easy to predict the incidence of metastasis and effectiveness of LN dissection for an individual patient, because these factors are co-related not only with tumor location but also with macroscopic type, depth of invasion, size of tumor, histological type, sex, and age. To resolve this complicated problem, a computer program was created at out department in 1984 [5, 6]. The initial database was provided from 3785 patients treated in 1969–1983. The seven above-mentioned variables were input preoperatively into the computer, which then predicted the 5YSR, incidence of metastasis at the 16 LN stations, likely cause of death, and probable curability by surgery (Fig. 5). A rational plan for optimal surgical approach could be made by reference to this report. The accuracy of the program was very high in a prospective study at our department: false negative results occurred in only 14 cases (1.8%) among 774 patients treated in 1984–1987. This program has been used at many hospitals abroad, and a study has revealed its high sensitivity and accuracy in patients treated in Germany [7] (Table 1).

```
PROGNOSIS AND LN-METASTASES OF THE PATIENTS WITH SAME BACKGROUND
treated by resection in National Cancer Center Tokyo, 1969-1983


   PATIENT           K.YAMAMOTO              92-352122
------------------------------------------------------------------
   SEX and AGE                      M    63 (+5/-5)
   MACROSCOPIC TYPE and DEPTH       B3   S1
   LOCATION                         A    L
   MAXIMAL DIAMETER                   6.0  cm  (+2.5/-2.5)
   HISTOLOGICAL TYPE                POR

[ DEPTH OF INVASION ] PM               S1                    S2
------------------------------------------------------------------
MACROSCOPIC TYPE       B3              B3                    B3
5 YEAR SURV. RATE      78.1%           50.1%                 42.8%
GREENWOOD 5% ERROR     22.6%           23.6%                 18.0%
NUMBER OF CASES        20              19                    34

[ LYMPH NODE METASTASIS ]  meta/dissect (meta% in group)
------------------------------------------------------------------
  LN- 1     1/20 (  5.0%)    3/18 ( 16.0%)     7/31 ( 21.0%)
  LN- 2     0/ 0 (  0.0%)    0/ 4 (  0.0%)     0/ 7 (  0.0%)
  LN- 3     6/20 ( 30.0%)   10/19 ( 53.0%)    28/33 ( 82.0%)
  LN- 4     1/20 (  5.0%)    8/19 ( 42.0%)    17/33 ( 50.0%)
  LN- 5     3/20 ( 15.0%)    2/18 ( 11.0%)     4/31 ( 12.0%)
  LN- 6     8/20 ( 40.0%)   10/18 ( 53.0%)    20/32 ( 59.0%)
  LN- 7     3/20 ( 15.0%)    7/19 ( 37.0%)    15/31 ( 44.0%)
  LN- 8     3/20 ( 15.0%)    7/19 ( 37.0%)    14/29 ( 41.0%)
  LN- 9     3/20 ( 15.0%)    3/18 ( 16.0%)     7/29 ( 21.0%)
  LN-10     0/ 0 (  0.0%)    0/ 3 (  0.0%)     0/ 0 (  0.0%)
  LN-11     0/ 8 (  0.0%)    2/ 7 ( 11.0%)     2/13 (  6.0%)
  LN-12     0/10 (  0.0%)    1/ 7 (  5.0%)     2/20 (  6.0%)
  LN-13     0/ 3 (  0.0%)    0/ 3 (  0.0%)     0/ 6 (  0.0%)
  LN-14     0/ 1 (  0.0%)    1/ 3 (  5.0%)     2/ 4 (  6.0%)
  LN-15     0/ 1 (  0.0%)    1/ 1 (  5.0%)     0/ 0 (  0.0%)
  LN-16     0/ 5 (  0.0%)    2/ 4 ( 11.0%)     1/ 7 (  3.0%)
------------------------------------------------------------------
[ CAUSE OF DEATH ]
LIVING NOW      15 ( 75.0%)      7 ( 37.0%)     10 ( 29.0%)
UNKNOWN          1 (  5.0%)      1 (  5.0%)      2 (  6.0%)
PERIT DISSEM     4 ( 20.0%)      4 ( 21.0%)      7 ( 21.0%)
HEPATIC META     0 (  0.0%)      2 ( 11.0%)      2 (  6.0%)
LOCAL RECURR     0 (  0.0%)      3 ( 16.0%)     10 ( 29.0%)
DISTANT META     0 (  0.0%)      1 (  5.0%)      0 (  0.0%)
RECURRENCE       0 (  0.0%)      0 (  0.0%)      0 (  0.0%)
DIRECT DEATH     0 (  0.0%)      0 (  0.0%)      0 (  0.0%)
OTHER CANCER     0 (  0.0%)      0 (  0.0%)      1 (  3.0%)
OTHER DISEASE    0 (  0.0%)      1 (  5.0%)      2 (  6.0%)
------------------------------------------------------------------
[ CURABILITY AT SURGERY ]
ABS CURATIVE    13 ( 65.0%)      8 ( 42.0%)     10 ( 29.0%)
REL CURATIVE     7 ( 35.0%)      6 ( 32.0%)     16 ( 47.0%)
REL NON-CURA     0 (  0.0%)      3 ( 16.0%)      2 (  6.0%)
ABS NON-CURA     0 (  0.0%)      2 ( 11.0%)      6 ( 18.0%)
------------------------------------------------------------------
```

Fig. 5. Example of a report from the computer system for preoperative estimation of the 5-year survival rate and lymph node metastasis of an individual patient. *5-Year surv*, 5-year survival; *LN*, lymph node; *meta*, metastasis; *dissect*, dissection; *Perit dissem*, peritoneal dissemination; *ABS*, absolute; *REL*, relative; *Non-cura*, non-curative

Table 1. Sensitivity, specificity, and accuracy of the computer program in 222 German patients with gastric cancer treated at Technical University, Munich (1986–89). (From [7]).

Lymph node station	No. 1–6	No. 7–12	No. 13–16
Sensitivity (%)	97	100	100
Specificity (%)	43	78	95
Positive predictive value (%)	80	83	86
Negative predictive value (%)	94	100	100
Accuracy (%)	82	89	96

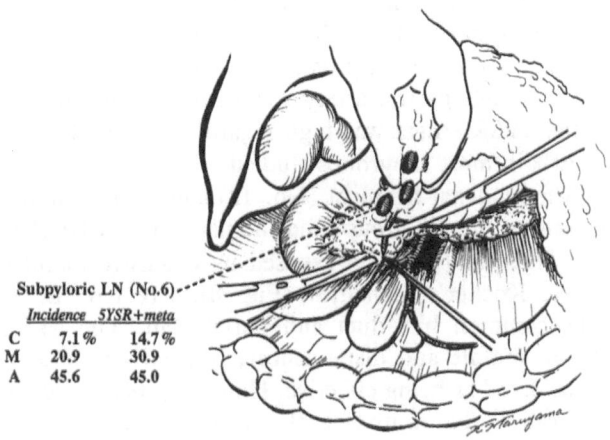

Subpyloric LN (No.6)

	Incidence	5YSR+meta
C	7.1%	14.7%
M	20.9	30.9
A	45.6	45.0

Fig. 6. Lymph node (*LN*) dissection of the subpyloric LN. *5YSR*, 5-Year survival rate; *meta*, metastasis; *C*, proximal third; *M*, middle third; *A*, distal third. (From [8] with permission)

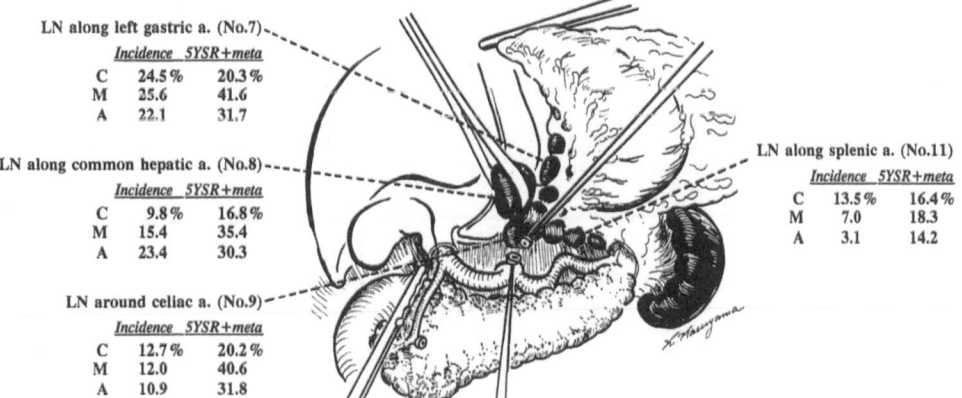

LN along left gastric a. (No.7)

	Incidence	5YSR+meta
C	24.5%	20.3%
M	25.6	41.6
A	22.1	31.7

LN along common hepatic a. (No.8)

	Incidence	5YSR+meta
C	9.8%	16.8%
M	15.4	35.4
A	23.4	30.3

LN around celiac a. (No.9)

	Incidence	5YSR+meta
C	12.7%	20.2%
M	12.0	40.6
A	10.9	31.8

LN along splenic a. (No.11)

	Incidence	5YSR+meta
C	13.5%	16.4%
M	7.0	18.3
A	3.1	14.2

Fig. 7. LN dissection along the upper border of the pancreas. *a*, Artery. Other abbreviations as in Fig. 6. (From [8] with permission)

Surgical Procedures Applicable for Systematic LN Dissection

The anatomical location and dissection technique of the subpyloric LN (No. 6) is shown in Fig. 6 [8]. The anterior sheet of the mesocolon was peeled off as the first step. Fatty tissue containing the LN was carefully removed from the middle colic and right gastro-epiploic veins, and then from the pancreatic parenchyma. Dissection of the LN No. 6 is very important for cancer of the middle and distal thirds, because the metastatic incidence and 5YSR+meta were 10.0% and 34.1%, respectively, in middle third cancer, and 26.4% and 47.2% in distal cancer.

LNs along the left gastric artery (No. 7), the common hepatic artery (No. 8), and the celiac artery (No. 9) are located along the upper border of the pancreas, and belong to the N2 group. The peritoneum is peeled off from the pancreas surface to expose these LNs. All fatty tissus was completely removed from these major arteries, and the left gastric artery was divided at its root (Fig. 7). It is noteworthy that the 5YSR+meta was high regardless of the location of tumor, being more than 30% in most subgroups studied.

LNs in the hepatoduodenal ligament (No. 12) and LNs behind the pancreas head (No. 13) belong to the N3 group, and the para-aortic LNs (No. 16) belong to the N4 group. These LNs can be exposed by extensive mobilization of the pancreas head, i.e., Kocher's maneuver (Fig. 8). LN No. 12 was detached carefully from the common bile duct and portal vein. The 5YSR+meta was 22.0% and 29.7% in middle and distal cancer, respectively, and the dissection was, therefore, considered as being effective. However, this dissection is not indicated for proximal cancer due to its lack of effectiveness , having a 5YSR+meta of 0%. The effectiveness of LN No. 13 dissection was also doubtful, because the

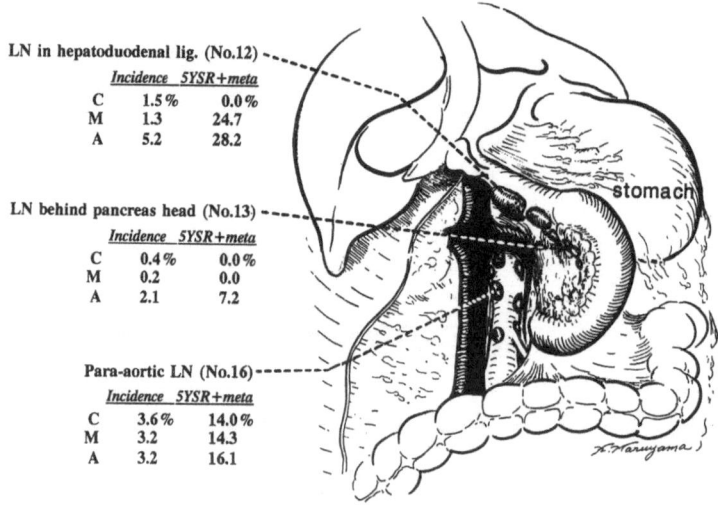

LN in hepatoduodenal lig. (No.12)

	Incidence	5YSR+meta
C	1.5%	0.0%
M	1.3	24.7
A	5.2	28.2

LN behind pancreas head (No.13)

	Incidence	5YSR+meta
C	0.4%	0.0%
M	0.2	0.0
A	2.1	7.2

Para-aortic LN (No.16)

	Incidence	5YSR+meta
C	3.6%	14.0%
M	3.2	14.3
A	3.2	16.1

stomach

Fig. 8. Mobilization of the pancreas head and lymph node (LN) dissection. *lig*, Ligament. Other abbreviations as in Fig. 5. (From [8] with permission)

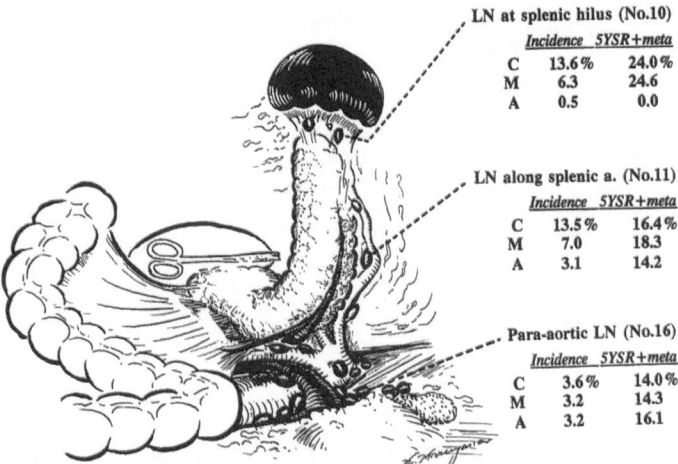

LN at splenic hilus (No.10)

	Incidence	5YSR+meta
C	13.6%	24.0%
M	6.3	24.6
A	0.5	0.0

LN along splenic a. (No.11)

	Incidence	5YSR+meta
C	13.5%	16.4%
M	7.0	18.3
A	3.1	14.2

Para-aortic LN (No.16)

	Incidence	5YSR+meta
C	3.6%	14.0%
M	3.2	14.3
A	3.2	16.1

Fig. 9. Mobilization of the pancreas-tail and LN dissection. *a*, Artery. Other definitions as in Fig. 5. (From [8] with permission)

incidence and 5YSR + meta were very low. The lower part of the para-aortic LN (No. 16b) can be observed after an extensive Kocher's maneuver, and can be removed by detachment from the surface of the vena cava, left renal vein, and abdominal aorta. The incidence of metastasis was low but the degree of effectiveness did not justify it. The incidence was 2.5%, 1.3%, and 1.4% in cancer of the proximal, middle, and distal thirds, respectively, and the 5YSR+meta was 13.8%, 12.0%, and 20.0%. It is noteworthy that these figures describing incidence and effectiveness are not altered by the location of the tumor.

In order to remove lymph nodes at the splenic hilus (No. 10), along the splenic artery (No. 11), and in the upper part of the para-aortic area (No. 16a), mobilization of the spleen and distal part of the pancreas is essential (Fig. 9). Splenectomy is necessary for the complete removal of LN No. 10, and the patients had no disadvantage from having undergone the procedure. Since the incidence of metastasis and effectiveness of LN dissection were very low in distal third cancer, splenectomy was not indicated. However, dissection of LN No. 10 is important for proximal and middle third cancer due to the high incidence of LN metastasis and satisfactory 5YSR+meta. Dissection of LN No. 11 is indicated for all gastric cancer regardless of the location, because the 5YSR+meta is similar: 15.9%, 19.0%, and 24.1% in cancer of the proximal, middle, and distal thirds, respectively.

Most nodes of the upper part of the para-aortic area (No. 16a) are located around the left renal artery and at the hilus of the left adrenal gland. For appropriate dissection of these LNs, the left kidney was sometimes mobilized and the left adrenal gland was frequently removed. The incidence of metastasis was

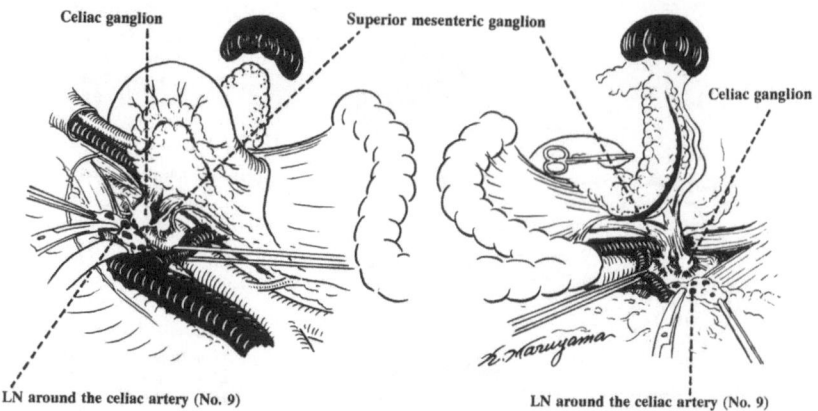

Fig. 10. Sparing of nerve ganglia around the celiac and superior mesenteric arteries. *LN*, Lymph node

low, 1.6% on the average. However, the effectiveness of dissection was moderate, with the 5YSR+meta having been 15.3%.

A new technique was introduced in 1986 to help assure complete LN dissection, "intra-operative lymphography" [9]. The staining medium is "India ink", which is simply an emulsion of fine particles of pure activated carbon (average particle diameter of 21 nanometer). When 0.5 ml of the solution is injected into a perigastric LN, all lymphatic vessels and LNs in the drainage area from the injection point are stained black within 1 min. All lymphatic tissues can be recognized easily by this staining, and it is very helpful for carrying out complete LN dissection. In addition, we could differentiate sympathetic nerve ganglions and major trunks from lymphatic tissue, and preserve the former (Fig. 10). This is effective in preventing postoperative disturbance of bowel movement and nutritional problems [10].

Advantages and Disadvantages of Systematic LN Dissection

The advantages and disadvantages of systematic LN dissection were studied using the previously described clinical material. The degree of LN dissection (R classification) correlated well with the survival rate. Complete removal of N1 and N2 was called "R_2 dissection", and was superior in terms of survival to R_1 and R_0 dissection. The 5YSR was 60.5% in the R_2 group, 31.4% in the R_1 group, and 15.1% in the R_0 group.

Table 2 shows that systematic LN dissection had a better 5YSR than non-systematic LN dissection in every stage.

The important prognostic factors for gastric cancer were studied by multivariate analysis (Fig. 11). The significance of each factor for prognosis is indicated

Table 2. Survival after systematic and non-systematic lymph node dissection of primary cancer excluding M1 (1972–1991).

Stage	Systematic (R₂, R₃)		Non-systematic (R₀, R₁)	
	5 y.s.rate (%)	Cases (n)	5 y.s.rate (%)	Cases (n)
I	93.1	1780	84.1[a]	477
II	73.9	461	64.0[a]	32
III	48.3	816	23.4[a]	58
IV	14.9	462	2.6[a]	398

[a] $P < 0.05$

5 y.s.rate, 5-Year survival rate (cumulative)

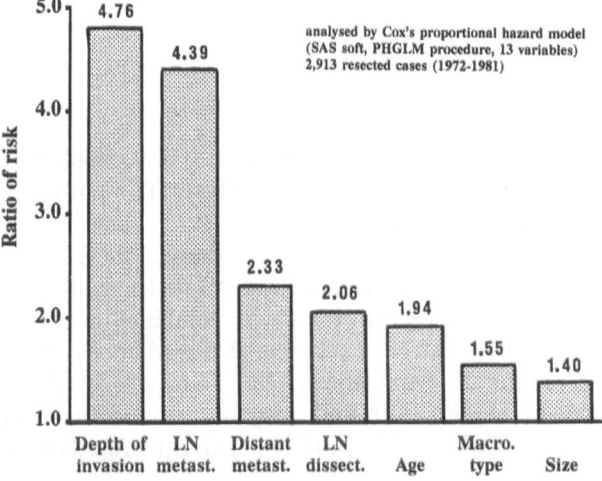

Fig. 11. Important prognostic factors in 2913 gastric cancer patients studied between 1972 and 1981 by multi-variate analysis by Cox's proportional hazard model (SAS soft, PHGLM procedure, 13 variables). *metast*, Metastasis; *LN*, lymph node; *dissect*, dissection; *Macro*, macroscopy

by the ratio of risk. The most important risk factor was depth of invasion, the second was LN metastasis, and the third was distant metastasis; the risk ratios were 4.76, 4.39, and 2.33, respectively. It was noteworthy that the "degree of LN dissection" occupied the fourth place. Its ratio of risk was 2.06; i.e., patients treated by systematic LN dissection have almost twice as good a survival rate as those treated by inadequate LN dissection.

The major effect of systematic LN dissection is in the reduction of local recurrence. The proportion of local recurrence has been decreased by the introduction of this procedure. It was 38% in the patients treated in the 5-year period from 1967 to 1971, but 16% in 1982–1986 (Fig. 12).

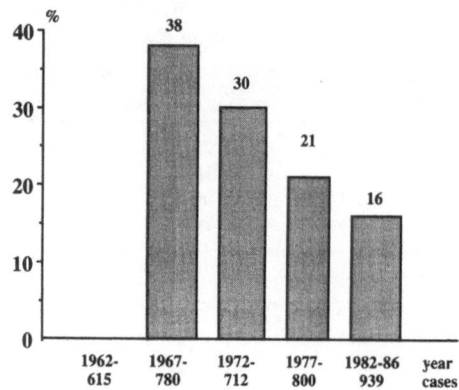

Fig. 12. Decrease of local recurrence over a 25-year period, excluding non-curative resection

What are the disadvantages of systematic LN dissection? It did not increase blood loss, postoperative mortality, or morbidity. The postoperative death rate was 2.3% in the first 10-year period (1962–1971), but improved to 0.4% in the last 10 years (1982–1991) (Fig. 1c). However, the procedure takes more operation time; we take 3 h and 15 min for distal gastric resection on the average, and 4 h and 55 min for total gastrectomy with combined resection of neighboring organs. The other disadvantage is subsequent disturbance of bowel function due to injury of nerves and the lymphatic system. To avoid such disturbance, we now try to preserve the nerve sheath and ganglions around the celiac and superior mesenteric arteries (Fig. 10). We think our current procedure is justified by its effectiveness.

Conclusion

The systematic LN dissection is one of the most effective procedures in the surgical treatment of gastric cancer. However, this treatment is not indicated for patients with distant metastasis. In addition, it does not increase postoperative mortality or morbidity. In our opinion, the minimal requirement for radical gastric resection is to completely remove the N1 and N2 lymph nodes.

Acknowledgments. This work was supported in part by a Grant-in-Aid for Cancer Research (91-03) from the Japanese Ministry of Health and Welfare, and by the Princess Takamatsu Cancer Research Fund (1992).

References

1. Inoue Y (1936) Lymphatic system around the stomach, duodenum, pancreas, and diaphragm. Jpn J Anat 9:35–117
2. Sawai K, Takahashi S, Kato G, Takenake A, Tokuda H (1985) Endoscopic injection of activated carbon particle (CH44) for extended radical lymphadenectomy of gastric cancer (in Japanese). Jpn J Gastroenterol Surg 18:912–917
3. Japanese Research Society for Gastric Cancer (1981) The general rules for gastric cancer study in surgery and pathology. Jpn J Surg 11:127–145
4. Maruyama K, Sasako M, Kinoshita T (1992) Role of systematic extended lymph node dissection, Japanese experience. Arch Chirurg Suppl (Kongressbericht) 130–135
5. Maruyama K, Gunven P, Okabayashi K, Sasako M, Kinoshita T (1989) Lymph node metastases of gastric cancer: General pattern in 1931 patients. Ann Surg 210:596–602
6. Kampschöer GHM, Maruyama K, van de Velde CJH, Sasoko M, Kinoshita T, Okabayashi K (1989) Computer analysis in making preoperative decisions: A rational approach to lymph node dissection in gastric cancer patients. Br J Surg 76:905–908
7. Bollschweiler E, Boettcher K, Hoelscher AH, Sasako M, Kinoshita T, Maruyama K, Siewert JR (1992) Preoperative assessment of lymph node metastases in patients with gastric cancer: Evaluation of the Maruyama computer program. Br J Surg 79:156–160
8. Maruyama K (1986) Surgical treatment and end results of gastric cancer. National Cancer Center Press, Tokyo
9. Maruyama K, Okabayashi K, Kinoshita T (1987) Progress in gastric cancer surgery in Japan and its limits of radicality. World J Surg 11:418–425
10. Maruyama K, Sasako M, Kinoshita T (1991) Preservation of sympathetic and vagal nerve system at gastric cancer surgery (in Japanese). Igaku-no Ayumi 159:898–900

Combined Resection

Mitsumasa Nishi, Keiichiro Ohta, and Toshifusa Nakajima[1]

Key words. Combined resection of gastric cancer—Lymphatic flow of the stomach—Lymph node metastases—Left thoracoabdominal approach—Pancreatoduodenectomy—Left upper abdominal evisceration—Survival rate

Introduction

The stomach is located adjacent to the pancreas, spleen, transverse colon and its mesenterium, and the diaphragm, and it is also connected directly with the esophagus and duodenum. Consequently, as gastric cancer progressively invades these organs. Metastasis of cancer into lymph nodes is often noted around or along the neighboring tissues or main blood vessels. (Fig. 1) [1]. Patients with such metastases in earlier times would not have had radical operations at all. As progress in surgical and anesthesiological techniques has, however, been made in recent years, radical operations to perform combined resection of gastric cancer and the neighboring organs can be safely conducted. The progress made in recent years in the control of respiration and parenteral nutrition has also contributed to the improvement of safety in these operations.

Combined resection is still important in gastric cancer despite the larger scale of operative aggression, since cancer infiltration metastasis are particularly notable in patients with gastric cancer and wide dissection and combined resection are effective and not so risky for bringing about improvements in therapeutic efficacy. Even if the excision of the gastric cancer is palliative, in not a few cases it can bring about improved symptoms and/or longer life expectancy. The combined resection of gastric cancer is technically easier and more worthwhile than is the case with cancers of other organs. The aim of combined resection in patients with gastric cancer is to ensure radicality so as not to overlook any carcinomatous cells. It is important in cancer operations to pay special attention

---

[1] Cancer Institute Hospital, 1-37-1 Kami-Ikebukuro, Toshima-ku, Tokyo, 170 Japan

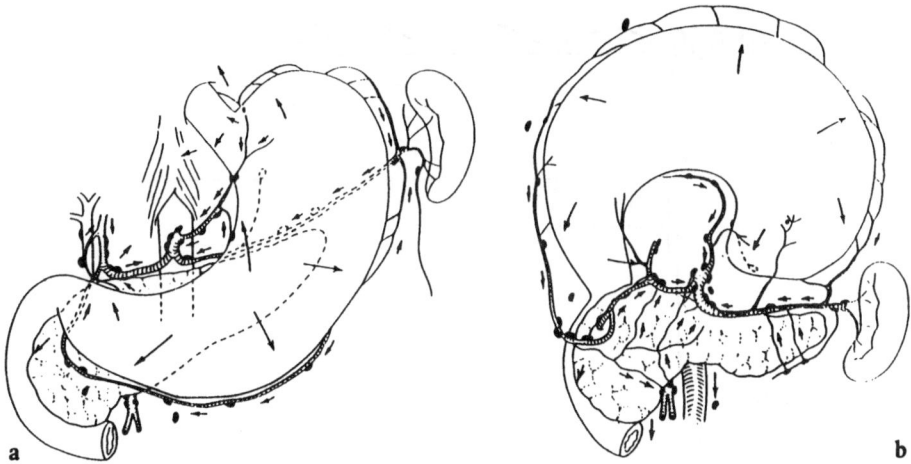

Fig. 1a,b. Lymphatic flow in stomach wall and perigastric lymphatic system. **a** Frontal view, **b** back view

to always keeping a balance among radicality, safety, and maintenance of organic function [2].

Combined Resection of Esophagus

Cancer of the upper stomach often infiltrates into the esophagus. In most cases of cancer of this kind, the cancer advances upward on the submucosal layer of the stomach, especially on the lower side of the mucosal muscle layer, while the outer side of the proper muscle layer is invaded subsequently (Fig. 2). For this reason, it is necessary to check the mucosal side for possible invasion by cancer cells even if the infiltration from the outer side is not distinct. It is also necessary to always pay attention to judgment of the upper limit of the advance of cancer cells on the oral side, not only before but also during the operation. On the other hand, patients in whom the cancer cells advance upward on the serosal side of the stomach tend to show infiltration in the scirrhous manner into the diaphragm and tend to be those for whom radical resection is not feasible. In patients with mucosal side infiltration by the gastric cancer, the resection should be made 2–3 cm away from the upper limit of grossly visible infiltration. In patients with the infiltrative type, the excision should be made more than 5 cm away from the upper limit of the cancer. In patients in whom resection of the esophagus is performed more than 4 cm from the esophagogastric junction, thoracotomy is absolutely necessary. Otherwise, neither the excision nor the dissection of lymph nodes can be fully attained, and thus the radical surgery cannot be fully completed and the safety of the anastomosis is endangered.

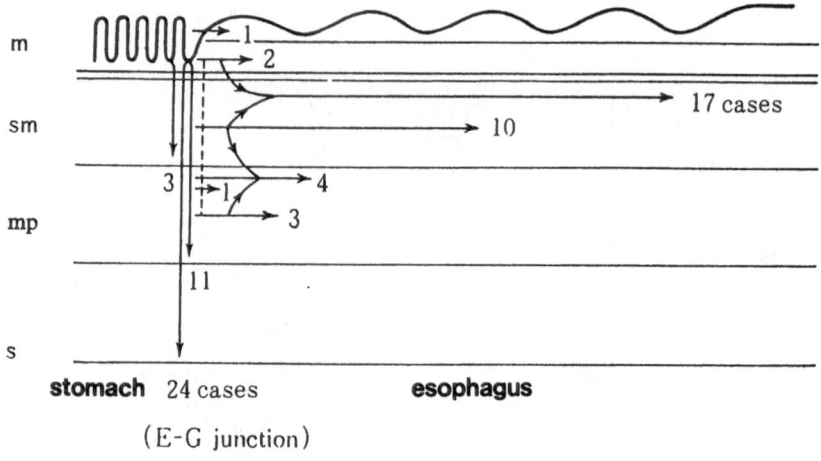

Fig. 2. Esophageal invasion of cardiac cancer in 38 cases (analysis of oral extension layer). *E-G*, esophagogastric; *m*, tunica mucosa; *sm*, tela submucosa; *mp*, tunica muscularis propria; *s*, tunica serosa

Generally, combined resection of the esophagus with gastric cancer is conducted by thoracotomy and laparotomy, providing a more aggressive approach. Therefore, the control of patients during and after the operation is of great importance.

We usually employ the following method, i.e., left-side thoracoabdominal approach with oblique incision of the trunk [3–5].

Body Position and Skin Incision

The body position should be 45° half right lateral decubitus, in which the left upper arm is stretched upward toward the right and is fixed onto a stand. The pelvic region is fixed with adhesive plaster. By revolving the operation table, the body position can also be changed to the dorsal decubitus and the fully lateral decubitus (Fig. 3).

The skin incision is made at the 6th or the 7th intercostal space, from the middle axillary line, traversing over the left costal arch and the median line of the upper abdomen in an arch style, and ending up on the right abdomen two finger widths downward from the right hypochondrium. The rectus abdominis muscle is cut traversely for laparotomy and the round ligament of the liver is ligatured. The thorax can thus be subjected to more extensive observation from the cardiac orifice to the diaphragm, which is positioned in the center of the observation range.

Fig. 3. Position and skin incision of
left thoracoabdominal approach

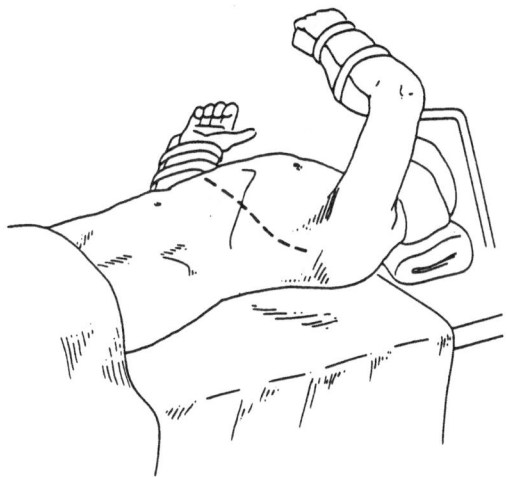

Incision of Diaphragm

With close care taken not to damage the left phrenic nerve, the diaphragm is incised in an arch style 3 cm forward and 7 cm backward from the outer side along the costal arch, by which even more extensive observation of the operative field is possible. In patients with cancer in the cardiac region, the hiatal muscle of the diaphragm around the esophageal hiatus is subjected to partial to combined as far as possible (Fig. 4).

Resection of Esophagus

The esophagus is resected 3–5 cm or more from the end of the oral side of the main focus. The resection can usually be made down to approximately 2 cm under the aortic arch. However, if metastasis into the esophageal wall can be seen extensively upward of the esophagus, the excision must be made in such a manner that the upper part of the esophagus over the aortic arch is resected up to around the neck by blunt dissection, thus finishing the total thoracoesophageal dissection. For cases of esophageal ablation, it is important to do the complete ligature of the proper esophageal artery branches branched from the aorta and to take enough care not to do an unnecessarily long ablation of the esophagus on the oral side that is to be left unoperated. In patients with lymph nodes metastasis up to the upper part of the mediastinum, metastasis is often also noted in the abdomen, and the extended spread of cancer inhibits the surgeon from performing a radical operation. Generally, in patients with infiltration of gastric cancer into the esophagus, in whom right thoracotomy is thus necessitated, the operation should proceed down to the esophageal hiatus while the lymph nodes in the paraesophageal area in the lower thorax and upper diaphragm are dissected,

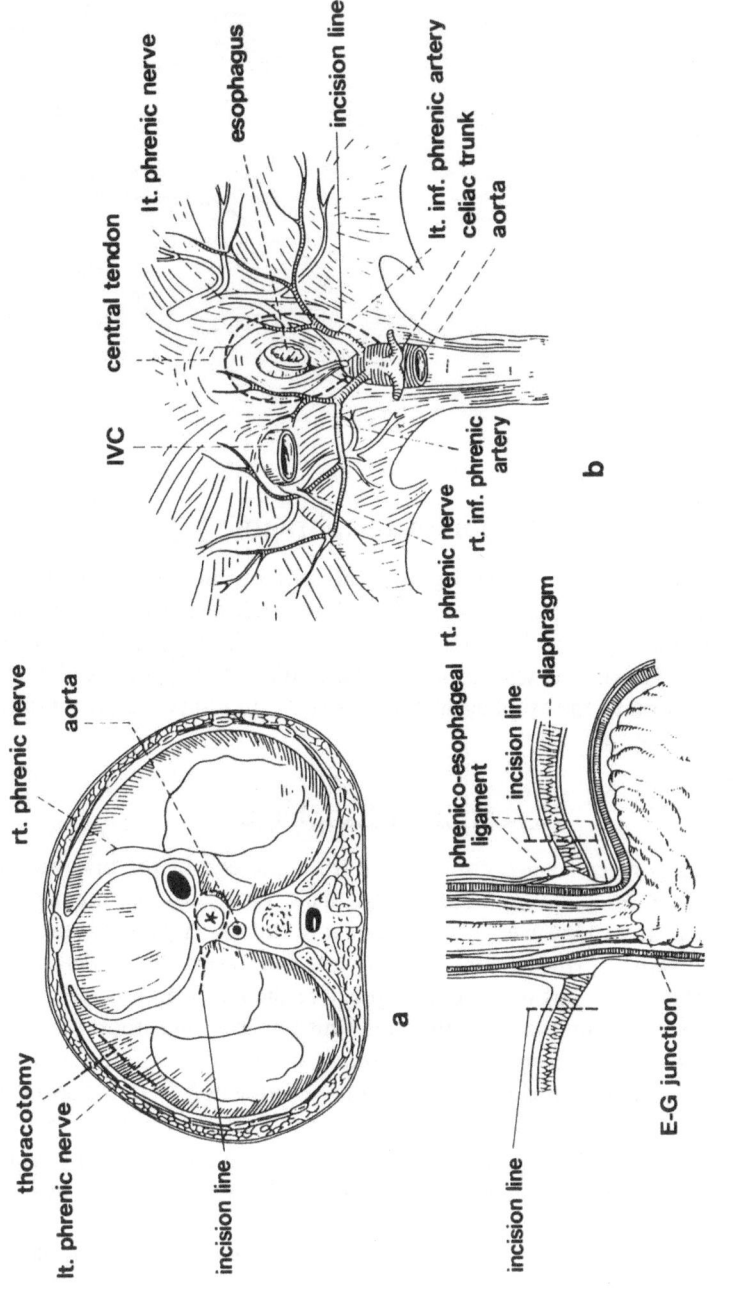

Fig. 4a–c. Incision of diaphragm. **a** pleural view, **b** abdominal view, **c** frontal view. *IVC* inferior vena cava

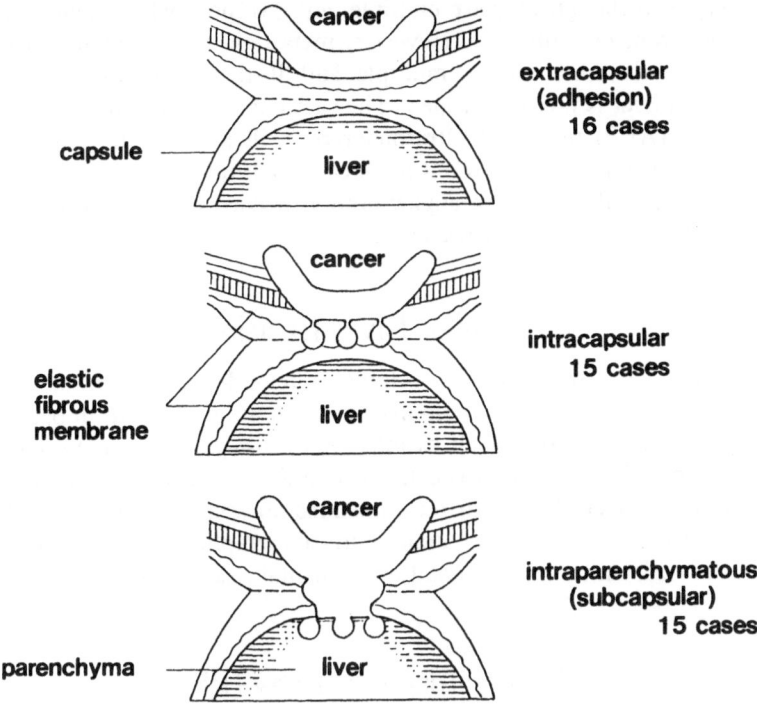

Fig. 5. Liver infiltration (analysis of combined hepatectomy cases)

and the muscles around the esophageal hiatus are subjected to partial combined resection.

Combined Resection of Liver

Because of its closeness to the liver, cancers in the gastric body or frontal cardiac wall tend to adhere to the left lobe of the liver and infiltrate into it. In patients with localized cancer, peritoneal dissemination occurs relatively rarely, and can be an indication for combined resection of the liver with the cancer. Our investigation of the adhesion or infiltration of gastric cancer into the liver revealed that in approximately one-third of cases the cancers remained outside the liver capsule, in one-third they infiltrated the capsule, and in one-third they had invaded the liver parenchyma (Fig. 5).

Indications for Combined Resection of Liver

Patients in whom this is indicated include (1) those whose general condition is still good and who could be expected to tolerate radical resection, (2) those whose metastatic foci are either isolated or localized within a certain region and are few in number, even though they are multiple, and (3) those whose cancers are only partially adherent or infiltrated. However, metastatic foci occurring in the liver via the blood flow are mostly multiple and if these are present, combined resection with liver is rarely indicated. The carcinoembryonic antigen (CEA) test, α-fetoprotein (AFP) test, and ultrasonography, in addition to general hepatic function tests, should be carried out in all cases. Also, CT scanning is needed for those with advanced cancer and angiography is needed for those in whom cancer spread into liver is strongly suspected.

Range of Liver Excision

Approximately 70% of total liver volume is regarded as the limit in normal treatments, but it is dangerous to do liver excision up to the limit in patients with large operative intervention such as total gastrectomy or that required in liver cirrhosis. Generally speaking, it is believed that the excision should be within two segments of the liver. It is also recommended to assess the blood vessels distributed in the operable region under ultrasonographic guidance and then to perform the excision as subsegmental or segmental resection [6].

Pancreatosplenectomy (PS)

The full length of the stomach is anatomically located adjacent to the pancreas. Consequently, gastric cancer infiltrates the pancreas either via the stomach-supporting tissues, both via anatomically connected organs and via the lymphatic flow, or by adhesion of the stomach to the pancreas. The large lymphatic flow from the stomach runs into the area of the celiac artery over the pancreatic body (head side) and over the mesenteric root under the pancreatic body. Lymph nodes around and behind the pancreas are frequently involved, and it is necessary to fully remove the metastatic lymph nodes in combination with pancreatectomy. If a radical operation is to be conducted in patients with locally advanced gastric cancer, combined resection of the pancreas with the stomach is often theoretically indicated.

This method (PS) is indicated for those patients with invasion of gastric cancer into the pancreas via its left side, and for those in whom metastasis is positive or strongly suspected in the splenic hilum or in the lymph nodes along the splenic artery. This PS is conducted, of course, in combination with total or proximal gastrectomy [7–9].

The resection of the pancreas in most cases will have to be over a wide region if there is direct invasion from the focus. If the metastasis into the lymph nodes around the splenic artery is not clear, the pancreas is separated on the central side just before the branching of the posterior gastric artery. The splenic veins are generally separated by a ligature on the periphery of the joint of the inferior mesenteric vein.

Pancreatoduodenectomy (PD)

Radical operation is often difficult in patients in whom the gastric cancer has infiltrated into the pancreatic head or into the duodenum. PD is theoretically indicated for producing extirpation of the cancer with sufficient surrounding normal tissues so that there is a surgical margin free of cancer. As metastasis in the lymph nodes takes place very close to the whole or dorsal surface of the pancreas, PD is conducted as an expanded operative method. To improve the late results of this operation, further elaboration is needed, in terms of the safety of the operation and preservation of postoperative digestive function.

Unlike the case with pancreatic cancer, ablation of the pancreas from important blood vessels like the portal vein is rather simple, and the operative intervention with such a procedure is not great. Histological examination of the resected specimens after PD revealed that the duodenum was involved in 28% of all cases and that 81% of dissected subpyloric lymph nodes (No. 6 in Fig. 6) were positive for metastasis, while 30% of dissected retropancreatic lymph nodes (No. 13 in Fig. 6) and 32% of dissected lymph nodes around the mesenteric root (No. 14 in Fig. 6) were positive for metastasis. Invasion into the pancreas was noted not only

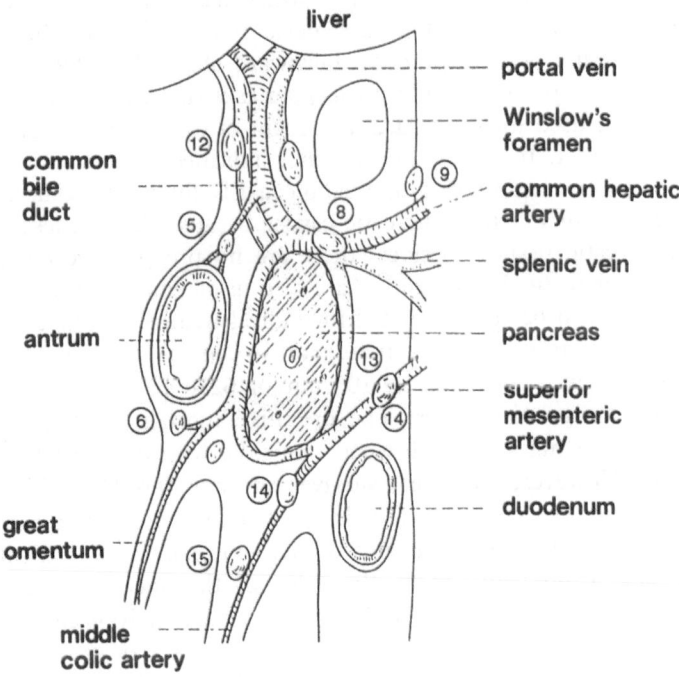

Fig. 6. Sagittal section of pancreas head region and lymph node: *5*, suprapyloric; *6*, subpyloric; *8*, retropyloric; *9*, around celiac trunk; *12*, intrahepatoduodenal ligament; *13*, retropancreatic; *14*, mesenteric root; *15*, around middle colic artery

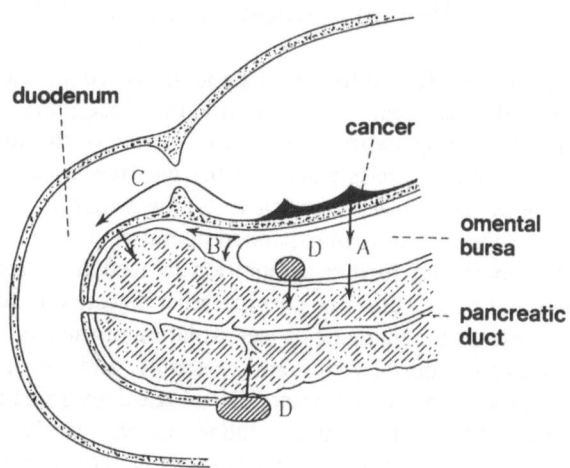

Fig. 7. Invasion into pancreas *A*, direct; *B*, subserosal via peritoneal reflection; *C*, extraluminal from duodenal invasion; *D*, secondary from nodal involvement

in the main focus but also in the secondary infiltration from the metastatic lymph nodes or via the veins (Fig. 7). Cancer which has invaded the pancreatic head area tends to invade from the mesenteric root to its periphery, and from the retropancreatic head upward or downward along the inferior vena cava or abdominal aorta; operative results are as poor as is the case for pancreatic cancer.

PD has been used for the radical treatment of cancers in the pancreatic head region or bile duct. In Japan, PD was first indicated for gastric rather than for pancreatic cancer. The process of ablation in PD for gastric cancer is generally easier than that in PD for pancreatic cancer because there is less invasion into the peripancreatic tissues. Besides, there are no preoperative complications of jaundice or pancreatic dysfunction as are seen in patients with pancreatic cancer. Therefore, PD can be recommended for radical treatment, but careful selection of its indications, technique, and postoperative control is mandatory.

This method was employed in 103 out of 6236 patients in our institution (1960–1989) for gastric cancer. The operative mortality within 1 month was 6.3%, which does not seem high when compared with the mortality of standard gastrectomy. However, the 5-year survival rate was only 8%, which was not as high as we had expected. Nevertheless, even in those patients who died, it brought about considerable elongation of life, and many of the patients so treated were liberated from pain. Thus, the value of this method as a conservative techniques can be accepted. Generally speaking, highly advanced cancer invading the pancreas adheres to or infiltrates the common hepatic or proper hepatic artery at the same time, which results in difficult ablation. Further, the infiltration of cancer into the lower edge of the pancreas and the mesenteric root of the transverse colon, and remarkable metastasis into lymph nodes often causes difficult ablation. Prognosis may be better if PD is employed in patients where it is properly indicated and in those who have no progression of cancer; however, assessment of such patients is difficult.

Left Upper Abdominal Evisceration

In order to resect gastric cancer foci which are exposed or which have infiltrated the serosal side or its surrounding tissues, in such a manner as to include the foci together with the surrounding organs, we have devised a method for total combined resection, including total gastrectomy, and for resection of the organs surrounding the stomach. This method was designated as left upper abdominal evisceration (LUAE) and has been employed since June of 1980 [10–12].

Organs to Be Resected by the Basic Method for LUAE

This method consists of combined resection of the transverse colon with its mesocolon, as well as total gastrectomy and pancreatosplenectomy. Organs to be resected concomitantly sometimes include the esophagus, diaphragm, left hepatic lobe, left adrenal gland, and left kidney.

Operative Technique

The skin incision is normally a reverse T-form incision produced by adding a median incision of the upper part to the oblique incision. The left thoraco-abdominal approach is recommended for the eradication of esophageal invasion. The standard technique consists of lifting the transverse colon, dividing the base of the mesocolon, proceeding to the splenic flexure and then to the retroperitoneum, and lifting the colon, pancreas, spleen, and stomach from the dorsal side to facilitate performing the total gastrectomy and pancreatosplenectomy. It is important to perform this total resection by wrapping up all the organs in the left upper abdomen and not by individually excising each of the organs.

Mobilization of the left kidney and adrenal gland is done by separating the peritoneum at the outer side of the left kidney and lifting up the left kidney and left adrenal gland toward the medial side. Extensive mobilization of the pancreas, spleen, and the organs in the posterior peritoneal lumen facilitates lymph node dissection around the aorta. The lymph nodes on the left renal vein are located less than 5 cm from the cardiac orifice, the posterior wall of the upper stomach, and the left cardiac lymph nodes, and they have a thick lymphatic canal running directly into the area to be operated. The lymph nodes above the left renal vein are important as sentinels over paraaortic node involvement; proper dissection of these nodes sometimes provides long survivors. If there is metastasis noted in this area, excision of the left adrenal gland will bring about higher radicality. The left kidney and the left renal artery and vein are left intact and returned to their original positions after the dissection. Figure 8a illustrates the range of the resection. In this Fig., the region outside the left hepatic lobe is also resected. In

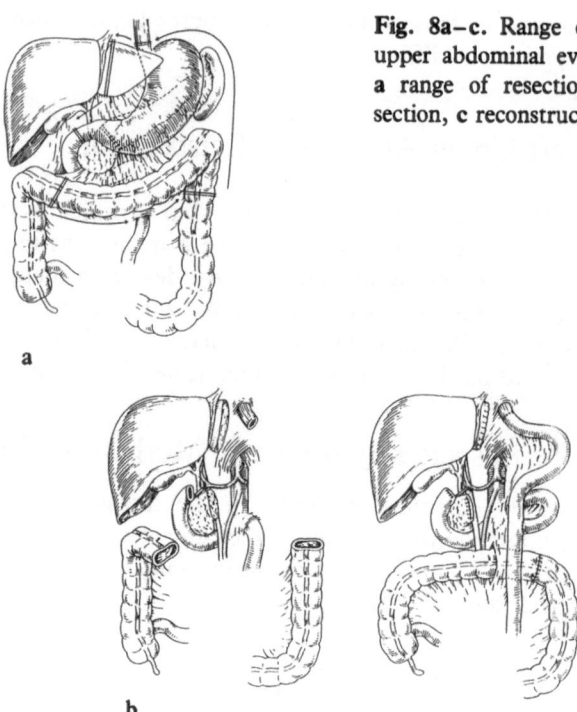

Fig. 8a–c. Range of resection of left upper abdominal evisceration (*LUAE*). **a** range of resection, **b** after the resection, **c** reconstruction

a

b   c

patients with upper gastric cancer, the esophagus is resected and the pancreas is excised at the superior mesenteric and portal veins. Figure 8 parts b and c illustrate views of the completed operation and the reconstruction method, respectively. The reconstruction is conducted in accordance with the double tract or Roux-en-Y method. The colon is treated by colo-colonic anastomosis via the retrojejunal way and via the jejunal mesenterium.

Postoperative Complications

The frequency of postoperative complications is as high as 57.0%; it is necessary to reduce the possible complications as far as possible. However, this method has greater safety and fewer postoperative complications and complaints from patients than PD or Appleby's method.

Indications

LUAE is mainly indicated for those gastric cancers located in the upper or middle parts of the stomach, and for those with (1) infiltration on the serosal side identified over a relatively large area, especially in the greater curvature or dorsal wall of stomach, (2) the beginning of lymphatic permeation into the tissues

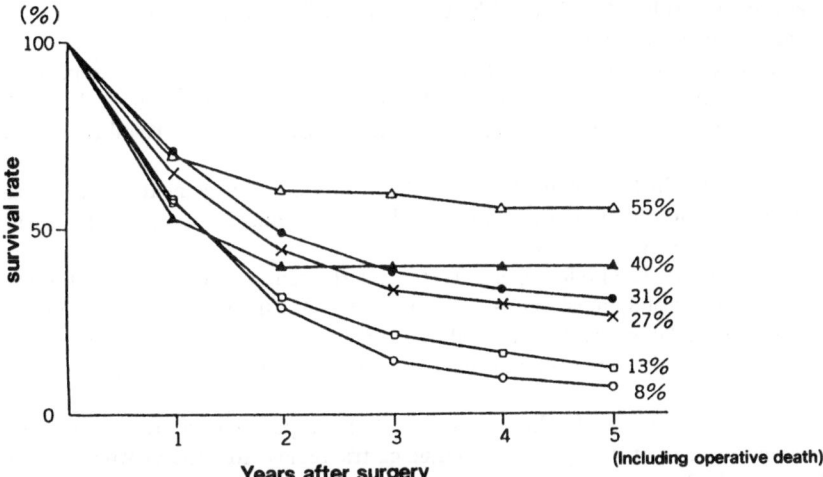

Fig. 9. Gastrectomy with combined resection of adjacent organs and survival rate (Total cases of single cancer resection, 1960–1989). *Open triangles*, Splenectomy (*n* = 105); *closed triangles* transverse partial pancreatectomy (*n* = 18); *crosses*, colonic resection (*n* = 164); *closed circles*, pancreatosplenectomy (*PS*; *n* = 1351); *open circles*, pancreatoduodenectomy (*PD*; *n* = 103); *open squares*, left upper abdominal evisceration (*LUAE*; *n* = 141)

surrounding the stomach, (3) direct infiltration of cancers or metastases into the stomach or neighboring lymph nodes or into the organs surrounding the stomach, or (4) the beginning of a small number of disseminations into the peritoneum, i.e., into the lesser, or greater omentum, or into the mesocolon, especially when the dissemination remains within the omental bursa. LUAE provides greater radicality than the standard gastrectomy in patients with S2, S3, or P1 disease.

Prognosis

The prognosis of LUAE is as shown in Fig. 9. Localized relapse is more or less prevented with LUAE, even though complete cure may not be possible. Proper evaluation of LUAE might require a greater number of cases to confirm its clinical significance.

References

1. Nishi M, Ohashi I, Ohta K, Kajitani T (1990) Cancer metastasis in lymphatic system. In: Nishi M, Uchino S, Yabuki S (eds) Progress in lymphology-XII, proceedings of the XII international congress of lymphology. Excerpta Medica, Amsterdam, pp 39–44
2. Nishi M, Nakajima T, Kajitani T (1986) The Japanese Research Society for Gastric Cancer—General rules for gastric cancer study and an analysis of treatment results

based on the rules. In: Preece PE, Cuschieri A, Wellwood JM (eds) Cancer of the stomach. Grune and Stratton, London, pp 107–121

3. Nishi M, Ohashi I, Ohta K (1986) Resection of cancer of the lower esophagus and cardia, reconstruction and left thoracoabdominal approach (in Japanese). In: Nishi M (ed) The lastest therapy 1, therapy of esophageal cancer. Igaku Kyoiku, Tokyo, pp 145–162

4. Nishi M, Ohashi I, Azekura K, et al (1985) Surgical management of gastric cancer infiltrating into the esophagus by left thoracoabdominal approach (in Japanese). Gastroenterol Surg 8:1469–1476

5. Nishi M, Ohta K (1988) Operation for gastric cancer with esophageal invasion: Oblique thoracoabdominal approach (in Japanese). Gastroenterol Surg 10:1582–1593

6. Makuuchi M, Hasegawa H, Yamazaki S (1983) Progress in hepatic surgery owing to intraoperative ultrasonic monitoring (in Japanese). Gastroenterolog Surg Semin 13:151–173

7. Nakajima T, Yamase H, Ohta H, et al (1983) Application of pancreatosplenic resection to cancer of the upper and middle gastric region from the viewpoint of radical lymph node dissection (in Japanese). Jpn J Gastroenterol Surg 16:1650–1655

8. Ohta K, Nishi M, Nakajima T, et al (1989) Indication of pancreatico-splenectomy for upper gastric cancer (in Japanese). Jpn J Gastroenterol Surg 22:2477–2481

9. Ohta K, Nishi M, Nakajima T, et al (1989) Indication for total gastrectomy combined with pancreaticosplenectomy in the treatment of middle gastric cancer (in Japanese). J Jpn Surg Soc 90:1326–1330.

10. Kajitani T, Takagi K, Ohashi I (1981) Radical surgery for gastric cancer (left side lymph node dissection) (in Japanese). Geka Shinryo 23:412–417

11. Nakajima T, Kajitani T, Nishi M, et al (1987) Left upper abdominal evisceration for gastric cancer (in Japanese). Prog Cancer Clin 14:140–145

12. Ohta K, Nishi M, Nakajima T (1988) Results of left upper abdominal evisceration for diffuse infiltrating carcinoma of the stomach (in Japanese). Jpn J Cancer Chemother 15 (Part II):1249–1255

Treatment Results of Gastric Cancer Patients: Japanese Experience

Taira Kinoshita, Keiichi Maruyama, Mitsuru Sasako, and Kazuo Okajima[1]

Introduction

The Japanese Research Society for Gastric Cancer (JRSGC) was established in 1962, and promoted actively, basic study as well as clinical management of the disease. Leading institutions of Japan, 311 in all, participated in the society; 214 were involved with surgical oncology, 54 medical oncology, 11 radiology, and 32 basic research. In order to standardize the documentation of diagnosis, treatment, and pathological findings, the society published a manual in 1962; "The General Rules for Gastric Cancer Study in Surgery and Pathology" [1]. The manual had been periodically improved and the 12th edition is now in use. The JRSGC and the National Cancer Center started a nationwide data collection of gastric cancer patients in 1963 using the mannual. Approximately 10 000 new patients had been registered annually from the member institutions. This registration was considered to cover approximately 16% of the gastric cancer patients in Japan. The collected data were analyzed by computer, and the results were published as annual reports (Fig. 1). The results showed the characteristics of gastric cancer as well as the latest situation of diagnosis and treatment of gastric cancer patients in Japan. Using the nationwide database, we revealed the results of gastric cancer treatments in Japan.

Patients and Methods: Patient Registration System in Japan

The 51 676 primary gastric cancer patients treated in the 16 years from 1963–1978 were registered in a nationwide database, and their analyses, including follow-up data, were published [2]. The data were collected from almost 130 leading institutions, mainly from Departments of Surgery. Each institution was requested to have surgical oncologists and a full time pathologist, and to report

[1] Department of Surgical Oncology, National Cancer Center Hospital East, 6-5-1 Kashiwanoha, Kashiwa, Chiba 7, 27 Japan

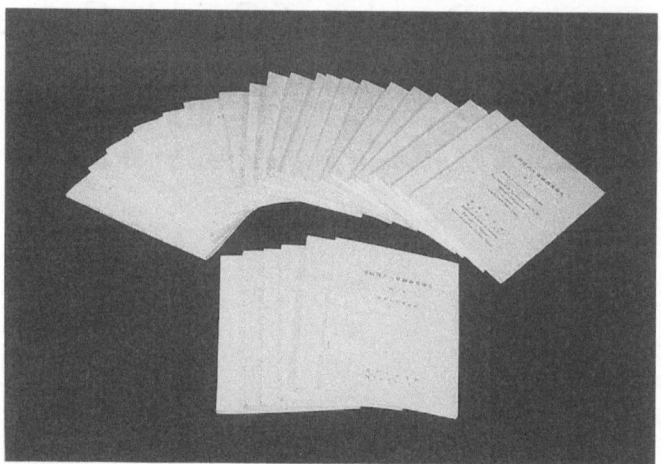

Fig. 1. Annual reports of nationwide registration of gastric cancer patients in Japan. Gastric cancer patients treated in 1962–1979 were registered and analyzed, and the results were published in 31 reports by the JRSGC. The losted to follow-up was only 1216 out of 51 674 patients, 2.4%

Table 1. 5 year survival rate and number of patients analyzed[a].

	First period (1963–1966) Nationwide	Second period (1969–1973) Nationwide	Third period (1974–1978) Nationwide	Fourth period (1979–1990) NCC
%	%	%	%	%
Registered cases	29.8 (8411)	45.4 (15 589)	47.4 (27 676)	69.2 (2987)
Resected cases	(6050)	(12 535)	(23 543)	72.0 (2824)
Available cases	44.3 (5706)	56.3 (11 845)	57.8 (21 976)	72.0 (2824)
Surgical death	(231)	(273)	(382)	(7)
Analyzed cases	44.3 (5475)	56.3 (11 572)	57.8 (21 524)	72.0 (2824)
Losted to follow-up	(48)	(244)	(767)	(19)

[a] The data were divided in four periods; The first period (1963–66), the second (1969–73), the third (1974–78) from the Nationwide registry, and the fourth (1979–90) from National Cancer Center Tokyo.

the detailed individual data using a special registration form. An important requirement for member institutions was a high follow-up rate. If the 5-year follow-up rate was less than 80%, the data were not accepted for the database.

In order to know trends of gastric cancer in Japan, the nationwide database was divided in three periods; the first was 1963–1966, the second 1969–1973, and the third 1974–1978. To know the latest treatment results, data from the National Cancer Center 1979–1990 were added as a fourth period (Table 1). Treatment results from the National Cancer Center might be a little superior to member hospitals, but not significantly different. Registered numbers were 8411, 15 589,

27 676, and 2987 in the first, second, third and fourth periods respectively. Excluding patients with no resection, double cancer, and surgical death, the analyzed patients were in total 5475, 11 572, 21 524, and 2824 in the first, second, third and fourth periods respectively.

Losted to follow-up cases were 48, 244, 767, and 19 (0.9%, 2.1%, 3.6%, and 0.7%), in the first, second, third, and fourth periods respectively. Survival was calculated by relative 5-year survival rate; i.e., the age and sex adjusted method. The categories were defined by the General Rules of the JRSGC. Nationwide registration included "unknown" data. We documented the number of cases and their 5-year survival rates in tables.

Results: Trends of Treatment Results in Japan

Figure 2 shows improvement of survival rate among the four periods. Five-year survival rate was 44.3% in the first period, but it was elevated to 72.0% by the fourth period. This improvement was produced both by early detection and progress of surgical treatment.

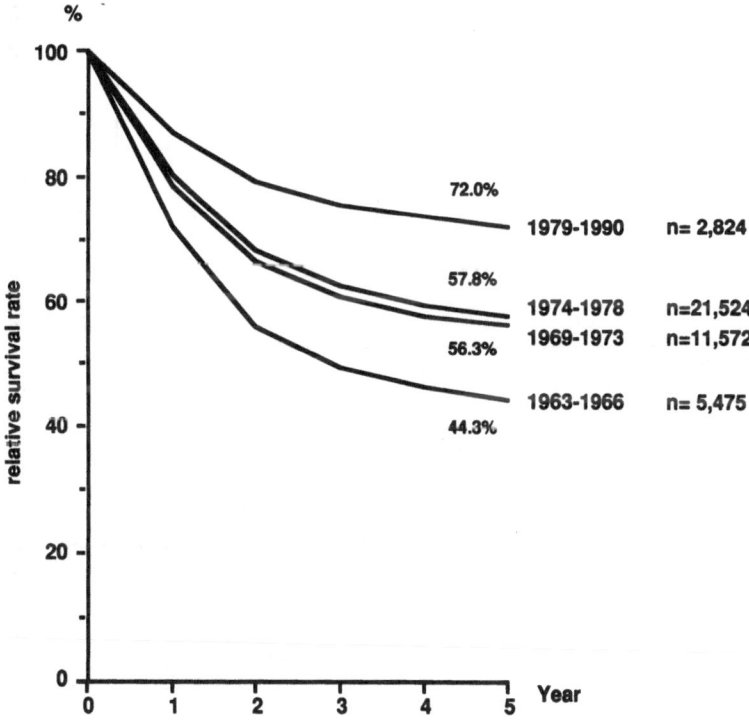

Fig. 2. Improvement of the survival rate for gastric cancer patients. Five-year survivial rates were elevated in a 28-year period. It was 44.3%, 56.3%, 57.8%, and 72.0% in the first (1962–1966), the second (1969–1973), the third (1974–1978), and the fourth (1979–1990) periods respectively

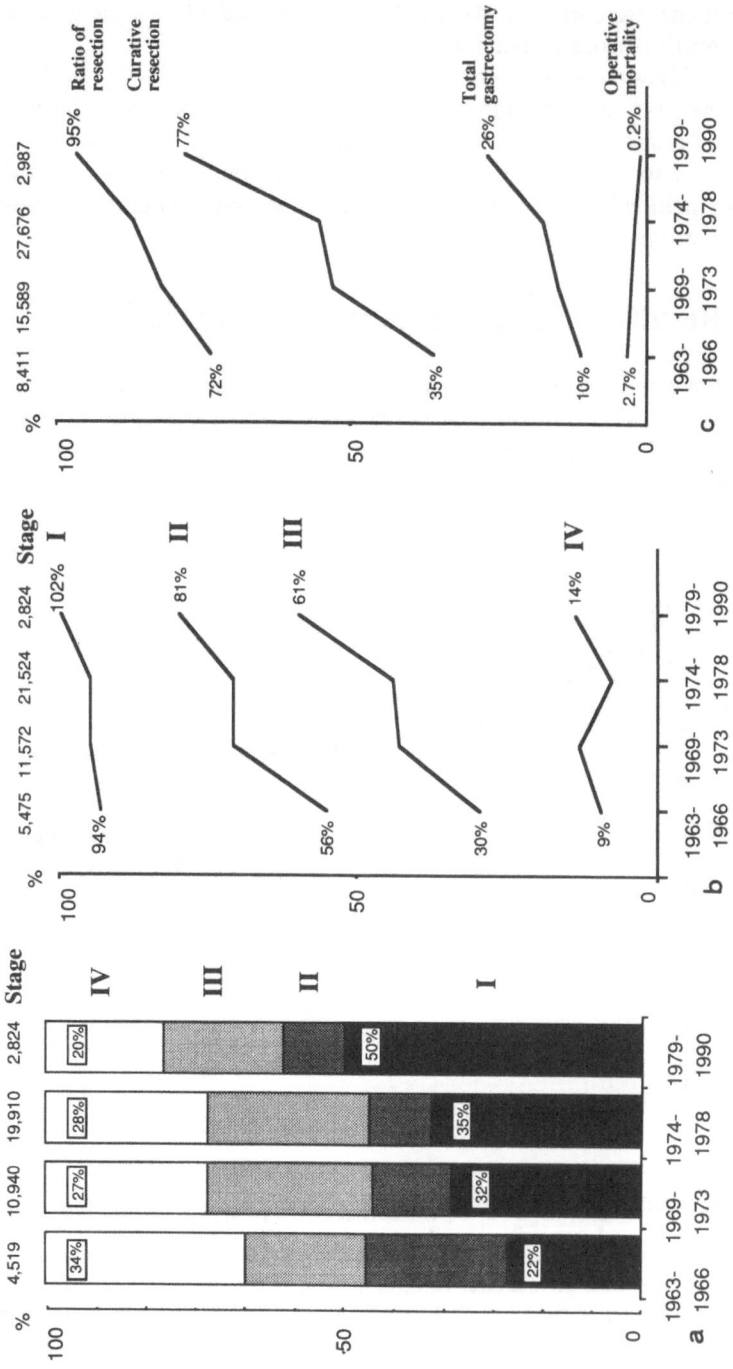

Fig. 3a–c. Trend of stage-proportion, 5-year survival rates by stage, surgical treatments, and operative mortality. These figures show increases in early stage cancer (**a**), improvement of treatment results by stage (**b**), increase of extended surgery, and decrease of operative mortality (**c**)

Figure 3a shows continuous increase of early stage cancer in Japan. Proportion of stage I cancer was only 27.2% in the first period, but increased to 49.6% by the last period. Proportion of early gastric cancer increased also from 14.6% to 47.4%. The improvement was produced by progress of diagnostic methods and establishment of a mass screening system in Japan.

Figure 3b shows elevation of 5-year survival rates in every stage. Five-year survival rates were remarkably elevated in stages II and III; from 60.6% to 87.4% in stage II and from 32.7% to 60.1% in stage III. It was also elevated in stage I; from 93.5% to 102.4%. However, the elevation was not significant in stage IV; from 5.8% to 13.9%. We considered that the improvement was produced mainly by progress of surgical treatment, particularly systematic lymph node (LN) dissection.

Figure 3c shows trends of surgical treatment in Japan. The resection rate has risen from 71.9% to 94.5%; the proportion of curative resection was also elevated from 35.2% to 76.6%. Total gastrectomy increased from 10.4% to 26.1%, and systematic lymph node dissection (R2 and R3 dissection) was also more frequently performed, rising from 37.0% to 73.6%. We were very much delighted to know that the mortality rate (death rate within the 30 post operative days) decreased from 2.7% to 0.2%. These data show the progress of surgical treatment, and that this progress was quickly and widely popularized.

Table 2 shows sex and age distribution; Fig. 4 shows from the nationwide registration 1974–78 in more detail. The male to female ratio was almost 2:1 in age groups more than 40-years old. In Fig. 4, the highest peak was observed in the 60- to 69-years age group in both sexes.

Survival of patients was significantly influenced by depth of invasion (Table 3). The table shows also the remarkable improvements of survival rates in the middle layers, but not in the other invaded organs. Five-year survival rate was strongly correlated with extension of LN metastasis, which was considered an important prognostic factor (Table 4). Improvements of survival rates were remarkable in cases with LN metastasis in the pN0, pN1, and pN2 nodes, but not in metastasis in the pN3 and pN4 nodes. Prognosis of patients with peritoneal and liver metastasis was very poor; less than 10% (Table 5).

Table 2. Sex and age distribution.

		First period (1963–1966) Nationwide	Second period (1969–1973) Nationwide	Third period (1974–1978) Nationwide	Fourth period (1979–1990) NCC
		%	%	%	%
Sex	Male	44.6 (3592)	56.9 (7528)	58.7 (13695)	74.0 (1917)
	Female	43.6 (1883)	55.2 (4044)	56.3 (7829)	70.9 (907)
Age	<50	45.7 (1562)	61.3 (3452)	63.0 (5837)	73.7 (597)
	50–69	44.4 (3482)	54.3 (6795)	57.7 (12186)	73.5 (1580)
	>70	41.7 (431)	50.8 (1325)	53.2 (3501)	73.3 (647)

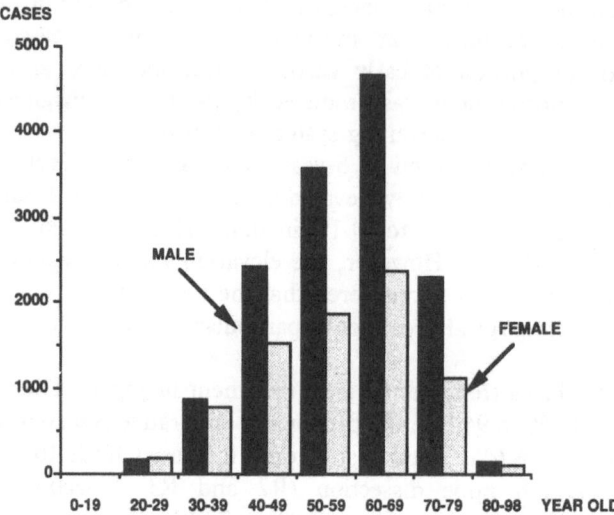

Fig. 4. Sex and age distribution in nationwide registration of gastric cancer patients in 1974–1978. Patients in the 60–69 age range were the highest both for male and female. The male to female ratio was almost 2:1. *Closed bars*, male; *Open bars*, female

Table 3. Five-year survival rates by depth of invasion.

	First period (1963–1966) Nationwide	Second period (1969–1973) Nationwide	Third period (1974–1978) Nationwide	Fourth period (1979–1990) NCC
	%	%	%	%
Mucosa	101.6 (356)	99.8 (1409)	100.1 (2889)	102.8 (743)
Submucosa	90.3 (421)	95.5 (1527)	94.8 (2984)	99.5 (596)
Muscularis propria	70.2 (632)	80.1 (1338)	78.9 (2541)	90.5 (281)
Subserosa	49.8 (766)	57.1 (1096)	51.9 (3669)	84.1 (192)
Serosa (suspected)	39.6 (725)	46.4 (1044)		74.9 (63)
Serosa (definite)	22.1 (1456)	30.0 (3776)	31.4 (6666)	42.0 (606)
Other organ	7.3 (526)	15.7 (1094)	15.1 (2100)	15.3 (343)
Unknown	29.2 (593)	46.3 (288)	47.9 (675)	— (0)

Five-year survival rates were closely correlated with stages (Table 6). In the period 1979–90, it was 101.8%, 81.2%, 61.0% and 14.0% in stage I, stage II, stage III, and stage IV respectively. The majority of tumors were located on the middle and distal third of the stomach and patient prognosis was superior to case with tumors located on the proximal third (Table 7). Proportion of proximal third cancer has gradually increased; from 11.6% to 17.4% in the period studied. The smaller size tumor has better prognosis (Table 8), and early gastric cancer, i.e., Type 0 cancer, has almost a 100% 5-year survival rate (Table 9). Prognosis of diffuse carcinoma, i.e., Type 4 cancer, was very poor, and has not improved in

Table 4. Five-year survival rates by lymph node metastasis.

	First period (1963–1966) Nationwide	Second period (1969–1973) Nationwide	Third period (1974–1978) Nationwide	Fourth period (1979–1990) NCC
	%	%	%	%
pN0	79.5 (1534)	87.4 (4761)	88.4 (9128)	97.6 (1557)
pN1	38.5 (1358)	45.4 (2923)	48.3 (4862)	76.0 (457)
pN2	22.8 (1068)	26.9 (2277)	27.7 (4231)	39.5 (536)
pN3	11.1 (249)	11.5 (490)	13.1 (1004)	5.0 (99)
pN4	8.5 (66)	1.5 (146)	1.9 (288)	5.9 (175)
Unknown	28.8 (1200)	33.9 (975)	33.0 (2011)	— (0)

Table 5. Five-year survival rates by in patients with peritoneal and liver metastsis.

	First period (1963–1966) Nationwide	Second period (1969–1973) Nationwide	Third period (1974–1978) Nationwide	Fourth period (1979–1990) NCC
	%	%	%	%
No peritoneal metastasis	53.5 (4325)	64.3 (9819)	65.0 (18 667)	79.2 (2599)
Peritoneal metastasis	9.1 (1065)	10.0 (1726)	2.5 (2802)	2.8 (225)
Unknown	16.5 (85)	41.8 (27)	28.8 (55)	— (0)
No liver metastasis	46.5 (5164)	58.2 (11 106)	60.2 (20 537)	75.0 (2740)
Liver metastasis	4.8 (262)	6.7 (444)	10.8 (933)	7.6 (84)
Unknown	22.5 (49)	34.7 (22)	31.5 (54)	— (0)

Table 6. Five-year survival rates by stage (histological).

	First period (1963–1966) Nationwide	Second period (1969–1973) Nationwide	Third period (1974–1978) Nationwide	Fourth period (1979–1990) NCC
	%	%	%	%
Stage I	94.4 (1016)	96.4 (3489)	96.6 (6952)	101.8 (1398)
II	56.1 (1070)	71.8 (1435)	72.0 (2179)	81.2 (303)
III	30.1 (910)	43.8 (3039)	44.8 (5292)	61.0 (565)
IV	9.3 (1523)	13.1 (2977)	7.7 (5487)	14.0 (558)
Unknown	40.2 (956)	58.1 (632)	58.8 (1614)	— (0)

Table 7. Five-year survival rates by location of tumor.

	First period (1963–1966) Nationwide	Second period (1969–1973) Nationwide	Third period (1974–1978) Nationwide	Fourth period (1979–1990) NCC
	%	%	%	%
Proximal third (C)	23.8 (637)	38.8 (1625)	43.6 (3102)	63.8 (490)
Middle third (M)	52.6 (2004)	63.4 (4552)	65.8 (8618)	87.9 (1047)
Distal third (A)	43.8 (2741)	57.2 (5177)	56.6 (9452)	78.4 (1032)
Total	10.9 (61)	9.1 (167)	8.5 (250)	22.4 (255)
Unknown	37.5 (32)	44.9 (51)	54.4 (102)	— (0)

Table 8. Five-year survival rates by size of tumor.

	First period (1963–1966) Nationwide	Second period (1969–1973) Nationwide	Third period (1974–1978) Nationwide	Fourth period (1979–1990) NCC
	%	%	%	%
<4.0 cm	75.1 (974)	85.2 (3089)	89.3 (5958)	98.7 (1489)
4.0–7.9 cm	44.9 (2509)	55.1 (5311)	58.1 (9648)	68.7 (854)
≥8.0 cm	27.7 (1478)	28.6 (2902)	28.3 (5449)	32.5 (481)
Unknown	26.7 (514)	40.8 (270)	44.8 (469)	— (0)

Table 9. Five-year survival rates by macroscopic type.

	First period (1963–1966) Nationwide	Second period (1969–1973) Nationwide	Third period (1974–1978) Nationwide	Fourth period (1979–1990) NCC
	%	%	%	%
Type 0 (early)	96.8 (790)	96.7 (3116)	97.8 (5835)	100.5 (1339)
Type 1	57.8 (180)	61.4 (325)	66.4 (564)	65.0 (64)
Type 2	48.0 (1535)	52.4 (2648)	54.7 (4457)	62.9 (384)
Type 3	29.8 (2063)	35.3 (3802)	36.7 (6988)	53.7 (746)
Type 4	15.0 (644)	15.0 (1139)	15.1 (2288)	9.8 (239)
Type 5	58.0 (102)	71.2 (416)	71.6 (1121)	53.7 (52)
Unknown	26.7 (161)	62.0 (126)	67.8 (271)	— (0)

Table 10. Five-year survival rates by histological type.

	First period (1963–1966) Nationwide	Second period (1969–1973) Nationwide	Third period (1974–1978) Nationwide	Fourth period (1979–1990) NCC
	%	%	%	%
Papillary ca.	48.5 (680)	55.3 (1489)	58.3 (1600)	73.1 (132)
Well diff. adenoca.			70.0 (3927)	92.9 (680)
Mod. diff. adenoca.	43.6 (3153)	58.7 (6643)	59.5 (5010)	72.0 (694)
Poorly diff. adenoca.			48.3 (6601)	52.8 (768)
Signet ring ca.	48.2 (934)	63.4 (2406)	69.8 (2291)	85.0 (467)
Mucinous ca.	43.6 (470)	47.3 (845)	47.3 (828)	38.2 (83)
Others	22.5 (26)	37.8 (52)	41.4 (511)	— (0)
Unknown	30.2 (212)	58.2 (137)	54.2 (756)	— (0)

the last 28 years. The Japanese histological classification system is almost the same as the WHO Classification, and the majority of cancers belonged to the adenocarcinoma type (Table 10). The survival rates were not correlated with histological type.

Surgical treatment in Japan is shown in Tables 11–13. It is characteristic that more than half of the patients were treated by distal gastrectomy, and very few

Table 11. Five-year survival rates by type of resection.

	First period (1963–1966) Nationwide	Second period (1969–1973) Nationwide	Third period (1974–1978) Nationwide	Fourth period (1979–1990) NCC
	%	%	%	%
Distal gastrectomy	50.3 (4187)	63.9 (8682)	65.1 (15 762)	83.1 (1944)
Proximal gastrectomy	23.1 (297)	43.6 (598)	48.2 (908)	83.1 (69)
Total gastrectomy	19.8 (875)	30.1 (2197)	35.5 (4622)	46.1 (781)
Other	72.1 (38)	68.0 (32)	44.6 (112)	89.2 (30)
Unknown	24.4 (78)	54.1 (63)	60.9 (120)	— (0)

Table 12. Five-year survival rates by lymph node dissection.

	First period (1963–1966) Nationwide	Second period (1969–1973) Nationwide	Third period (1974–1978) Nationwide	Fourth period (1979–1990) NCC
	%	%	%	%
R0	26.0 (381)	20.5 (582)	18.4 (1665)	32.5 (118)
R1	42.4 (1885)	46.0 (2420)	49.8 (4345)	62.1 (507)
R2 + R3	48.1 (3107)	61.6 (8510)	64.2 (15 383)	76.9 (2199)
Unknown	27.5 (102)	30.0 (60)	43.6 (131)	— (0)

Table 13. Five-year survival rates by curability of surgery.

	First period (1963–1966) Nationwide	Second period (1969–1973) Nationwide	Third period (1974–1978) Nationwide	Fourth period (1979–1990) NCC
	%	%	%	%
Curative resection	64.2 (2963)	73.3 (8100)	74.2 (14 934)	87.5 (2289)
Palliative resection	10.4 (1641)	11.6 (3056)	13.4 (5260)	11.2 (535)
Unknown	34.1 (871)	44.1 (416)	45.7 (1330)	— (0)

were by proximal gastrectomy (Table 11). Systematic LN disssection, called R2 LN dissection, was standardized and popularized in Japan. The proportions of R2 and R3 operations increased from 56.7% to 77.9% in analyzed cases, and their 5-year survival rates also improved from 48.1% to 76.9% (Table 12). Due to progress of early detection methods and extended surgery, patients with curative resection increased from 35.2% to 76.6% (Fig. 3c), and 5-year survival rates were elevated from 64.2% to 87.5% (Table 13). However survival rates of palliative resection has not improved; from 10.4% to 11.2%.

Discussion

Death rate of gastric cancer was extremely high in Japan. The Japanese Research Society for Gastric Cancer was established in 1962, and promoted both clinical and basic studies. The Society contributed to standardizing and popularizing double contrast X-ray examination, endoscopy and biopsy, ultrasound examination, mass screening systems, systematic LN dissection, and extended operations. To collect high quality data, the Society organized a committee for the nationwide registration of gastric cancer patients, and also published a manual for the registry. Data of 180 978 patients treated in 1963–1983 were collected and analyzed, and the results were published in 30 reports up till 1990.

In these reports, studies on treatment results in 1963-1978 were included. In order to keep the accuracy of the study, data from the institutions with less than 80% follow-up rates were excluded. Data of 51 676 patients accepted. To study the end results of surgical treatment, nonresectable and double cancer cases were excluded and data of 39 527 patients were selected. To calculate relative survival rates, 886 surgical deaths were excluded, and data of 38 571 patients were finally analyzed.

The recent nationwide database was not completed. To cover the lack of latest treatment results, data of the National Cancer Center were added as a reference. The number of the registered cases, evaluable cases, analyzed cases, surgical death, and losted to follow-up was 2987, 2824, 2824, 7, and 19 respectively.

The committee of the nationwide registration published the results with survival data in the three consecutive periods: 1963–66, 1969–73, and 1974–78. To know the trends of gastric cancer in Japan, the data in these three periods were separtely presented in this paper, and the last 12 years of data from the National Cancer Center were compared as a fourth period. The results showed clearly remarkable changes in tumors, and treatments. All data were documented, following the Japanese manual.

Following is the characteristics of gastric cancer in Japan. The male to female ratio was 2:1 in Japan, and was not different from western countries [3, 4]. However it is notable that the largest population of cancer patients belonged to the 60- to 69-years age group which was 10 years younger than western patients [3, 4]. Mucosal and submucosal cancer were called "early gastric cancer". The proportion had increased to 44.8% (1339 out of 2987 patients) in 1979–90. However, the proportion was only 9.2% in Germany in 1982–89 [5], and 7.4% in the United States in 1977–79 [4]. The relative 5-year survival rate was almost 100%.

Classification of LN metastasis was a little diferent between the Japanese and the TNM manual [6]. N3 and N4 were classifed together in Japan, but they were regarded as distant metastasis in the TNM due to low survival rate. Five-year survival rate was 5.0% in N3 LN metastasis along the hepatoduodenal ligament, behind the pancreas head, and along the superior mesenteric artery. It was only 5.9% in N4 LN metastasis in the para-aortic lymph node.

Distant metastasis was described separately in peritoneal and liver metastasis in Japan. Its prognosis was very poor, and no improvement of the survival rates was observed in the last 28 years. Japanese Staging System determined stage by depth of invasion, serosal involvement, LN metastasis, and peritoneal and liver metastasis. The Staging system was not the same for the former TNM Staging system, and the results could not be comparered directly. To remove such difficulty of international comparison, the Japanese Staging System and the TNM Staging System were unified in 1993. However, prognosis was well correlated with stage. It was notable that The 5-year survival rate of the proximal third cancer was poorer than the other thirds. The proportion of proximal cancers was not large in Japan gradually increasing from 11.6% to 17.4%, compared with western countries, for example, 37.9% in Germany [3]. With early detection, small size tumor numbers were increasing, and the proportion of tumors less than 4.0 cm rose from 17.8% to 52.7%. The 5-year survival rate was strongly correlated with tumor size. Proportion of diffusely infiltrating cancer, Type 4, was almost 10% in Japan, but was larger in western countries [7]. Its prognosis was strikingly poorer when compared with that of other types. This cancer type is characterized by rapid growth, high incidence of peritoneal metastasis and is never found in the early stages [8].

Surgical treatment was also characteristic in Japan. Total gastrectomy is not frequent in Japan, and its proportion was 27.7% in the last period. In Germany, total gastrectomy was performed in 50.9% of patients with curative resection [9]. The difference was caused by the high incidence of proximal, diffuse tumor, and advanced cancer, indicated by the use of total gastrectomy in Germany. Complete removal of the N1 lymph nodes is called "R1 dissection", and that of N1 and N2 is defined as "R2 dissection". Effectiveness of the R2 dissection was noticed internationally, and was evaluated in several multi-center trials. Some studies reported its ineffectivenes in prognosis [10], but many studies reported that prognosis of "R2 dissection" was superior to that of conventional dissection [5, 11, 12]. Japanese nationwide data showed the R2 an R3 dissection had been increasing from 56.7% to 77.9%, and 5-year survival rates were also elevated from 48.1% to 76.9%. The fact showed that the R2 systematic LN dissection was accepted as standard and effective treatment in Japan. Philosophies of "curability" in the Japanese manual and "residual tumor, R classification" in the TNM manual were the same. However, the Japanese manual defined the "curability" in detail by residual tumor at surgical margine, distant metastasis, relation between LN metastasis, and dissection. The Japanese results could therefore not be compared with the TNM residual tumor. However, the 5-year survival rate of patients with curative resection was 87.5% in Japan and 51.8% in Germany [13], and that with palliative resection was 11.2% in Japan and 11.5% in Germany.

Conclusion

Trends of gastric cancer in Japan were studied in this paper in the period from 1963 to 1990 using the nationwide database of Gastric Cancer from the JRSGC and data of the National Cancer Center Tokyo. It was noteworthy that early stage cancer increased remarkably and the treatment results were also significantly improved. The rise in early stage detection was produced by progress of the early detection system, and the unproved treatment results by developments in surgical treatment.

Characteristics of gastric cancer in Japan were as follows: the largest population of cancer patients belonged in the 60- to 69-years age group which was 10 years younger than western patients. The proportion of proximal cancer and diffuse carcinoma was smaller than the western proportion, and distal gastrectomy and systematic LN dissection were more popular in Japan.

Acknowledgments. This work was supported in part by the Grant-in-Aid for Cancer Research (91-03 and 91-05) from the Japanese Ministry of Health and Welfare, and by the Princess Takamatsu Cancer Research Fund (1992).

References

1. JRSGC (1985) The general rule for the gastric cancer study in surgery and pathology. Jpn J Surg 11:127–139
2. JRSGC (1966–1993) Annual reports of gastric cancer patients treated in 1963–1989, Reports 1–31, National Cancer Center Press, Tokyo
3. Rohde H, Gebbensleben B, Bauer P, Stützer H, Zieschang J (1989) Has there been any improvement in the staging of gastric cancer? Findings from the German Gastric Cancer TNM Study Group. Cancer 64:2465–2481
4. Curtis RE, Kennedy BJ, Myers MH, Hankey BF (1983) Evaluation of AJC stomach cancer staging using the SEER population. Semin Onco 12:21–31
5. Rohde H, Stützer H, Bauer P, Heitmann K, Gebbensleben B, and the German Gastric Cancer TNM Study Group (1991) Early gastric cancer in comparison to advanced gastric cancer. Langenbeacks Arch Chir 376:16–22
6. UICC: TNM Classification of malignant tumours, ed. 4, Springer-Verlag, Berlin, 43–46, 1987
7. Meyer WC, Damiano RJ, Postlethwait RW, Rotolo FS (1987) Adenocarcinima of the stomach, changing patterns over the last 4 decades. Ann Surg 205:1–8
8. Maruyama K, Okabayashi K, Kinoshita T (1987) Progress in gastric cancer surgery in Japan and its limits of radicality. World J Surg 11:418–425
9. Rohde H, Bauer P, Stützer H, Heitmann K, Gebbensleben B, and the German Gastric Cancer TNM Study Group (1991) Proximal compared with distal adenocarcinoma of the stomach: Difference and consequences. Br J Surg 78:1242–1248
10. Dent DM, Madden MV, Price SK (1988) Randmized comparison of R1 and R2 gastrectomy for gastric carcinoma. Br J Surg 75:110–112
11. Shiu MH, Moore E, Saunders M, Huvos A, Freedman B, Goodbold J, Chaiyaphruk S, Wesdorp R, Brennan M (1987) Influence of the extent of resection on survival after curative treatment of gastric carcinoma. Arch Surg 122:1347–1351
12. Siewert JR, Lange J, Böttcher K, Stier A (1986) Lymphadenektomie beim Magenkarzinom. Langenbecks Arch Chirur 368:137–148
13. Gall FP, Hermanek P (1985) New aspects in the surgical treatment of gastreic carcinoma—a comparative study of 1636 patients operated on between 1969 to 1982. Eur J Surg Oncol 11:219–225

End Results of Surgical Treatment of Gastric Adenocarcinoma: American Experience**

*Man H. Shiu**, Martin Karpeh, Jr.[1], *and Murray F. Brennan*[1]

Key words. Gastric cancer—Surgical treatment results—United States

Introduction

The incidence of carcinoma of the stomach has been declining for the last 40 years in the United States. The disease ranks eighth as a cause of death from cancer, accounting for 13 700 (2.7%) of the 510 000 cancer deaths in 1990 [1]. There are no mass screening programs for the early detection of gastric cancer in this country, and most patients present for treatment at an advanced stage of disease.

According to the Surveillance, Epidemiology, and End Results (SEER) Program of the National Center for Health Statistics, 16% of gastric cancers were localized to the stomach, 34% had lymph node metastases, 37% had distant metastases, and 13% had unknown stage during the years 1979–1984. Unlike the experience of Japan, early gastric cancer is relatively uncommon. However, many American clinics began to use flexible fiberoptic gastroscopy in the 1970s, and by the 1980s it had become a standard tool of gastric surgeons and gastro-enterologists. As a result, early gastric cancers are diagnosed with increasing frequency, particularly in patients with vague symptoms. Since 1990, the frequency of early gastric cancers has reached 10% or higher in most centers.

Development of Surgical Treatment in the United States

Historically, surgeons in several American centers laid the foundation for the technique of radical resection of gastric carcinoma in the 1940s and 1950s.

** Supported by a grant from the Wells Foundation
* Present address: Room 501, Central Building, Pedder Street, Hong Kong
[1] Department of Surgery, Memorial Sloan-Kettering Cancer Center, 1275 York Avenue, New York, NY 10021, USA

Table 1. Pattern of failure in reoperation series after curative resection of gastric carcinoma (Minnesota University Hospitals).

	Only site of recurrence[a]		As part of any component	
Local or regional + localized peritoneal	24	29%	72	88%
	44	54%		
Peritoneal	3	4%	44	54%
Localized			20	24%
Diffuse			24	30%
Distant metastases (mostly liver)	5	6%	24	30%

(Adapted from [8])

[a] Of 107 evaluable patients, 86 had recurrence; this was totally documented in 82.

Among these were McNeer and Pack [2–4] at the Memorial Hospital for Cancer and Allied Diseases (now known as Memorial Sloan-Kettering Cancer Center); Wangensteen and his co-workers [5] at the University of Minnesota, and Priestley, Remine, and others [6, 7] at the Mayo Clinic. These workers emphasized the importance of radical resection and the need for extensive lymphadenectomy in the curative treatment of gastric cancer. Sunderland, McNeer, and their co-workers documented the pathway and frequency of lymphatic spread of gastric carcinoma at different sites [3]. McNeer and Pack [4] further reported these pioneering studies on the lymphatic spread of gastric cancer and described the technique of resection by radical subtotal and total gastrectomy.

Despite these early efforts at radical resection, the results of treatment have been poor in the United States. Most of the cancers have been unresectable and those that were resected were often large tumors with extensive lymph node metastases or invasion of adjacent organs. Recurrence and metastases were common, despite apparent curative resections.

Gunderson and Sosin [8] reported on their prospective study of 109 (107 evaluable) patients who underwent reoperation after resection of gastric carcinoma at the University of Minnesota Hospitals. Tumor recurrence was documented in 80% of these patients. Local or regional recurrence, or both, occurred in 29% as the sole site of recurrence, and in 88% as a component of more generalized recurrence (Table 1). Peritoneal metastases were noted in 54%, and distant metastases, mostly in the liver, in 29%. The extent of the initial gastric resection bore little relationship to the incidence or type of subsequent recurrence. A more recent study from the Massachusetts General Hospital [9] also revealed a high incidence (38%) of local/regional recurrence in 130 patients, the site of recurrence being mostly at the anastomosis, in the gastric stump, or in the stomach bed.

These reports and the unreported local experience of many centers have led surgeons to regard the treatment of gastric cancer with pessimism. This disillusionment has occurred despite continuing efforts at radical resection in some centers.

Current Surgical Treatment

In many American hospitals, most of the surgical treatment of gastric cancer consists of palliative operations for advanced disease. For less advanced cancers which are relatively uncommon, surgical resection does not routinely include wide lymphadenectomy, either because of the lack of training and experience of the surgeon, or lack of belief that such resection can offer real benefit. However, in some university hospitals and other specialized referral centers, curative surgical resections of gastric cancer are performed according to the principles of wide removal of the tumor with lymph node dissection [10, 11]. Data from these centers [6, 11], as well as from numerous Japanese clinics, continue to confirm that long-term survival can be achieved in many patients with early as well as advanced stage cancers.

The extent of lymphadenectomy varies considerably. According to an unofficial questionnaire (Department of Surgery, Memorial Sloan Kettering Cancer Center, unpublished data) sent to selected surgical departments, only 55% of the responding departments performed lymphadenectomy in all or most of their curative gastric resections, 20% performed it in half, and 25% in few of these operations.

At the Memorial Sloan-Kettering Cancer Center (MSKCC), there has been a long tradition of radical resection for gastric cancer. In the 1940s and 1950s, the cancers were mostly large and locally advanced. McNeer and his co-workers attempted to control many of these tumors by extended radical total gastric resection, which consisted of en bloc removal of the entire stomach, spleen, and body and tail of the pancreas, as well as the perigastric, celiac, and other upper abdominal lymph nodes [12]; later analyses suggested that this operation did yield survival benefit for some patients [12–14]. For tumors that invade adjacent organs such as the colon, pancreas, liver, or spleen, experience at the MSKCC has also indicated that resection of the stomach en bloc with the affected organ(s) can offer a substantial cure rate in carefully selected patients [15].

In recent years, the standard recommended surgical procedure at the MSKCC for a potentially curable gastric carcinoma has been subtotal or total gastrectomy with en bloc dissection of at least two echelons of the draining lymph nodes (R2 resection) for early as well as advanced cancers [11, 16].

Survival After Treatment

The SEER program, which consists of a large sample of selected hospital centers in the United States, reported that for patients treated in the years 1979–1984, the 5-year survival rates were 58% for tumors recorded as localized to the

Table 2. Five-year survival according to stage in 434 patients who survived operation (1963–1983) (Charity Hospital experience).

Stage	No. of patients	Five-year survivors
0-I	48	13 (27%)
I-II	40	10 (25%)
III-IV	346	21 (6%)

(Adapted from [10])

Table 3. Five-year survival according to stage in 244 patients (Duke University Medical Center [1953–1983]).

Stage[a]	No. of patients	Five-year survivors
I	2	0
II	25	11 (40%)
III	41	5 (11%)
IV	176	3 (1%)

(Adapted from [18])
[a] TNM staging according to [33]

stomach, 16% for those with lymph node metastases, 2% for those with distant metastases, and 11% for those of unknown stage. The overall 5-year survival rate was 17%. These are crude 5-year survival rates. The SEER program does not require the reporting center to use a uniform clinico-pathologic staging method and standardized surgical treatment, such as is used by the Japanese Research Society for Gastric Cancer. The SEER program also does not take into account whether or not the patients were curatively treated. Several centers have analyzed and reported their accumulated results of treatment of gastric carcinoma in recent years.

Breaux [17] and his coworkers at the Louisiana State University reported the cumulative results of treating 1710 patients with gastric adenocarcinoma at the Charity Hospital in New Orleans from 1948 to 1983. Resection was performed in 835 (49%) of the patients; 526 had only a bypass or biopsy. The 5-year survival rate was 17.9% for patients who underwent resection and 7.9% for the entire group of patients. Of 434 patients who underwent and survived an operation in 1963–1983, the 5-year survival rates were 27% for stages 0–I, 25% for stages I–II, and 6% for stages II–IV (Table 2). Radical subtotal gastrectomy, which the authors described as 75% gastric resection with removal of the omentum and lymph nodes along the right and left gastric arteries, and extended in selected patients to include the celiac and portal nodes, was performed in 165 patients. This operation yielded 46 5-year and 26 10-year survivors, plus 13 patients still alive at less than 10 years.

The Duke University Medical Center reported their experience of treating 255 patients with gastric carcinoma from 1953 to 1983 [18]. Advanced lesions predominated; 17% and 72% of the lesions were recorded as stage III and stage IV, respectively. The 5-year survival rate was 6% for the entire group, and 24% for curatively-treated patients ($n = 65$). Table 3 shows the survival according to the TNM stage, which was available in 244 of the patients.

Between 1960 and 1980, 1464 patients with gastric carcinoma were treated at MSKCC; 210 of these patients underwent curative resection [11]. The overall 5-year survival rate after curative resection was 30% (Table 4). Multivariate analysis of data from this retrospective review suggested a survival benefit consequent to extended lymphadenectomy. Recurrence and metastases were

Table 4. Five-year survival after curative resection of gastric cancer (Memorial Sloan-Kettering Cancer Center [1960–1980] retrospective series).

Nodal stage	No. of patients[a]	Five-year survivors
N_0	79	44 (56%)
N_1	93	15 (16%)
N_2	30	1
N_3	3	1

(Adapted from [11])
[a] Total of 205 patients evaluable.

documented in 77 of 150 patients who died of the disease. Metastases or recurrence occurred in the peritoneum or omentum in 49, the liver in 36, the lung in 11, and the gastric remnant or gastric bed in nine. The results of treating early gastric cancer in 60 patients were recorded in a separate review [16]. The disease-free 5-year survival rate after resection was 76%. Three of eight patients with nodal metastases survived 5 or more years, including one who had second-echelon deposits.

Since 1985 a prospective gastric cancer database has been maintained at MSKCC. From July 1 1985 to December 31, 1990, a total of 744 patients were admitted to the Center for treatment of gastric adenocarcinoma. Adequate staging information is currently available on 681 patients. The resection rate was 74% and 53% of the resections were performed with curative intent. Figure 1 shows the survival distributions of these patients according to the tumor, nodes, metastases (TNM) staging. The overall projected 5-year survival rates were 86% for stage IA, 91% for IB, 47% for stage II, 28% for stage IIIA, 8% for stage IIIB, and 3% for stage IV.

Complications of Surgical Treatment

Operative mortality rates of 10% to 15% were commonly experienced during 1950–1960 [17, 18] and even higher mortality rates occurred with extended gastric resections in these early years [13, 15]. However, these authors all quoted much lower operative death rates in more recent years. Thus at MSKCC from 1960 to 1984, out of a total of 392 curative gastric resections, 16 patients (4%) died of the operation [19]. Splenectomy, which was performed as part of the operation in 163 of the patients, did not seem to independently affect survival in this retrospective analysis. However, patients who underwent splenectomy had a higher incidence of septic complications. A recent study comparing the morbidity and mortality of extended lymph node dissection has shown an overall operative mortality of 1.1% and no increase in morbidity by the more extended lymph node dissection [20].

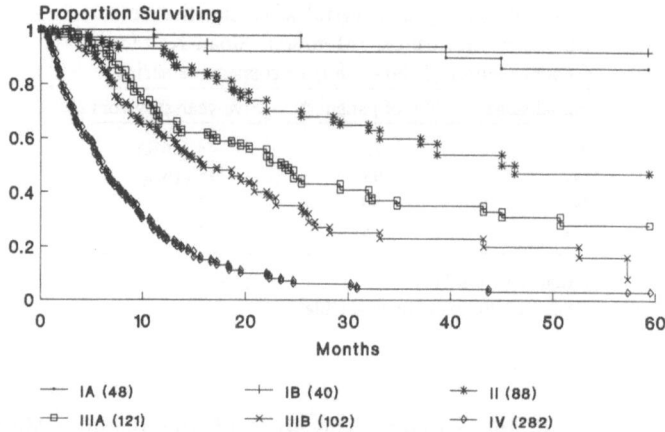

Fig. 1. Survival of 681 patients treated for gastric adenocarcinoma by stage, Memorial Sloan-Kettering Cancer Center (*MSKCC*) prospective database (1985–1990). There was a resection rate of 74%, 53% curatively resected

Adjuvant Chemotherapy

In the 1960s the Veterans Administration Cooperative Research Adjuvant Study Group [21] tested thiotepa, and Serlin and coworkers [22] similarly used 5-fluorodeoxyuridine for the adjuvant chemotherapy of gastric cancer, without benefit. The Gastrointestinal Tumor Study Group (GITSG) reported in 1984 the preliminary results of a trial in which patients were randomly assigned to receive either methyl CCNU and 5-FU for 18 months following potentially curative resection or no treatment after surgery [23]. This study showed a survival benefit of borderline statistical significance for the treated patients. However, two other randomized trials using the same chemotherapy regimen have not shown any benefit [24, 25]. During the 1970s and 1980s some surgeons used the FAM (5-FU, doxorubicin, and mitomycin C) regimen for the adjuvant treatment of gastric cancer. However, a multi-center randomized trial of adjuvant chemotherapy of gastric cancer using FAM has been completed, again showing no survival benefit [26]. Because of the negative results obtained in these trials, most centers in the United States today do not routinely recommend adjuvant chemotherapy for gastric cancer. However, adjuvant chemotherapy trials continue to be performed for this disease, using different drugs and different routes of administration. Ongoing trials at MSKCC consist of intraperitoneal 5-FU and cisplatin plus intravenous 5-FU and intraoperative chemotherapy for T_3 lesions staged by endoscopic ultrasound (EUS) [27].

Changing Pattern of Gastric Cancer in the United States

During the last 40 years there has been a dramatic increase in the ratio of proximal to distal gastric cancers seen in many centers in the United States. Meyers and his colleagues [18] reviewed the records of the Durham Veterans Administration Hospital in Durham, North Carolina from 1953 to 1983 and found that this ratio had increased from 16% in the 1960s to 44% in the 1980s. A similar increase has been noted in the Lahey Clinic [28], and at MSKCC. This change is mostly due to a decrease in the incidence of the antral cancers [29].

Surgical treatment of the increasingly common proximal gastric cancers poses a greater challenge to the surgeon, because of the need to perform total gastrectomy or esophagogastrectomy for most of these lesions. Fortunately, with improvements in surgical technique and perioperative surgical care, these operations are now performed with an operative mortality rate below 4% in most centers.

Flow cytometry studies have indicated that these proximal tumors are biologically different. Nanus and coworkers [30] studied the DNA ploidy of 50 gastric cancers at MSKCC and found that 96% of cancers of the cardia or gastro-esophageal junction were aneuploid, compared with only 48% for body or antral lesions. Lymph node metastases were more common with aneuploid tumors, and the median disease-free survival for patients with diploid tumors was 18.5 months, as compared with only 5.4 months for patients with aneuploid tumors.

Discussion

Overall results of treatment of gastric cancer in the United States are far inferior to those in Japan. One major reason is the remarkable increase in, and the very high proportion of, early gastric cancer in Japan. Stage for stage, however, the results of treatment in the United States are inferior by comparison.

Noguchi and coworkers [31, 32] have reviewed the factors that may account for this difference. In Japan, radical resection with extensive lymph node dissection is the standard surgical treatment in practically every hospital center, while in the United States, radical resection and lymph node dissection are not as commonly practiced, and not to the same extent as in Japan. This aggressive resection of the potentially curable gastric cancer should add to the survival rate, although this has yet to be proven by a randomized clinical trial.

Extensive resection and lymphadenectomy also permit much more accurate staging of the cancer, as compared with less extensive resections. Thus a patient with metastasis in a celiac lymph node would be accurately staged as N_2 after radical lymphadenectomy, but a less radical resection would have missed the affected lymph node(s) so that the patient would be recorded as having only node-negative (N_0) disease. The survival rates of N_0 gastric cancer, as published in many American studies, therefore, are much lower, because many of the so-called N_0 patients probably had N_1 or N_2 tumors. The same can be said for the reported survival rates of N_1 and N_2 stages of gastric cancer. How much of the difference in survival rates, stage for stage, is due to this phenomenon of mis-staging cannot be ascertained, until data from a prospective randomized trial of radical lymphadenectomy versus no lymphadenectomy become available.

Surgeons and oncologists must continue to face the challenge of the more advanced gastric cancers currently seen in the United States. Because of the relative infrequency of gastric cancer in this country, early diagnosis by mass screening is not cost-effective and will not be performed. Fortunately, patients with symptoms of gastric cancer are seeking earlier medical attention today compared to patients two or three decades ago. Surgeons and gastroenterologists have also been diagnosing an increasing number of early gastric cancers in recent years, by endoscopic examination of patients with vague symptoms. This gradual increase of less advanced cancers, and advances in surgical technique and medical care in general will, hopefully, lead to a gradual improvement of the end results of treatment in future years.

References

1. Silverberg E, Boring CC, Squires TS (1990) Cancer statistics. CA 40:9–26
2. McNeer G, Sunderland DA, McInnes G, Vandenberg HJ Jr, Lawrence W Jr (1951) A more thorough operation for gastric cancer; anatomical basis and description of technique. Cancer 4:957–967
3. Sunderland DA, McNeer G, Ortega LG, Pearce LS (1953) The lymphatic spread of gastric cancer. Cancer 6:987–996
4. McNeer G, Pack GT (eds) (1967) Neoplasms of the stomach. Lippincott, Philadelphia
5. Lewis FJ, Wangensteen OH (1950) Exploration following resection of the colon, rectum or stomach for carcinoma with lymph node metastases. Surg Forum, 1950, pp 535–540
6. Remine WH, Priestley LT (1952) Late results after total gastrectomy. Surg Gynecol Obstet 94:519–525
7. Remine WH, Gomes MMR, Dockerty MB (1969) Long-term survival (10–56 years) after surgery for carcinoma of the stomach. Am J Surg 117:117–184
8. Gunderson LL, Sosin H (1982) Adenocarcinoma of the stomach—areas of failure in a reoperation series, second of symptomatic looks. Clinicopathologic correlation and implications for adjuvant therapy. Int J Radiat Oncol Biol Phys 8:1–11
9. Landry J, Tepper JE, Wood WL, Moulton EO, Koerner F, Sullinger J (1990) Patterns of failure following curative resection of gastric carcinoma. Int J Radiat Oncol Biol Phys 19:1357–1362
10. Breaux JR, Bringaze W, Chappuis C, Cohn I Jr (1990) Adenocarcinoma of the stomach: a review of 35 years and 1710 cases. World J Surg 14:580–586
11. Shiu MH, Moore E, Sanders M, Huvos A, Freedman B, Godbold J, Chaiyaphruk S, Wesdorp R, Brennan MF (1987) Influence of the extent of resection on survival after

curative treatment of gastric carcinoma: A retrospective multivariate analysis. Arch Surg 122:1347–1351

12. McNeer G, Bowden L, Booher RJ, McPeak CJ (1974) Elective total gastrectomy for cancer of the stomach; end results. Ann Surg 108:252–256
13. Shiu MH, Papachristou DN, Kosloff C, Eliopoulos G (1980) Selection of operative procedure for adenocarcinoma of the midstomach. Ann Surg 192:730–737
14. Papachristou DN, Fortner JG (1980) Adenocarcinoma of the gastric cardia; choice of gastrectomy. Ann Surg 192:58–64
15. Papachristou DN, Shiu MH (1981) Management by en bloc multiple organ resection of carcinoma of the stomach invading adjacent organs. Surg Gynecol Obstet 152:483–487
16. Lawrence M, Shiu MH (1991) Early gastric cancer: 28-Year experience. Ann Surg 213:327–334
17. Breaux JR, Bringaze W, Chappuis C, Cohn I (1990) Adenocarcinoma of the stomach: A review of 35 years and 1710 cases. World J Surg 14:580–586
18. Meyers WC, Damiano R Jr, Postlethwait RW, Rotolo FS (1987) Adenocarcinoma of the stomach: Changing patterns over the last four decades. Ann Surg 205:1–8
19. Brady MS, Rogatko A, Dent L, Shiu MH (1991) Effect of splenectomy on morbidity and survival following curative gastrectomy for carcinoma. Arch Surg 126:359–364
20. Smith JW, Shiu MH, Kelsey L, Brennan MF (1991) Morbidity of radical lymphadenectomy in the curative resection of gastric carcinoma. Arch Surg 126:1469–1473
21. VA Cooperative Research Adjuvant Study Group (1965) Use of thiotepa as an adjuvant to the surgical management of carcinoma of the stomach. Cancer 18:291–297
22. Serlin O, Wolkoff J, Amadeo J (1969) Use of 5-fluorodeoxyuridine as an adjuvant to the surgical management of carcinoma of the stomach. Cancer 23:223–228
23. Gastrointestinal Tumor Study Group (1982) Control trial of adjuvant chemotherapy following curative resection for gastric cancer. Cancer 49:1116–1112
24. Engstrom P, Lavin P, Douglass H (1985) Postoperative adjuvant 5-fluorouracil plus methyl-CCNU therapy for gastric cancer patients. Cancer 55:1868–1873
25. Higgins G, Amadeo J, Smith D (1983) Efficacy of prolonged intermittent therapy with combined 5-FU and methyl-CCNU following resection for gastric carcinoma. Cancer 52:1105–1112
26. Shein P, Coombes R, Chilvers C (1986) A controlled trial of FAM chemotherapy as adjuvant treatment for resected gastric carcinoma: an interim report. Proc Am Soc Clin Oncol 5:79
27. Atiq O, Kelsen D, Shiu MH, Saltz L, Coit D, Turnbull A, Niedzwiecki D, Smith J, Trochanowski B, Toomasi F, Brennan MF (1991) Postoperative adjuvant intraperitoneal and intravenous chemotherapy in poor-risk gastric cancer patients (abstract). Proc Am Soc Clin Oncol, 1991
28. Cady B, Rossi RL, Silverman ML, Piccone W, Heck TA (1989) Gastric adenocarcinoma: A disease in transition. Arch Surg 124:303–308
29. Correa P (1985) Clinical implications of recent developments in gastric cancer pathology and epidemiology. Semin Oncol 1:2–10
30. Nanus DM, Kelsen DP, Niedwzwieki D, Chapman D, Brennan MF, Cheng E, Melamed M (1989) Flow cytometry as a predictive indicator in patients with operable gastric cancer. J Clin Oncol 7:1105–1112
31. Noguchi Y, Imada T, Matsumoto A, Coit D, Brennan MF (1989) Radical surgery for gastric cancer: A review of the Japanese experience. Cancer 64:2053–2062

32. Brennan MF (1989) Radical surgery for gastric cancer: A review of the Japanese experience (editorial). Cancer 64:2063
33. American Joint Committee for Cancer Staging and End Results Reporting (1983) End results of surgical treatment of gastric adenocarcinoma: American experience. Lippincott, Philadelphia

End Results of Surgical Treatment: British Experience

John L. Craven[1]

Key words. British—Stomach cancer—Trials—Surgery

Brief Historical Survey

The overall incidence of gastric cancer in England and Wales has not changed over the past 30 years, but mortality from the disease has fallen significantly in both sexes—from $34/10^5$ to $22/10^5$ in males and $25/10^5$ to $14/10^5$ in females. This, at first sight, is a surprising finding, suggesting, as it does, an improvement in treatment results [1]. Throughout much of that period, most British cancer registries record that only about 50%–60% of patients were treated initially by surgery, the most common operation performed being a simple partial gastrectomy without particular attention being paid to adjacent lymph nodes, omenta, or adjoining structures.

Although the overall survival rate has increased slightly throughout the decades, it is still depressingly close to 5% [2]. Perhaps it is understandable that all British clinicians, outside of a small but, fortunately, growing group of doctors have viewed the subject of gastric cancer with great pessimism, and that the standard British undergraduate surgical textbook still refers to gastric cancer as "captain of the men of death" which "at presentation is usually too advanced for attempts at surgical cure" [3].

Such pessimism springs from the results of gastric cancer treatment that were published in the 1950s and 1960s. From the Oxford hospitals [4], it was reported that of 375 patients with gastric cancer, only 30% had a surgical resection. The overall 5-year survival rate for those resected cases was no greater than 23%, and no more than 5.6% of the whole group survived that length of time. The surgeons and epidemiologists in Birmingham have long been interested in gastric cancer and, in the first of their large reviews [5], they painted a depressingly similar picture. They reviewed 5441 cases of gastric cancer obtained from the (then)

---

[1] York District Hospital, Wigginton Road, York YO3 7HE, UK

hospital-based regional cancer registry over the 10-year period of 1950–1959. The majority of patients presented with an advanced stage of the disease. Less than 60% justified surgical exploration and only 1444 (25%) underwent attempted curative resections. They reported an average survival rate of no more than 4.9% and of those who had undergone that procedure, a 5-year survival rate of only 15.6%. Neither of these reviews contained pathological criteria that enabled staging of the cancers to be made or the potential adequacy of the resection to be determined. There was no sign in the prospective multicenter international study organized by the International Federation of Surgical Colleges, to which British surgeons contributed, that either British or European surgeons had, at that time, any concept of pathological staging or en bloc resection by a defined surgical protocol. Their report of the surgical treatment of 901 patients dwelt once again on the high frequency of advanced disease at the time of presentation, low resectability rates, high postoperative mortality (20% after gastric resection), and poor long-term survival rates (9% overall, 23% after "radical" surgery).

This, then, was the picture in Britain up to the mid 1970s—one of little change and no improvement in either the rate of earlier diagnosis or in the results of surgical treatment. It was then, however, that the developments emanating from Japan, especially those of double contrast barium meals and flexible fiberoptic endoscopy, began to be adopted in the UK, and this was followed by a reawakening in the concept of earlier diagnosis of gastric cancer. Slowly, too, the large amount of experimental and clinical work being reported in Japan became available to UK surgeons through translation and visits between the two countries. There was some initial resistance to accepting that the rate of diagnosis of early gastric cancer could be improved. In 1975, a group of surgeons, oncologists, pathologists, and statisticians joined to form the British Stomach Cancer Group (BSCG). This was merely one manifestation that the depressingly black years of the previous three decades, insofar as gastric cancer treatment was concerned, were thought by some to be lagging behind. The pace of British clinical epidemiological and laboratory investigation into gastric cancer began to quicken, and I shall now try to summarize the results since reported on the surgical treatment of gastric cancer in the UK.

Current Experience

The BSCG has completed two multicenter randomized trials on the surgical treatment of gastric cancer. Its first tested the efficacy of two adjuvant chemotherapy regimens in operable gastric cancer [7]. All patients had undergone resection for proven adenocarcinoma of the stomach, although patients with Stage I and Stage II disease were excluded. A total of 411 patients were entered, stratified by surgeon, stage of disease, age and sex and randomized into 130 patients with surgery alone (Group A), and 140 (Group B) and 141 patients (Group C) who received 5 fluorouracil (5FU) 15 mg/kg and mitomycin C (MMC) 150 mg/kg, respectively, three times weekly. In addition to a 5-day induction

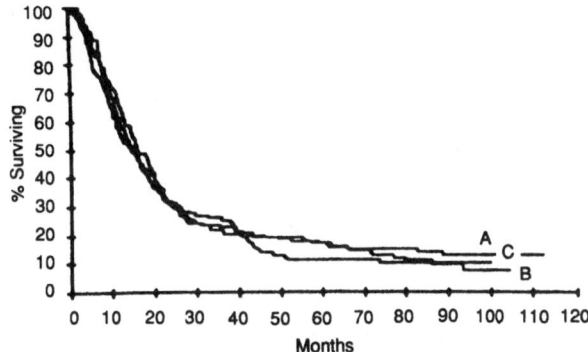

Fig. 1. Survival data of control (group *A*) and patients treated with surgery and adjuvant chemotherapy (groups *B* and *C*)

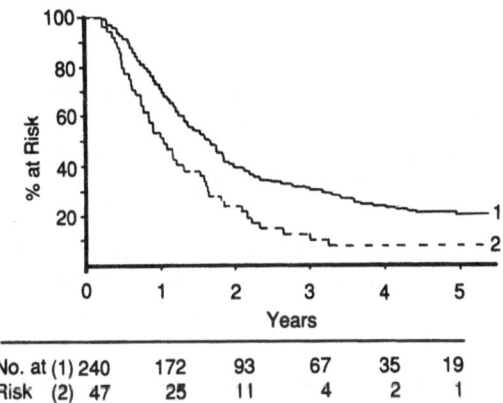

No. at (1)	240	172	93	67	35	19
Risk (2)	47	25	11	4	2	1

Fig. 2. Survival by resection line status for "curative" cases: (*1*) resection line uninvolved, (*2*) resection line involved

course of cyclophosphamide 5FU, Group B received vincristine and methotrexate. A 5.5-year follow-up study revealed no survival advantage for either group receiving adjuvant chemotherapy (Fig. 1). Of the 366 deaths, 22 were from chemotherapy-related conditions among which hemolytic uremic syndrome was prominent.

This was the first British paper on the surgical treatment of gastric cancer that was supported by a pathological study comparable in detail with that which is usual in Japanese literature on the subject. Multivariate analysis revealed that pathological staging and its contributing factor, nodal involvement, together with resection line involvement, were major prognostic determinants. This, in itself, is not a surprising result—Japanese work had many times demonstrated this fact— but since among the 86 patients who had resection line involvement, 47 were in

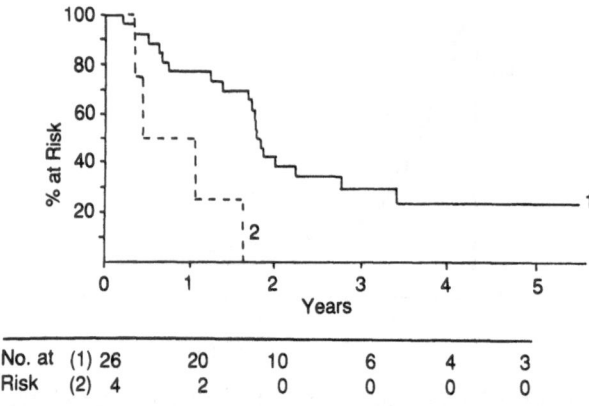

Fig. 3. Survival by resection line status for serosa negative, node positive patients: (*1*) resection line uninvolved, (*2*) resection line involved

a group that had been clinically staged as having had a "curative" gastrectomy, it did mean that the British surgeons working in 10 centers in this multicenter study were frequently unable to achieve the macroscopic clearance that they were aiming for [8]. Not surprisingly, resection line involvement resulted in a worse prognosis (Fig. 2), and this effect was particularly noted in those patients who were serosa negative (Fig. 3). It was recommended that more frequent use should be made of intra-operative microscopic assessment of the resection line if wide resection margins cannot be achieved. Resection line involvement has decreased in subsequent BSCG trials.

Its second trial began in 1981 and, as before, was a multicenter prospective randomized control trial of adjuvant chemotherapy and radiotherapy after gastric resection, based on careful documentation of the surgery performed and detailed pathological staging. Stage I disease and disease with distant metastases were excluded. It had 3 arms: surgery alone, surgery and radiotherapy to the tumor bed, and surgery followed by adjuvant MMC, adriamycin, and 5FU (MAF). There were 436 patients entered, and the interim report [9] published after a minimum follow-up of 2 years revealed neither form of adjuvant therapy to have conferred any survival advantage (Fig. 4). This study, while revealing that large groups of clinicians can combine their efforts in complex adjuvant studies, did show the logistic difficulties that followed this: only 45% of chemotherapy patients began treatment in the first postoperative month as planned and only 62% completed six or more of the recommended eight cycles of treatment. Both of these factors may have contributed to the failure to translate the proven efficacy of these chemotherapeutic agents in advanced disease into a survival benefit when used in an adjuvant setting.

The disappointing results of both these trials have convinced the BSCG that while, at present, surgery offers the only proven prospect of cure for gastric

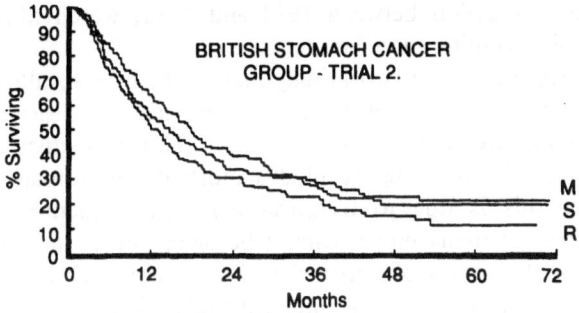

Fig. 4. Survival by treatment group. Surgery (S) 110/145 deaths, radiotherapy (R) 123/153 deaths, chemotherapy (M) 101/138 deaths

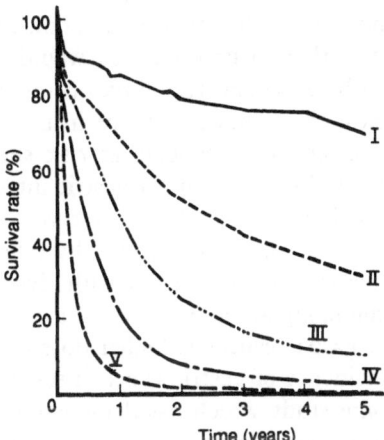

Fig. 5. Overall survival by stage of disease

cancer, the benefits of future adjuvant regimens can only be tested in randomized trials where the surgical procedure is standardized and clinico-pathological staging is rigorously employed.

In 1989 there appeared another report from the Birmingham Regional Cancer Registry [2] describing a population-based survey of all registered gastric cancer cases from 1957 to 1981. They reported on 31 716 cases, recording a fall in age-standardized mortality from 17.42 to 15.30 per 100 000 during the study, with an apparent increase of proximal tumors (11.3% to 21.2%) occurring alongside a decrease in distal tumors (45.9% to 33%) during this time. Throughout the study, the stage of the disease at presentation remained constant; 80% had disease too advanced for curative surgery, less than 1% had Stage I disease, and, as a result, the curative resection rate was 21% with the mean overall postoperative mortality remaining high at 13% (partial gastrectomy) and 29% (total gastrectomy) throughout the period. The overall survival data are gloomy and are summarized in Fig. 5, but there is, encouragingly, a significant increase in survival time for those treated by curative resection between 1972 and 1981, which hints that more radical surgery was becoming more common.

The postoperative mortality is worryingly high. When the results of individual surgeons were examined, the importance of experience was clearly emphasized, particularly in total gastrectomy. Even so, none of the Birmingham surgeons can approach the overall Japanese figure of 3% mortality after total gastrectomy, although whether this is due to technical expertise, patient-related factors, or perioperative patient management cannot be determined. It should be noted that some recent publications of personal series of radical resections from UK surgeons report much lower operative mortality rates, being at 5% [10] and 0% [11].

Another point where this major review from Birmingham is at variance with other smaller reports is in its incidence of Stage I gastric cancer which remained in that study at 0.7% throughout. Other reports from the UK describe rates of Stage I cancer of 10% [12], 12% [13], and 26% [14], but these reports are from hospital- rather than population-based case data and this suggests that expertise in earlier diagnosis is, as would be expected, improving faster in areas where enthusiasm and techniques co-exist than in the country overall. It was becoming clear that clinical practice in the UK should change, and that early endoscopic assessment of patients at risk should be encouraged. Patients with symptoms referrable to the upper gastric intestinal tract require early endoscopy rather than the investigation being reserved only for those with established symptoms of gastric cancer—which usually reflect advanced incurable disease. Detailed investigation of all patients with dyspepsia is impractical because the symptom is commonplace and many of its causes are evanescent; yet, those in whom the risk of gastric cancer is higher do require investigation. In Britain, as elsewhere, the incidence of gastric cancer rises with age. Hallisey et al. [15] have undertaken a pilot study which has demonstrated an effective low cost approach to the earlier diagnosis of gastric cancer. The aim of the study was to endoscope *all* dyspeptics over 40 years of age within 3 weeks of their first presenting to their general practitioner. Among the 2659 patients referred, 2584 (97.1%) required endoscopy. Malignant disease was identified in 115 (4%) patients, of which 58 were found to be arising in the stomach. Of the 57 gastric adenocarcinomas diagnosed, 36 (63%) with no evidence of distant metastases, residual local disease, or N3 node involvement were suitable for curative surgery (Table 1). Of the 15 cases (26%) of early

Table 1. Stage of gastric cancers (57 cases[a]).

Stage	I	II	III	IVA	IVB
Number	12	7	17[b]	8	12
% of Total	21	12	30	14	21

[a] One patient refused surgery
[b] Includes three patients with node-positive early gastric cancer

gastric cancers, 12 had no lymphatic involvement. It is of interest to note that of the 14 patients with Stage I or II of the disease who were treated symptomatically prior to surgery, all but one had had complete resolution of their symptoms.

In addition to diagnosing patients with established disease, it has been possible to identify patients with high risk mucosal changes and undertake follow-up measures. This has yielded one cancer which is clearly a case of progression being diagnosed on the 5th annual follow-up endoscopy for type III intestinal metaplasia. While it has been possible to change the stage of disease among the patients entered into the study, it is as yet impossible to determine the impact of such a program on mortality from gastric cancer. In order to demonstrate an improvement in mortality rates, a larger study is required with a defined control population. The age after which investigation is recommended also needs to be examined. In the Birmingham study, only one patient aged under 55 years was found to have gastric carcinoma, and it may be appropriate to raise the age at which investigation is undertaken. This paper has received much attention, and there is now an increasing awareness that dyspepsia appearing after middle age should be investigated rather than palliated.

It would be remiss to conclude without mention of the British Medical Research Council (MRC) trial on the surgical treatment of gastric cancer. We in Britain are aware of the Japanese experience with gastric cancer and of their vastly improved 5-year survival rate for all stages of the disease with a higher resectability rate, a lower operative mortality rate, and their commitment to the more radical R_2 resection. Nonetheless, the Japanese have not compared it with the less radical R_1 resection and their case for adopting R_2 remains uproven. The MRC Surgical Gastric Cancer trial aims to examine the case for radical resection. Eligible cases are those having up to Stage III and are randomized once curative resectability has been ascertained at laparotomy into an R_1 or R_2 resection while also having been stratified according to clinical stage and surgeon. The resection is undertaken by a method agreed to in the protocol, and pathological staging is undertaken and confirmed by a panel of pathologists.

Some 25 surgeons contribute cases to the trial where recruitment target is 400 patients. More than 380 patients have been randomized, and it is expected that recruitment will cease before the end of 1993. No report has yet been published.

The declared intent of this trial is to define the radicality of curative gastric cancer surgery, but the clinicians involved in it also hope it will revive interest in improving surgical treatment of the disease. We cannot afford to be complacent in the UK. As the reader may have learned, operative staging is not widely practiced, gastric resections are not standardized, and probably, in many cases, the measures taken are less than those required for cure. The operative mortality is unacceptably high and, in most hospitals, the pathological examination of resected specimens is limited and often affords too little information either to stage the disease or to assess curability. If the MRC trial succeeds in changing surgeons' and pathologists' attitudes to this disease, still too aptly called "captain of the men of death", it will have been a very successful trial indeed.

References

1. Ashton-Key M, Hammersley S, Johnson CD (1991) Incidence and mortality of gastric and pancreatic cancer in England and Wales 1961–1988. Gut 32:A580
2. Allum WH, Powell DJ, McConkey CC, Fielding JW (1989) Gastric cancer: A 25 year review. Br J Surg 75:535–540
3. Mann CV, Russell RCG (eds) (1992) Bailey and Love's short practice of surgery, 21st edn. Chapman and Hall, London
4. Swynnerton BF, Truelove SC (1952) Carcinoma of the stomach. BMJ I:287–292
5. Brookes VS, Waterhouse JAH, Powell DJ (1965) Carcinoma of the stomach: A 10-year survey of results and of factors affecting prognosis. BMJ I:1577–1583
6. Lundh G, Burn JI, Kolig G, Richard CA, Thomson JWW, van Elk PJ, Oszacki J (1974) A cooperative international study of gastric cancer. Ann R Coll Surg Engl 54:219–228
7. Allum WH, Hallisey MT, Kelly KA (1989) Adjuvant chemotherapy in operable gastric cancer. Lancet I:571–574
8. Hockey MS, Fielding WL, Kelly KA, Brookes VS, Craven JL, Mason MC, Winsey HS (1984) Resection line disease in gastric cancer. BMJ 289:601–603
9. Allum WH, Hallisey MT, Ward LC, Hockey MS (1989) A controlled prospective randomised trial of adjuvant chemotherapy or radiotherapy in resectable gastric cancer: Interim report. Br J Cancer 60:739–744
10. Diggory RT, Cuschieri A (1985) R2/3 Gastrectomy for gastric carcinoma: An audited experience of a consecutive series (1985) Br J Surg 72:146–148
11. Irvin TT, Bridger JE (1988) Gastric cancer: An audit of 122 concecutive cases and the results of R_1 gastrectomy. Br J Surg 75:106–109
12. Evans DMD, Craven JL, Murphy F, Cleary BK (1978) Comparison of "early gastric cancer" in Britain and Japan. Gut 19:1–9
13. Houghton PWJ, Mortensen NJ McC, Allan A, Williamson RCN, Davies JD (1985) Early gastric cancer: The case for longterm surveillance. BMJ 291:305–308
14. Sue-Ling H, Lansdowne MRJ, Martin I, Dixon MF, Axon ATR, Johnson D (1992) Gastric cancer—a curable disease. Gut [Suppl] 1:S6
15. Hallisey MT, Allum WH, Jewkes AJ, Ellis DS, Fielding JWL (1990) Early detection of gastric cancer. BMJ 301:513–515

End Results of Surgical Treatment: German Experience

Henning Rohde[1] and The German Gastric Cancer TNM Study Group

Key words. Gastric cancer—Surgery—Lymphadenectomy—TNM system—Gastrectomy

Introduction

The cure rate for gastric carcinoma in Germany continues to be poor. Maximal 5-year survival rates, as a valid indicator of curability, are 10% [1], 11% [2], 13% [3], 16% [4], 17% [5], 22% [6], and 24% [7] and, in many cases, even worse. Japanese surgeons however, report survival rates at 5 years of 45% [8], 46% [9], 50% [10], and 62% [11]. It appears that the survival differences are due mainly to a greater frequency in diagnoses of early gastric cancer in Japan [12–14] and meticulous histopathologic evaluation of the surgical specimens [12], resulting in more accurate surgical and pathologic staging [6, 15–18], and the presumed benefit of systematic lymphadenectomy [11–14].

Earlier diagnostic intervention including fiberoptic gastrointestinal endoscopy and a need for a change of attitude on the part of Western surgeons is necessary [6, 19], since the dismal prognosis of gastric cancer in the Western hemisphere is certainly related to late presentation (with already advanced disease) and is also the result of an inadequate surgical effort [14, 19–21].

I present here-in data from a large prospective multicentre surgical-pathological observational study of 1420 stomach cancer patients [6, 14, 21–23] with a short recruitment time (2.5 years, 1982–1984) and a high 5-year follow-up rate (99.6%, 1987–1989) which describe the end results of surgical treatment of this disease in Germany.

---
[1] Friesenplatz 17a, D-50672 Köln 1, Germany

Patients and Methods

A protocol for patients with carcinoma of the stomach was prepared which permitted the staging of gastric cancer. The stomach was divided into thirds (upper, middle, and lower) and the extent of involvement, i.e., invasion of contiguous structures, was classified according to the TNM system [24, 25]. Lymph node involvement was categorized as N0–N2 according to the AJCC [24] and UICC [25] definitions and as N1–N16 as described in the Japanese General Rules [18]. The resected specimen was subjected to detailed pathological examination, which identified the depth of penetration of the stomach wall, whether the margins were free of tumor, and the presence of secondary deposits in the various nodal groups and tiers; the histological type of the primary was established according to Laurén (diffuse or intestinal) [26]. The tumor was finally staged by the TNM system [24, 25] and the operation categorized. Because the 1978 UICC-TNM classification [27], which was valid when we started our study, uses the terms "radical resectable" and "not radical resectable" without any definition of radicality, we decided that whenever the pathologist found microscopic residual tumor (R_1) [24] in a given patient, no radical resection had been performed [6]. When the surgeon's classification was R_2 (macroscopic residual tumor) [24], we accepted the surgeon's statement because only he was able to identify residual tumor within the opened abdomen [6]. All data were prospectively recorded on special patient record forms and follow-up information was obtained every 3 months after surgery during the first year, every 6 months during the second, and then once a year, or until death [6]. In order to obtain a broad sample of patients with gastric cancer, 11 university departments of surgery and 11 affiliated hospitals with 14 departments of pathology in various regions of the Federal Republic of Germany joined the study. Each patient with untreated histologically verified carcinoma of the stomach who was admitted to these surgical units between April 1, 1982 and October 31, 1984 was included. The surgeon's TNM staging procedures were mandatory, whereas type and extent of surgical therapy was completely discretionary. Participating surgeons and pathologists met at a study center at 3 monthly intervals to be instructed, tested, retested, informed, and motivated to conduct good clinical practice and documentation. After having passed extensive error and plausibility checks by special computer programs, all data were stored in a SIR data base (Institute of Scientific Information, Deerfield, II). Statistical analyses were performed along the lines of hierarchical log-linear model, product-limit, and estimation of survival according to Kaplan-Meier, and the multivariate proportional hazards regression model of Cox by using BMDP (Statistical Software Inc., Los Angeles, Calif.) [28].

Results

Findings on patient age and sex (Fig. 1) showed a preponderance of males in comparison to females predominantly in the age groups of 50 to 60 and 70

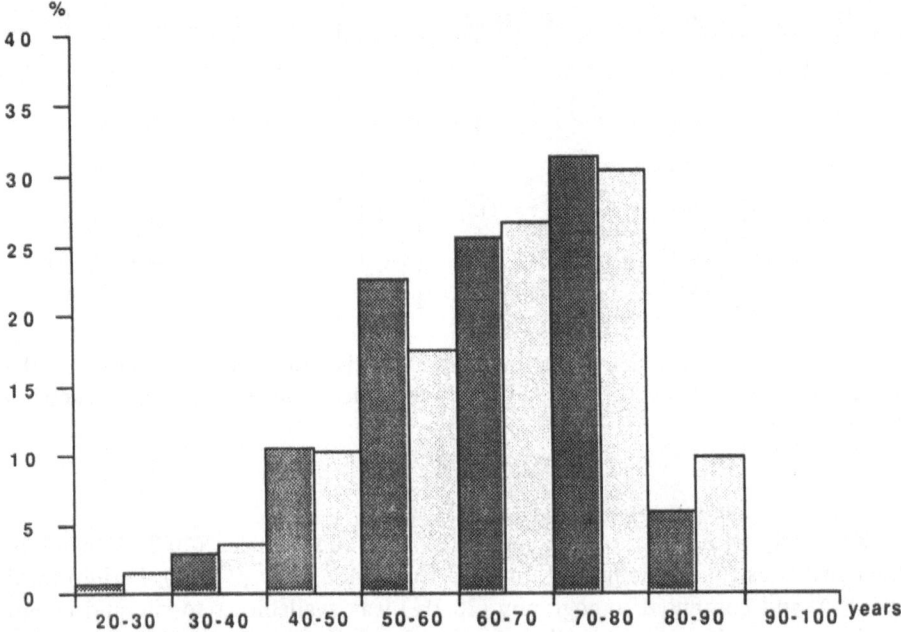

Fig. 1. Age and sex of 1420 patients (914 males, *darker columns*; 506 females, *lighter columns*) with cancer of the stomach of the German Gastric Cancer TNM Study

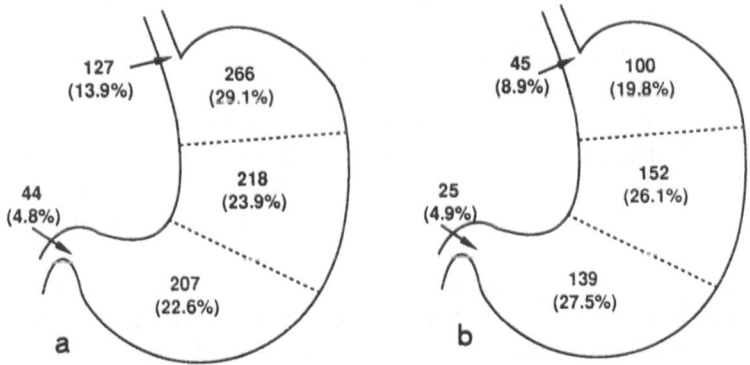

Fig. 2. Site of the primary tumor as judged by surgeons after opening the abdomen in **a** 914 males and **b** 506 females with cancer of the stomach (German Gastric Cancer TNM Study). The primary tumor filled the stomach in 44 male patients (4.8%) and in 44 female patients (8.7%). The extent of the lesion was not specified in 8 (0.9%) and 1 (0.2%), respectively

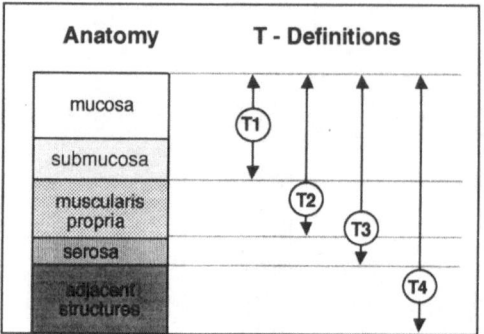

Fig. 3. Degree of penetration of the stomach wall by the primary tumor according to the T-definitions of the AJCC [24] and UICC [25] with the results of T-stagings of surgeons and pathologists

to 80 years, with most of the males (37.4%) and females (40.3%) being in their seventies [6]. Although information from endoscopy (98.5%), barium meal (84.2%), and computed tomography (20.1%) was available as to site and extent of the primary lesion within the stomach [6], only the surgeon's view of the localization of the primary lesions is presented here. It is my opinion that after opening the abdomen, the surgeon is able to give the most reliable information on the site of the primary tumor (Fig. 2). A high proportion of proximal gastric cancers was found in more than one-half of the males in this study (53%) and in almost one-half of the females (45.9%).

Adequate operative staging is not widely practiced in the Western hemisphere [16, 20, 23, 29], in contrast to Japan [8, 10, 11, 15, 18]. It should result in better planning and performance of treatment and, therefore, in better results [16, 17, 25, 27, 29]. The results of staging of the primary tumor (T) according to the TNM system [24, 25, 27] by surgeons and pathologists are given in Fig. 3. The majority of patients (58.8%) were those with advanced stomach cancers (T3- and T4-tumors), whereas the proportion of early gastric cancers was low (12.9%). Reliability of surgical T-staging was very good compared with the results of pathologic T-staging (Fig. 3) followed by distal subtotal gastrectomy (28.5%) (Table 1). The large number of patients with advanced disease is illustrated by a number of palliative operations which accounts for almost one-third (27%) of the study patients.

Although a broad spectrum of postsurgical complications were seen (Table 2), proximal subtotal gastrectomy was found to be a much more dangerous operation than total gastrectomy (13.3% vs 8.7% 30-day mortality).

Only 299 out of 1420 patients (22%) had extended systematic lymphadenectomy. Astonishingly, this surgical procedure has been performed slightly less frequently in patients with early gastric cancers than in patients with advanced stomach cancer (27.5% vs 30.4%) [14], illustrating that German surgeons do not seem

Table 1. Treatment of primary tumor.

	n	%
Total gastrectomy	527	38.8
Subtotal distal gastrectomy	386	28.4
Subtotal proximal gastrectomy	75	5.5
Exploratory laparotomy	194	14.3
Gastroenterostomy	83	6.1
Gastrostomy, tube insertion	44	3.2
Local excision	4	0.3
Endoscopic polypectomy	1	0.1
Other procedures	44	3.2
Total	1358	99.9

Table 2. Postoperative complications and death in correlation to surgical procedure (German Gastric Cancer TNM Study, 1982–1984; n = 1420).

Surgical procedure	n	%	Complications n	%	Death n	%
Gastrostomy/tube ins./loc. excision/polypect.	49	3.6	10	20.4	8	16.3
Expl. laparotomy/GE	277	20.4	20	7.2	32	11.5
Subtotal distal gastrectomy	386	28.4	89	23.1	26	6.8
Subtotal prox. gastrectomy	75	5.5	33	44.0	10	13.3
Total gastrectomy	527	38.8	203	38.5	46	8.7
Other procedures	44	3.2	14	31.8	8	18.2
Total	1358	100.0	369	27.2	130	9.6

ins., Insertion; *Loc.*, local; *Polypect.*, polypectomy; *Expl.*, exploratory; *GE*, gastroenterostomy; *prox.*, proximal

convinced of the possible benefit of this type of surgical procedure especially in low-stage stomach cancers [6, 14, 23]. However, its results in the hands of German surgeons performing systematic lymphadenectomy were excellent in this study: the 5-year survival of 36 patients with early gastric cancer and systematic lymphadenectomy was better than that of 95 patients with early gastric cancer without this procedure ($P = 0.0916$) [14].

That surgery may cause high mortality rates even in low-stage carcinomas when they are located in the upper part of the stomach is impressively demonstrated by the survival curves of patients with early stages of proximally localized gastric adenocarcinomas (PGA) in comparison to distally located adenocarcinomas (DLA). Compared with the survival curves for the same tumor stages of DLA, the patients with PGA show an initial dramatic drop, illustrating their high perioperative death rates. Thus, a patient with an early-stage PGA may be expected to be a much higher surgical risk than a patient with the same tumor stage located distally (Fig. 4).

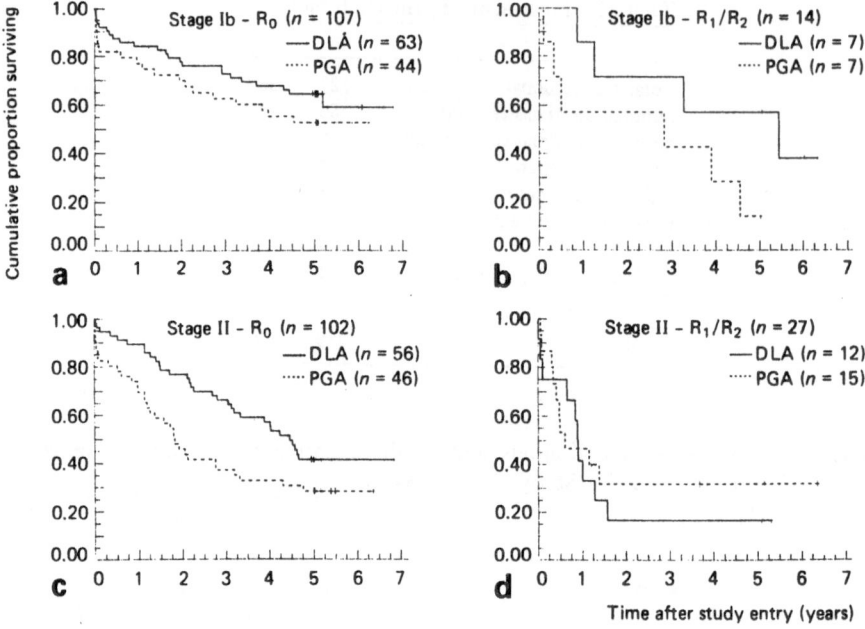

Fig. 4a–d. Survival according to stage, site, and residual tumor (**a, c** without residual tumor, **b, d** with residual tumor). R_0, No residual tumor; R_1, microscopic residual tumor; R_2, macroscopic residual tumor [24]; *PGA*, proximally localized gastric adenocarcinoma; *DLA*, distally located adenocarcinoma. (From [22] with permission)

Table 3. Histologic typing according to Laurén.

| Histologic types | Patients | | No. of patients and age | | | |
| | | | <65 years | | >65 years | |
	n	%	n	%	n	%
Intestinal type	624	52.2	271	45.2	353	59.3
Diffuse type	525	43.9	309	51.6	216	36.3
Mixed type	36	3.1	14	2.4	22	3.7
Not classified	9	0.8	5	0.8	4	0.7
Total	1194	100.0	599	100.0	595	100.0

Results of histologic typing according to Laurén [26] including age differences are given in Table 3. Laurén's diffuse type [26] was found more frequently in patients younger than 65 years than in the older age group. The multivariate structure of the data as evaluated by a log-linear model is shown in Fig. 5. Strong partial association ($P = 0.001$) was observed for age and site (more distal tumors for elderly patients), age and depth of penetration (older patients showed deeper penetration of the primary lesion), age and Laurén histologic type [26] (more intestinal tumors being found in elderly patients), depth of penetration and

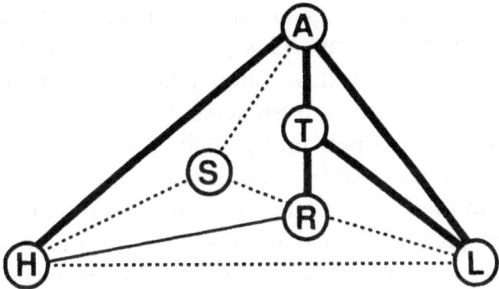

Fig. 5. Multivariate structure of the influencing factors. T, Depth of penetration of primary tumor; A, age of patients; S, sex of patient; L, localization of primary tumor; H, histologic type according to Laurén [26]; R, residual tumor. Using the measure of the partial association in the log-linear model: ____ $P = 0.001$; ___ $P = 0.01$; . . . $P = 0.05$. (From [22] with permittion)

residual tumor (the deeper the penetration of the primary lesion the more residual tumors that were found), and depth of penetration and site (more advanced in patients with proximal adenocarcinomas). An intermediate partial association ($P = 0.01$) was found for the Laurén type and residual tumor (diffuse types were associated with more residual tumors). Weak associations ($P = 0.05$) were found for residual tumors and site (more residual tumors were found in proximal gastric cancers), Laurén type and site (there were more intestinal type tumors with proximal gastric cancers), sex and age (females were older), sex and Laurén type (females more often had a diffuse type according to Laurén), and sex and residual tumor (females more often had residual carcinoma).

Comment

Patients of this study were diagnosed during 1982–1984 and followed-up for 5 years (until 1989). They came from various parts of Germany and from different institutions and, therefore, were reflective of current clinical practice in Germany. Although our male to female ratio is identical to Japanese findings, Japanese stomach cancer patients are younger [11]. The proportion of proximal gastric cancers in our series is higher than that of the lower third, and very similar to the findings of Maruyama and coworkers from Japan [11]. However, this is in contrast to most published series from Western countries [30–32]. Site is a prognostic factor, even in patients with low-stage carcinomas. This is impressively demonstrated by the survival curves of patients with early stages of proximal gastric adenocarcinomas compared with the survival curves for the same tumor stages of distally located adenocarcinomas of the stomach [22]. Although the general rules of the Japanese Research Society for Gastric Cancer were published in English in 1981 [18] and their translation into German was published as early as 1985 [33], German surgeons do not seem to have become familiar with systematic lymphadenectomy. This procedure was performed in only one-fifth (22%) of the patients of this study, and not even in all patients with early gastric cancer. In contrast, systematic lymphadenectomy is part of the multicenter randomized trials now under study in the United Kingdom [20] and in the Netherlands [34], and will become accepted practice not only in Japan but also in Europe and in the United States [19]. In the future, only radical extended surgery, defined as partial or total gastrectomy (according to the site of the primary lesion), routinely performed systematic lymphadenectomy, and distal pancreatico-splenectomy with splenic vessel lymph node dissection will provide the chance to cure a patient with cancer of the stomach. This, it seems to me, is the lesson to be learned by Western surgeons.

Acknowledgements. I would like to thank the participants of this multicenter observational study. Without their interest, effort, and indulgence it would have been impossible to perform this study. The study was supported by a grant of the German Ministry of Science and Technology No. 070 1908 A.

References

1. Becker HD (1981) Chirurgie des Magenkarizinoms. Therapiewoche 31:3494–3500
2. Hildebrand J, Wündrich B, Herrmann U (1988) Chirurgische Verfahrenswahl beim Magenkarzinom in fortgeschrittenen Alter—eine retrospektive Untersuchung. Akt Chir 23:202–206
3. Braun I (1988) Zur Prognose des Magenkarzinoms. Dtsch Med Wschr 113:672–677
4. Bittner R, Schirrow H, Butters M, Roscher R, Krautzberger W, Oettinger W, Beger HG (1985) Total gastrectomy. Arch Surg 120:1120–1125
5. Gall FP, Altendorf A, Hermanek P, Gentsch HH (1982) Chirurgische Therapie des Magenkarzinoms—Stagnation oder Fortschritt? Fortschr Med 100:1876–1882
6. Rohde H, Gebbensleben B, Bauer P, Stützer H, Zieschang J (1989) Has there been any improvement in the staging of gastric cancer? Cancer 64:2465–2481
7. Slislow W, Marx G, Seifart W, Staneczek W (1987) Argumentation für eine regionale Behandlung beim Magenkarzinom. Zentralbl Chir 112:27–33
8. Kodama Y, Sugimachi K, Soejima K, Matsusaka T, Inokuchi M (1981) Evaluation of extensive lymph node dissection for carcinoma of the stomach. World J Surg 5:241–248
9. Koga S, Kaibara N, Kishimoto H, Nishidoi H, Kimura O, Okamoto T, Tamura H (1982) Comparison of 5- and 10-year survival rates in operated gastric cancer patients. Langenb Arch Chir 356:37–42
10. Soga J, Kobayashi K, Saito J, Fujimaki M, Muto T (1979) The role of lymphade-nectomy in curative surgery for gastric cancer. World J Surg 11:418–425
11. Maruyama K, Okabayashi K, Kinoshita T (1987) Progress in gastric cancer surgery in Japan and its limits in radicality. World J Surg 11:418–425
12. Noguchi Y, Imada T, Matsumoto A, Coit DG, Brennen MF (1989) Radical surgery for gastric cancer. Cancer 64:2053–2062
13. Fielding JWL (1989) Gastric cancer: Different diseases. Br J Surg 76:1227

14. Rohde H, Stützer H, Bauer P, Heitmann K, Gebbensleben B, und die Deutsche Magenkarziom TNM Studiengruppe (1991) Das Magenfrühkarzinom im Vergleich zum fortgeschrittenen Magenkarzinom. Langenbecks Arch Chir 376:16–22
15. Maruyama K, Miwa K (1987) Japanese staging system for gastric cancer. Evaluation and documentation of tumor extension. Scand J Gastroenterol 22 [Suppl 123]:22–26
16. Carr D (1983) Is staging of cancer of value? Cancer 51:2503–2505
17. Kennedy BJ (1987) The unified international gastric cancer staging classification system. Scand J Gastroenterol 22 [Suppl 123]:11–13
18. Japanese Research Society for Gastric Cancer (1981) The general rules for the gastric cancer study in surgery and pathology. Jpn J Surg 11:127–145
19. Brennan MF (1989) Radical surgery for gastric cancer. Cancer 64:2063
20. Cuschieri A (1986) Gastrectomy for gastric cancer: Definitions and objectives. Br J Surg 73:513–514
21. Rohde H, Bauer P, Stützer H, Vierzig A, Gebbensleben B (1987) Radikalität und Prognose: Ergebnisse der multizentrischen chirurgisch-pathologischen Magenkarzinom-TNM-Studie. Langenbecks Arch Chir 372:599–602
22. Rohde H, Bauer P, Stützer H, Heitmann K, Gebbensleben B, and the German Gastric Cancer TNM Study Group (1991) Proximal compared with distal adenocarcinoma of the stomach: Differences and consequences. Br J Surg 78:1242–1248
23. Rohde H, Troidl H (eds) (1984) Das Magenkarzinom. Methodik klinischer Studien und therapeutischer Ansätze. Thieme, Stuttgart
24. AJCC (1987) Manual of staging of cancer, 3rd edn. J.B. Lippincott, Philadelphia
25. UICC (1987) TNM classification of malignant tumors, 4th edn. Springer, Heidelberg New York Tokyo
26. Laurén P (1965) The two histologic main types of gastric carcinoma: Diffuse and so-called intestinal type carcinoma. Acta Pathol Microbiol Scand 64:31–49
27. UICC (1978) TNM classification of malignant tumors, 3rd edn. Springer, Heidelberg Berlin New York Tokyo
28. BMDP Statistical Software (1985) University of California Press
29. Rohde H (ed) (1987) Gastric cancer. Importance of surgical staging, tumor pathology and quality of life. Scand J Gastroenterol 22 [Suppl 123]:1–106
30. Allum WH, Roginski C, Fielding JWL (1986) Adenocarcinoma of the cardia: A ten year regional view. World J Surg 10:462–467
31. Weed TE, Nuessle W, Ochsner A (1981) Carcinoma of the stomach: Why are we failing to improve survival? Ann Surg 193:407–413
32. Nielsen J, Aagaard J, Toftgard C (1985) Gastric cancer with special reference to prognostic factors: A review of 799 cases. Acta Chir Scand 151:49–55
33. Japanese Research Society for Gastric Cancer (1985) Allgemeine Richtlinien für Chirurgie und Pathologie der Japanischen Magenkarzinomstudie. Der Chirurg 56:539–546
34. Plukker JTM, Kampschöer GHM (1990) Extended lymph node dissection for gastric cancer: A challenge for better survival results. Neth J Surg 42:3–7

Results of Surgery on 6589 Gastric Cancer Patients Indicating Immunochemosurgery as Being the Best Multimodality Treatment for Advanced Gastric Cancer

Jin-Pok Kim[1]

Key words. Gastric cancer—Immunochemosurgery—Survival rate—Postoperative recurrence

Summary. The surgical results of 6589 cases of gastric cancer treated at the Department of Surgery, Seoul National University Hospital from 1970 to 1990 were reported. About two-thirds (76.6%) were advanced gastric cancer (Stages III and IV), and the 5-year survival rate of operated stage III gastric cancer was only 30.6%, with frequent recurrence. On the other hand, cell-mediated immunities of advanced gastric cancer patients were significantly decreased.

Therefore, to improve the cure rate and to prevent or delay the recurrence of malignancy, real curative surgery with confirmation of free resection of margins and systematic lymph node dissection of perigastric vessels was performed and followed by early postoperative immunotherapy and chemotherapy (immunochemosurgery) in stage III patients.

To evaluate the effect of immunochemosurgery, two randomized trials were conducted, in 1976 and 1981. In the first one, 5-FU, Mitomycin C, and Cytosine Arabinoside for chemotherapy and OK 432 for immunotherapy were used. The 5-year survival rates of surgery alone ($n = 64$) and immunochemosurgery ($n = 73$) were 23.4% and 44.6%, respectively, showing a significant difference.

In the second trial there were 3 groups: group I, immunochemosurgery ($n = 159$), group II, surgery and chemotherapy ($n = 77$), and group III, surgery alone ($n = 94$). The drugs 5-FU and MMC were used for chemotherapy and OK-432 for immunotherapy and were administered for 2 years. The 5-year survival rate of group I was 45.3%, significantly higher than the 29.8% of group II and than the 24.4% of group III. The postoperative 1-chloro-2,4-dinitrobenzene (DNCB) test, T-lymphocyte percent, phytohemaglutinin (PHA)- and concavalin-A (con-A)-stimulated lymphoblastogenesis, and antibody-dependent cellular cytotoxicity (ADCC) test showed more favorable values in the immunochemosurgery group.

---

[1] College of Medicine, Seoul National University Hospital, 28 Yongon-Dong, Chongno-Gu, Seoul 110-744, Korea

Consequently, immunochemosurgery is considered to be the best multimodality treatment for advanced gastric cancer.

Results of Surgery on 6589 Gastric Cancer Patients

Introduction

Gastric cancer is the most frequent malignancy and the primary cause of cancer death in Korea [1–3]. One of four patients with malignant tumor has gastric cancer. During the period from July 1, 1989 to June 30, 1990, a total of 10 511 newly diagnosed cases of gastric cancer were registered [1], and 663 new gastric cancer patients were treated at Seoul National University Hospital (SNUH) in 1991.

Table 1. TNM stages of 6589 gastric cancer patients at the Department of Surgery, Seoul National University Hospital (1970–1990).

	No. of cases	Stages			
		I	II	III	IV
1970–1979	1209	42 (3.5)ᵃ	140 (11.6)	547 (45.2)	480 (39.7)
1980–1984	1858	158 (8.5)	175 (9.4)	957 (51.5)	568 (30.6)
1985–1987	1512	224 (14.8)	212 (14.0)	728 (48.1)	348 (23.0)
1988	710	94 (13.2)	91 (12.8)	364 (51.3)	161 (22.7)
1989	660	106 (16.1)	99 (15.0)	304 (46.1)	151 (22.9)
1990	640	106 (16.6)	96 (15.0)	305 (47.7)	133 (20.8)
Total	6589	730 (11.1)	813 (12.3)	3205 (48.7)	1841 (27.9)

ᵃ (%)

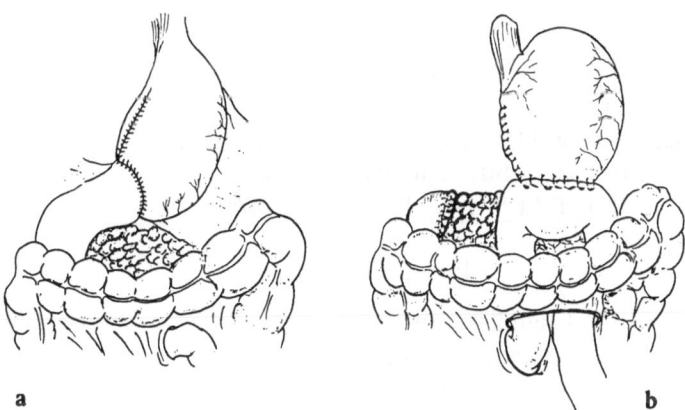

a   b

Fig. 1a,b. a Gastroduodenostomy (Billroth I) and **b** retrocolic gastrojejunostomy (Billroth II) after subtotal gastrectomy

Despite the fact that endoscopical diagnostic techniques have been developed and are in widespread use, over 70% of the Korean patients are still being initially diagnosed as having advanced cancer (Table 1). Thorough and extensive radical operations have been performed on patients with stage III gastric cancer, but recurrent diseases are found in many of them within 2–3 years postoperatively, and the reported 5-year survival rate varies from only 6% to 33.2% [4–9]. Survival curves of 1207 patients who underwent surgery for gastric cancer at SNUH during a 7-year period are shown in Fig. 4.

The more effective radical curative surgical treatment such as: (1) radical resection of primary tumor with an adequate enough resection margin, (2) complete systematic lymph node dissection, and (3) carefully thought out anastomotic techniques must be considered to increase surgical cure rate in advanced gastric cancer patients.

Materials and Methods

A total of 6589 gastric cancer patients were treated at the Department of Surgery, Seoul National University Hospital for 21 years during the period from 1970 to 1990.

Clinical Stage

UICC TNM Classification of these 6589 cases was Stage I: 11.1% (16.6% in 1990), Stage II: 12.3% (15.0% in 1990), Stage III: 48.7% (47.7% in 1990), and Stage IV: 27.9% (20.8% in 1990) (Table 1). The incidence of early gastric cancer in 1990 was 23% among all resected gastric cancer patients. The male to female ratio was 2:1 and the peak age incidence was the 6th decade, with the average age being 54 years.

The Frequency of Pathologic Characteristics of 6589 Cases of Gastric Cancer Were

1. Location: antrum-pylorus 61.6%
2. Depth: m 9.0, sm 7.4, s 36.6, ss 27.4%
3. Borrmann classification: III 57.2, II 28.0, I 3.2%
4. Differentiation: poor 43.3, moderate 25.2, well 14.1%
5. Laurén type: int. 52.3, diff. 42.0, Mixed 5.7%
6. LN Meta: N 38.1, P 61.9 (1–3, 19.3, ≥4, 42.6)%

Prognostic Factors

To determine the most significant prognostic factors affecting gastric cancer, first univariate analysis of prognostic factors was done and showed some significance except for age and sex. Then, multivariate analysis carried out by a multiple regression method with a SAS software/life regression procedure showed two significant factors, lymph node metastasis ($P = 0.001$) and depth of invasion ($P = 0.004$) (Table 2).

Table 2. Multivariate analysis of 1488 resected gastric carcinomas (1981–1986, Seoul National University Hospital by multiple regression with SAS software/life-regression procedure).

Variables	Category						Statistics	
	1	2	3	4	5	6	χ^2	P
Sex	M	F					0.30	0.580
Age	<30	30	40	50	60	>69	10.93	0.054
Location	A	m	C				4.07	0.130
Gross type	I	II	III	IV	EGC		9.41	0.051
Histology	W	M	P	sig	muc	pap	8.11	0.229
Depth	MM	SM	PM	SS	S	organ	16.81	0.004[a]
Lymph node	n1	n1	n2	n3			73.59	0.001[a]
Resection	ST	T	ET				3.86	0.144

[a] Significant

A, antrum; m, body; C, cardia and fundus; W, well differentiated; M, moderately differentiated; P, poorly differentiated; sig, signet ring cell; muc, mucinous; pap, papillary; MM, mucosa; SM, submucosa; PM, proper muscle; SS, subserosal; S, serosa; ST, subtotal; T, total; ET, extended total

Table 3. Procedures performed in 6589 patients with adenocarcinoma of stomach (Seoul University National Hospital, 1970–1990).

	No. of cases	Operation (% op./total)	Resection (% res./op.)	ST (% ST/op.)	T and ET (%/op.)
1970–1979	1209	1105 (91)	790 (71)	663 (60)	127 (11)
1980–1984	1858	1768 (95)	1364 (77)	1094 (62)	273 (15)
1985–1987	1512	1408 (93)	1166 (83)	910 (65)	256 (17)
1988	710	646 (91)	514 (80)	388 (60)	126 (20)
1989	660	624 (95)	520 (83)	381 (61)	139 (22)
1990	640	617 (96)	507 (82)	359 (58)	148 (24)
Total	6589	6168 (94)	4861 (79)	3795 (62)	1069 (17)

ST, Subtotal; T, total; ET, extended total; op., operation; res., resection

Recently, epidermal growth factor receptors, oncogenes, suppressive oncogenes, and other prognostic factors have been undergoing careful investigation and the results will be clinically useful in the future.

Operability and Resectability (Table 3)

In 6589 cases of gastric cancer, the average rate of operability was 94%, which was an improvement from 87% in early 1970 to 96% in 1990. Resectability was possible 79% of the time, which was an improvement from 70% in early 1970 to 82% in 1990. Of the gastric cancer patients who underwent surgery in 1990, 58% had subtotal gastrectomy and 24% had total or extended total gastrectomy. Total gastrectomy has become a more popular procedure for Borrmann type IV, cardia, or fundus cancer as well as for signet-ring cell or poorly differentiated cancers.

Curative Surgery

Three Essential Surgical Techniques in Curative Surgery

The resection margin should be more than 6 cm from the cancer margin in advanced stomach cancer and at least 2 cm in early gastric cancer, on the proximal site 2–3 cm from the pylorus on a distal site.

Complete systematic lymph node dissection including the lymph nodes around the celiac axis LN (9), common hepatic LN (8) and proper hepatic artery and portal vein LN (12), must be dissected out in addition to the retropancreatic LN (13) and splenic artery lymph nodes (so-called skeletonization of vessels). Modified R_3 (R_2 + α) resection of LN (8, 9, 11, 12, and 13) are highly recommended because there were high incidences of lymph node metastasis in the N3 node. We adopted the Japanese Gastric Cancer Study Group's classification [10] of 18 regional lymph nodes, (LN 1, right cardia; LN 2, left cardia; LN 3, lesser curvature; LN 4, greater curvature; LN 5, suprapyloric; LN 6, subpyloric; LN 7, left gastric a.; LN 8, common hepatic a.; LN 9, celiac a.; LN 10, splenic hilum; LN 11, splenic a.; LN 12, hepatoduodenal; LN 13, retropancreatic; LN 14, mesenteric a.; LN 15, mid-colic a.; LN 16, aortic a.; LN 110, lower thoracic paraesophageal; LN 111, diaphragmatic).

The choice of anastomosis after subtotal or total gastrectomy must be carefully weighed (Fig. 1).

Billroth I or II?

Billroth I anastomosis is usually done after subtotal gastrectomy in distal gastric cancer especially in an early stage, and Billroth II anastomosis is done in most cases of advanced cancer located in the body of the stomach.

Retrocolic or Antecolic Anastomosis?

Whenever feasible, retrocolic gastrojejunostomy is performed (1) because there are no cancer cells in the mesocolon, (2) to create a short afferent (blind) loop, (3) it can absorb more nutrients and iron absorption occurs in the duodenum and proximal jejunum, and (4) there is less postoperative retrostomal herniation.

However, if the mesocolon is congenitally short or absent, antecolic anastomosis becomes necessary.

Loop Esophagojejunostomy with EEA Stapling

Loop, end-to-side esophagojejunostomy was commonly used in the past. However, reflux esophagitis following loop esophagojejunostomy was one annoying postoperative complication. Therefore, many reconstruction methods including Roux-en-Y, reverse 6, β or ρ anastomisis, and jejunal interposition were tested

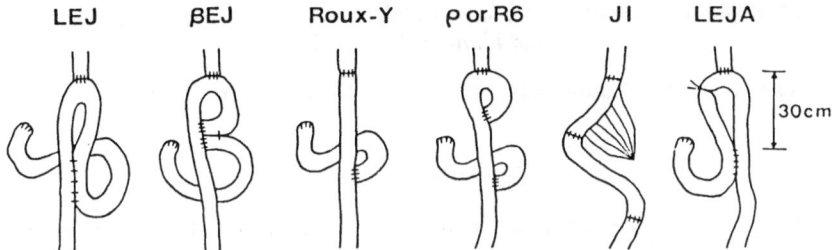

LEJ   βEJ   Roux-Y   ρ or R6   JI   LEJA

30cm

Fig. 2. Various methods of reconstruction after total gastrectomy

Table 4. Comparison of Roux-en-Y and loop esophagojejunostomy.

	Roux-en-Y ($n = 68$)	Loop esophagojejunostomy ($n = 122$)
Operating time (min)	254 ± 37	209 ± 53 ($P < 0.001$)
Postoperative leakage (%)	2 Patients (2.9)	2 Patients (1.8)

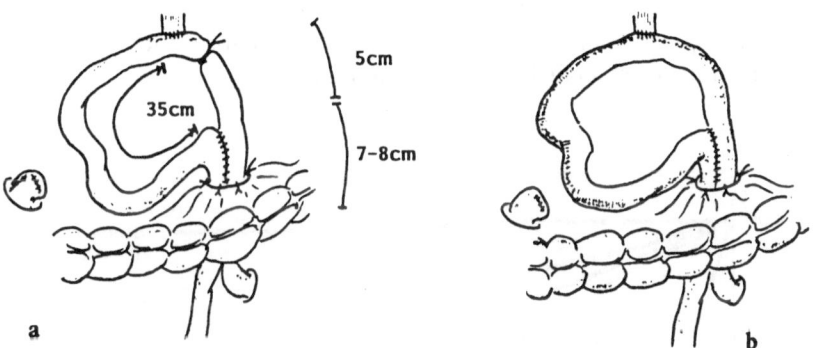

35cm   5cm   7-8cm

a

b

Fig. 3a,b. Esophageal reflux study **a** on the patients who received loop esophago-jejunostomy with ($n = 9$) or **b** without ($n = 5$) afferent loop obstruction after total gastrectomy

for many years, and the long-term results were similar among the various techniques for anastomosis (Fig. 2). The author then used a loop end-to-side esophagojejunostomy with the afferent loop obstruction method because it is easy, safe, has a shorter operation time (209 vs 254 min), and involves less postoperative leakage (1.9% vs 2.9%) (Table 4, Fig. 3). More recently, we have been using the disposable EEA stapler anastomosis which enables a markedly shorter operation time and entails less leakage problems.

A Comparative Study of Esophageal Reflux Between Afferent Loop Ligation and Unligated Group [11]

The results showed significant preventive effects in the afferent loop ligated group.

Quality of Life Study

The items which were evaluated included reservoir function (number of meals, weight), investigation of symptoms (appetite, dysphagia, vomiting, dumping regurgitation), and Spitzer's quality of life index (activities of daily living, health, support, and outlook). These aspects were acceptable and improving in 100 consecutive patients who underwent total gastrectomy with loop esophagojejunostomy and afferent loop occlusion.

Therefore, it was concluded that the method of loop esophagojejunostomy with afferent loop obstruction provides a good enough anastomosis after total gastrectomy.

Postoperative Complications and Mortality

Major postgastrectomy complications were fistulas from the esophagojejunostomy site, pancreatic fistulas, bleeding, and intestinal obstructions.

Postoperative complication rates after subtotal, total, and extended total gastrectomy were 3%, 9%, and 18%, respectively, and the overall complication rate was 5%.

The overall operative mortality rate was 0.34% (0.3% for subtotal gastrectomy and 0.4% for total or extended total gastrectomy).

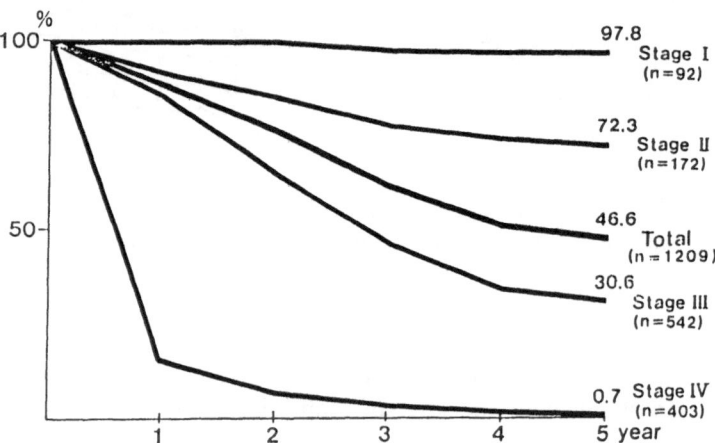

Fig. 4. Survival curves of patients with gastric cancer according to TNM stage (Seoul National University Hospital, 1975–1981). Number of follow-up cases/total: 1209/1387 (87.1%)

Results

Postoperative Survival Rate

The overall 5-year survival rate of resectable gastric cancer was 46.6%, which was well correlated with primary tumor location, number of lymph node metastasis, depth of invasion, and UICC TNM clinical stage. It was especially well correlated with the number of lymph node metastases and depth of invasion, but not with age or sex.

Five-year survival rates according to TNM clinical staging were 97.3% for Stage I and 73.5% for Stage II, but only 30.6% for Stage III gastric cancer patients, which is still a very dismal result (Fig. 4). Since the condition of the majority of our gastric cancer patients is advanced more than Stage III, we have to consider how to develop a more effective treatment modality geared for them.

Immunochemosurgery (Postoperative Immunochemotherapy)

Introduction

Why is immunochemosurgery necessary? The majority of gastric cancer patients are still in either Stage III or IV when they are first diagnosed. The 5-year survival rate for Stage III gastric cancer was only 30.6%, which is disappointing. Therefore, the question arises, "Can surgery alone cure gastric cancer patients?". My answer is affirmative, but only for patients in Stages I and II. Surgery alone, no matter how radical it is, can not cure patients with gastric cancer in an advanced stage. Stomach cancer in Stage III is already a systemic disease. To improve the prognosis of advanced stomach cancer, we need systemic treatment such as immunotherapy or chemotherapy in the early postoperative period to eradicate the micrometastatic or residual cancer cells even after curative resection (Fig. 5).

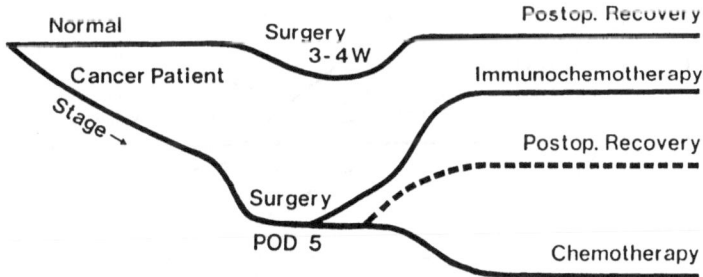

Fig. 5. Cell-mediated immunity of gastric cancer patients decreased according to clinical stage and further decreased by surgery and postoperative (*postop.*) chemotherapy. Simultaneous immunochemotherapy may revive the immunity to the near-normal level. *POD*, Postoperative day

There have been some encouraging reports of prolonged survival and disease-free interval. Taguchi et al. [12] reported improved survival in patients with Stage III gastric carcinoma who received mitomycin C and 5-fluorouracil (5-FU) after surgery. Macdonald et al. [13] reported a prolonged disease-free interval and survival following curative resection for gastric carcinoma using adriamycin and mitomycin C. Although the results of primary chemotherapy in advanced cases are generally poor, a combined administration of mitomycin C, 5-FU, cytosine arabinoside (MFC), or 5-FU and methyl-CCNU (FME) was documented as being efficacious [14, 15].

In the late 1960s, Mathé carried out a study, published in 1971 [16], in which he reported an immunotherapeutic effect of BCG and allogenic tumor cell vaccine with an increase in the duration of remission and survival in a child with leukemia, and Morton et al. [17] reported an immunotherapeutic efficacy of intradermal BCG inoculation on metastatic cutaneous malignant melanoma. Since then, the interest in immunotherapy has greatly increased. Rosenberg [18] and many others [19–27] have shown that immunotherapy can be effective against certain malignancies, including gastric cancer. Immunotherapy alone is rarely effective against clinically measurable cancer. It would be an important means of therapy, however, to attack cancer cells and to improve the host's immune status in conjunction with the other treatment modalities.

Kim and others [28–30] have shown that both cell-mediated immunity, measured by T-lymphocyte quantitations, and the positivity of DNCB delayed cutaneous hypersensitivity in patients with malignancy are decreased significantly, and that the level of immunosuppressive acid protein (IAP) is significantly higher than that of normal individuals. The further the clinical stage of gastric cancer has progressed, the more depressed is the cell-mediated immunity of the host [31, 32] (Fig. 6). In view of this finding, enhancement of the depressed immune status

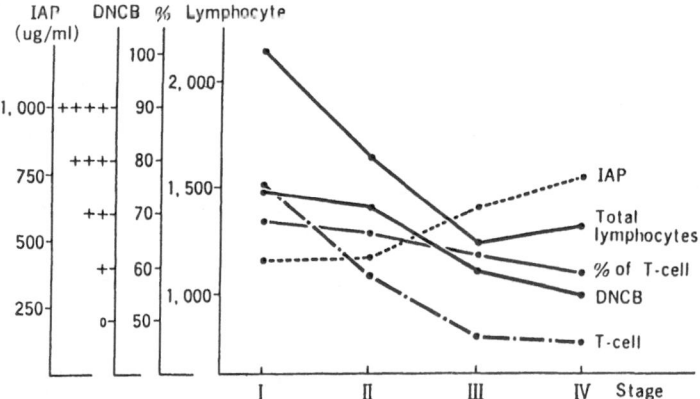

Fig. 6. Levels of various immune parameters in each clinical stage of gastric adenocarcinoma. *T cell % and 1-chloro-2,4-dinitrobenzene (DNCB)* positivities were decreased, whereas immunosuppressive acidic protein (*IAP*) levels were increased according to the advancement of clinical stage

of the host is thought to be an important aspect in the treatment of cancer patients.

The purpose of this study is to evaluate the therapeutic effectiveness of post-operative immunochemotherapy in advanced, but resectable, adenocarcinoma of the stomach. Survival rate and immune status of patients with Stage III gastric carcinoma who received postoperative immunochemotherapy were compared with those of patients who received surgery with no adjuvant therapy.

Materials and Methods

First Trial

This study was comprised of 138 patients who had received radical subtotal gastrectomy for Stage III gastric cancer from 1976 to 1980 at the Department of Surgery, Seoul National University Hospital (Table 5). Prior to surgery, all patients with stomach cancer underwent a complete case history and physical examination with measurements of disease, the immune parameters detailed below, performance status, routine laboratory tests, and liver scanring. Two groups were found to be comparable. Following the previously described curative surgery, patients who were specifically chosen with histologically confirmed lymph node-positive Stage III adenocarcinoma of the stomach were randomized to receive postoperative immunochemotherapy or not after their results for the routine examinations including hemogram, liver function test, and renal function test were shown to be within the normal range. Patients were ineligible for study if they had a previous history of chemotherapy or radiation therapy or if their age was over 70 years. The initial performance status of 0–2 in all patients was within the range of the Eastern Cooperative Oncology Group (ECOG).

Immunological Studies

The following immunological tests were performed before surgery and in the 3rd–4th postoperative month.

In the *DNCB cutaneous hypersensitivity test.* 0.1 ml of 2% DNCB (J.T. Baker Chemical Co., Phillipsburg, N.J.) solution in acetone (sensitizing dose) and

Table 5. Method (immunochemosurgery)

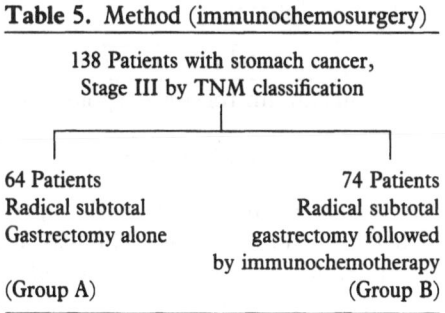

138 Patients with stomach cancer,
Stage III by TNM classification

64 Patients	74 Patients
Radical subtotal	Radical subtotal
Gastrectomy alone	gastrectomy followed
	by immunochemotherapy
(Group A)	(Group B)

0.05% DNCB solution in acetone (challenge dose) were smeared over a 2-cm area of the inner surface of the arm. The flare-up reaction was measured between 7 and 14 days after application and was evaluated as follows: (a) erythema on both sides of the sensitizing dose area and challenge dose area, $++++$, (b) erythema on the sensitizing dose area only, $+++$ (if there was no reaction by 14 days, 0.1 ml of 0.05% DNCB solution was smeared again and the reaction was evaluated 48 hours later), (c) extent of erythema and induration exceeding that of challenge dose area smeared, $++$, (d) erythema and induration not exceeding one-half of the challenge dose area smeared, $+$, and (e) no response, 0.

For testing *T-lymphocytes (percent and count)*, lymphocytes were isolated by the Ficoll-Hypaque method from the heparinized peripheral blood of the patients. Isolated lymphocytes were washed with saline and Hank's solution and then mixed with washed sheep erythrocytes and incubated for 18 h at 37°C. After incubation, the number of rosette-forming cells with at least 3 sheep erythrocytes was counted among 200 lymphocytes and was represented as the percentage of T-lymphocytes.

In the evaluation of *lymphoblastogenesis by phytohemagglutinin (PHA) and concanavalin-A (con-A) stimulation*, lymphocytes were prepared by the Ficoll-Hypaque method from the peripheral blood of the patients. The prepared lymphocytes were adjusted to $1.5 \times 10^6/0.2$ ml with Tissue Culture-199 media. PHA (0.1 ml) and 50 µg con-A were added to the mixture of 0.2 ml of cell suspension and 3 ml of media, respectively, and incubated for 72 h in the presence of 5% CO_2. Four hours before harvest, 0.5 µCi tritiated thymidine was added to each culture tube. After culture, the tubes were centrifuged at 4°C and washed with cold saline. A 5% trichloroacetic acid solution (5 ml) was added to the precipitates and centrifuged at 4°C, and 90% formic acid solution (0.5 ml) was added and kept overnight. Radioactivity was determined by using a scintillation counter.

The investigation of *antibody-dependent cellular cytotoxicity (ADCC)* used lymphomononuclear cells isolated from the peripheral blood of the patients. ^{51}Cr-labeled chicken red blood cells, anti-chicken red blood cell antibody from rabbit, and 10% fetal calf serum-RPMI (Roswell Park Memorial Institute, New York) media were mixed together and incubated for 18 h at 37°C. After culture, the radioactivity of the supernatant was determined. The lymphomononuclear cells (effector cell) to ^{51}Cr-labeled chicken red blood cells (target cell) ratio was 10:1. Cytotoxicity was calculated as follows:

$$^{51}\text{Cr release}(\%) = \frac{\text{experimental release} - \text{spontaneous release}}{\text{maximum release} - \text{spontaneous release}} \times 100$$

Survival Rate

Survival rates were calculated from the day of the operation, and the immune status was compared between the two groups. Statistical comparisons of patient characteristics and immune parameters were performed utilizing the chi-squared (χ^2) test or Student's *t*-test. The differences were considered significant when

$P < 0.05$. The difference in survival rate between the two groups was determined using the Cox-Mantel test.

Postoperative Immunochemotherapy

Patients in the immunochemosurgery group received the following therapy.

For *immunotherapy*, OK 432 (*Streptococcus pyogenes* preparation) was given intramuscularly with a dosage of 1.0 KE (Klinische Einheit) every week from the 4th or 5th postoperative day.

Chemotherapy consisted of a MFC (mitomycin C, 5-FU, and cytosine arabinoside) regimen which was selected at random for the patients and started at the 8th to 10th postoperative day. The dosage administration schedule was as follows: MFC-mitomycin C, 4 mg/50 kg; 5-FU, 500 mg/50 kg; cytosine arabinoside, 40 mg/50 kg, given intravenously twice a week for the first 2 weeks and then every week for the next 6 weeks. Then, oral 5-FU was given daily at a dosage of 600 mg/50 kg for 18 months after surgery if the patients tolerated it. Just prior to each cycle of chemotherapy, white blood cell and platelet counts were obtained, and liver function tests were checked if indicated. The control of drug dosage was based on the parameters of hematologic toxicity and other adverse reactions.

Second Trial

Postoperative Immunochemotherapy

After undergoing the previously described curative subtotal gastrectomy between 1981 and 1985, 370 histologically proven Stage III gastric cancer patients, with a 30- to 70-year age range, a performance status of 0–2, and without systemic disease, were randomly assigned to three groups: 170 for immunochemosurgery, 100 for postoperative chemotherapy, and 100 for surgery alone (Table 6). Because they altered or discontinued treatment, 40 patients were excluded from the study.

Table 6. Randomization of gastric cancer patients.

Criteria: Age >30, <70 (years)
Stage III, performance status: 0–2
Subtotal gastrectomy with lymph node
dissection
Billroth II gastrojejunostomy

Treatment	Subjects (*n*)	No. evaluated
Immunochemosurgery	170	159[a]
Postop. chemotherapy	100	77[a]
Surgery only	100	94[a]
Total	370	330 (89%)

[a] Discontinued or altered treatment cases were excluded from evaluation
Post op., Postoperative

Table 7. Postoperative immunochemotherapy programs.

Immunotherapy—starts at the 4th or 5th postoperative day Picibanil (*Streptococcus pyogenes* preparation); 1.0 Klinische Einheit (*K*E), I.M. weekly

Chemotherapy—starts at the 8th to 10th postoperative day

MF $\left\{ \begin{array}{l} \text{Mitomycin-C; 4 mg/50 kg} \\ \text{5-Fluorouracil; 500 mg/kg} \end{array} \right\}$ I.V. × 2/week for 2 weeks then weekly 6 times

followed by oral 5-FU (futrafur); 600 mg/50 kg, daily

Duration: 24 months (PMF/2 months, PF/22 months)

Prior to surgery, all patients with stomach cancer underwent a complete physical examination with staging of the disease, determining immune parameters (as mentioned above) and performance status, routine laboratory testing, and liver scanning. Patients were ineligible for the study if they had a previous history of chemotherapy or radiation therapy, or if their age was over 70 years. The initial performance status (0–2) was within the range of the Eastern Cooperative Oncology Group (ECOG) in all patients.

Postoperative immunotherapy was started from the 4th or 5th postoperative day with OK-432, and chemotherapy was started from the 8th to 10th postoperative day with mitomycin and 5-FU. Both immunotherapy and chemotherapy were carried out for 2 years. The three groups were comparable in terms of age, sex, performance status, preoperative immune parameter data, number of lymph node metastasis, and Laurén's classification. The protocol of immunochemotherapy in the 2nd trial was essentially the same as for the 1st trial, except for the omission of cytosine arabinoside in chemotherapy because of toxicity and that the treatment duration was 24 months (Table 7).

Survival Rate and Immunoparameter Studies

Survival rates, calculated from the day of the operation, and immune statuses were compared among the three groups. A statistical comparison of patient characteristics and immune parameters was performed utilizing the chi-squared (χ^2) test or Student's t-test. Differences were considered significant when $P < 0.05$. Differences in survival rates between the three groups were determined using the Cox-Mantel test.

Results

Results of the First Trial

A total of 138 patients were randomly divided into two groups and followed-up for at least 5 years. Of these 138 patients, 74 received postoperative immunochemotherapy and 64 received no further anticancer therapy after surgery. Patient characteristics, preoperative value of immune parameters, and the proportion of histologic type and extent of lymph node involvement of the two groups of patients were similar.

Curative surgery for gastric cancer performed in our center inclucdes subtotal gastric resection, complete dissection (so-called skeletonization) of regional lymph nodes along the celiac axis, hepatic artery, splenic artery, portal vein, and retropancreatic lymph node as well as perigastric lymph nodes and removal of the omentum with adjacent tissues. All the tissues were removed in an en bloc fashion. A frozen biopsy of both resection margins was done in all cases.

Survival Rates

Survival curves of the two groups of patients are shown in Fig. 7. The 5-year survival rate of the postoperative immunochemotherapy group was 44.6% and that of the surgery alone group was 23.4%. The difference in survival rate as determined by the Cox-Mantel test is statistically significant ($Z = 2.09$, $P < 0.05$).

Immunoparameter Studies

In the DNCB cutaneous hypersensitivity test, preoperative DNCB positivity was 47.4% in the surgery alone group and 54.8% in the postoperative immunochemotherapy group. DNCB positivity at the 4th postoperative month was 73% in the surgery alone group and 92.9% in the immunochemotherapy group. More patients were converted from negative to positive after postoperative immunochemotherapy.

The T-lymphocyte percent and count in the surgery alone group were decreased from $58.8 \pm 7.8\%$ and $1142 \pm 344/mm^3$ to $56.4 \pm 6.9\%$ and $985 \pm 495/mm^3$, respectively, following surgery. In the postoperative immunochemotherapy group, preoperative T-cell percent and count, $55.2 \pm 5.6\%$ and $1133 \pm 509/mm^3$, respectively, were increased to $58.4 \pm 5.9\%$ and $1179 \pm 537/mm^3$, after therapy.

Postoperative degrees of lymphoblastogenesis by PHA and con-A stimulation ation were $3653 \pm 403\,cpm$ and $4304 \pm 463\,cpm$, respectively, in the surgery

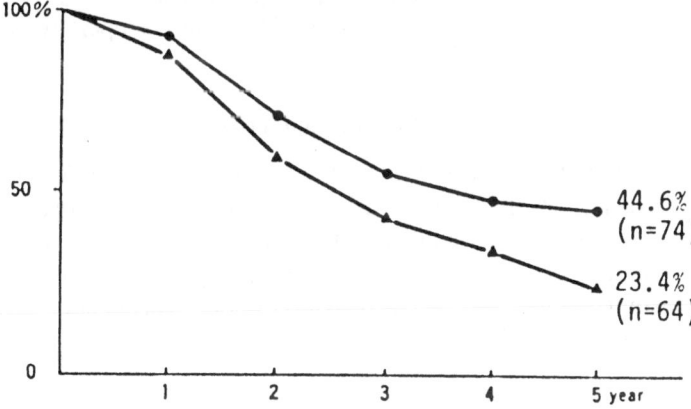

Fig. 7. Survival curve of immunochemosurgery group and surgery alone group in Stage III stomach cancer. *Solid circles*, Immunochemosurgery; *solid triangles*, surgery alone

Table 8. Pre- and postoperative values of immune parameters.

Immune parameter	Control		Immunochemotherapy	
	Preoperative	Postoperative	Preoperative	Postoperative
DNCB positivity (%)	47.4 (9/18)	73.0 (14/19)	54.8 (24/42)	92.9 (40/42)
T Cell (%)	58.8 ± 7.8	56.4 ± 6.9	55.2 ± 5.6	58.4 ± 5.9
T Cell (count/mm³)	1142 ± 344	985 ± 495	1133 ± 509	1179 ± 537
Blastogenesis (cpm)				
PHA-stimulated	5535 ± 1315	3653 ± 403	5183 ± 852	4779 ± 559
Con-A-stimulated	8547 ± 1301	4304 ± 463	8882 ± 1336	5412 ± 476
ADCC activity (%)	36.9 ± 11.6	37.7 ± 12.9	37.2 ± 12.1	39.6 ± 11.4

DNCB, 1-Chloro-2,4-dinitrobenzene; *ADCC*, antibody-dependent cellular cytotoxity; *PHA*, phytohemagglutinin; *Con-A*, concavalin A

Table 9. Pre- and postoperative values of immune parameters.

Immune parameter	Immunochemosurgery		Postoperative chemotherapy		Surgery alone	
	Preoperative	Postoperative	Preoperative	Postoperative	Preoperative	Postoperative
DNCB postivity (%)	52.5 (41/78)	85.9 (67/78)	48.9 (14/29)	72.5 (21/29)	46.8 (15/32)	75.0 (24/32)
T Cell (%)	56.4 ± 6.1	59.7 ± 5.8	59.2 ± 7.4	57.3 ± 6.8	58.7 ± 7.9	56.1 ± 6.8
T Cell (count/mm³)	1.135 ± 507	1.182 ± 541	1.146 ± 352	974 ± 496	1.154 ± 440	1.152 ± 364
Blastogenesis (cpm)						
PHA-stimulated	5.279 ± 759	4.638 ± 602	5.567 ± 1.872	2.302 ± 290	5.536 ± 1.321	3.654 ± 411
Con-A-stimulated	8.879 ± 1.301	5.327 ± 494	8.624 ± 1.312	2.872 ± 340	8.502 ± 1.321	4.409 ± 472
ADCC activity (%)	37.8 ± 11.9	40.2 ± 11.2	36.7 ± 11.0	37.8 ± 11.3	36.8 ± 11.4	37.9 ± 12.8

Definitions as in Table 8

alone group and 4779 ± 559 cpm and 5412 ± 476 cpm in the immunochemo-therapy group. They were much less decreased in the postoperative immuno-chemotherapy group.

Antibody-dependent cellular cytotoxicity activity at the 3rd postoperative month was 37.7 ± 12.9% in the surgery alone group and 39.6 ± 11.4% (not significant) in the immunochemotherapy group. Pre- and postoperative values of immune parameters are shown in Table 8.

Results of the Second Trial

A follow-up study of the 2nd trial was performed on 330 of 370 (89%) patients for at least 5 years. Of these, 159 patients received postoperative immuno-chemotherapy, 77 conventional adjuvant chemotherapy postoperatively, and 94 had no further therapy. The patient characteristics, preoperative values of immune parameters, histologic type, and extent of lymph node involvement of the three groups of patients were similar.

Survival Rates

Survival curves of the three groups of patients are shown in Fig. 8. The 5-year survival rate of the immunochemosurgery group was 45.3%, that of the chemo-

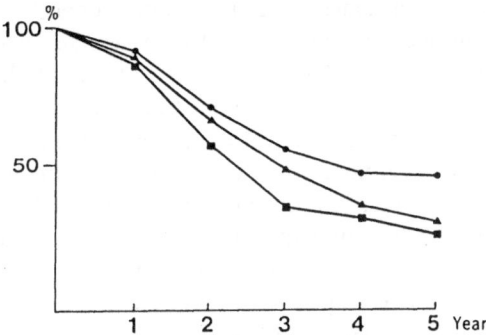

Fig. 8. Survival curve of the immunochemosurgery group, the surgery and postoperative chemotherapy group, and the surgery alone group in Stage III stomach cancer (330 cases, 1981–1985). *Solid circles*, Immunochemosurgery: 45.3%, n = 159; *solid triangles*, surgery and postoperative chemotherapy: 29.8% (n = 77); *solid squares*, surgery alone: 24.4%, n = 94

therapy group was 29.8%, and for the surgery alone group it was 24.4%. The difference between the immunochemosurgery group and the other two groups is statistically significant.

Immunoparameter Studies

The postoperative T cell percentage was increased in the immunochemosurgery group after immunochemotherapy, but was decreased in both postoperative chemotherapy and surgery alone groups. The positive conversion rate of DNCB-negative patients after treatment was 85.9% in the immunochemosurgery group compared to 72.5% in the postoperative chemotherapy group and 75% in the surgery alone group. Lymphoblastogenesis and ADCC activity were also favorable in the immunochemosurgery group (Table 9).

Discussion

The outcome of gastric cancer surgery is dependent primarily on clinical stage and the radicality of surgery, but is also affected by the patient's immunity and other biological characteristics. Certainly the depth of invasion, presence of lymph node metastases—especilly multiple involvement in more than 4 lymph nodes—and distant metastases are the most important prognostic factors in gastric carcinoma [32]. Kim and Choi [31] recently analyzed 448 cases of stomach cancer in order to evaluate the prognostic value of Laurén's histologic classification. The 5-year survival rate of the intestinal type (43.7%, n = 190) was higher than that of the diffuse type (30.4%, n = 138) (P < 0.05). The distribution of these histologic types was similar among the three groups in this study. Furthermore, the extent of lymph node metastases as well as the presence or absence of metastatic lymph nodes were significant prognostic indicators. It was demonstrated in the author's previous study that 5-year survival rates of patients with from one to three metastatic lymph nodes is significantly higher than that of patients with more than four metastatic lymph nodes [32].

Although adjuvant therapy after radical gastric resection had been expected to be the most promising treatment for stomach cancer, there is no long-term follow-up report to demonstrate improvement of survival with the use of adjuvant therapy. Several regimens for adjuvant chemotherapy have been suggested and evaluated clinically. The MFC [12, 14] FAM [13] and FME [15] regimens were reported to have good response rates in advanced gastric cancer. The Gastrointestinal Tumor Study Group [6] reported long-term follow-up results of adjuvant chemotherapy with 5-FU and methyl-CCNU following curative resection of gastric cancer. Nissen-Meyer et al. [33] reported decreasing recurrences and death rates when adjuvant chemotherapy was started in the early postoperative period for breast cancer, but that there was no improvement when it was initiated 3 weeks after mastectomy. A survival advantage was associated with adjuvant treatment and lasted up to 24 months after surgery. The survival difference between the control and adjuvant therapy groups was nearly 20% after 4 years of follow-up. The survival benefit of the present study is similar to that of GITSG [6].

There have been many reports on the effectiveness of immunotherapy for certain malignancies such as acute myeloblastic leukemia, lymphoma, breast cancer, malignant melanoma, ovarian cancer, childhood neuroblastoma, head and neck cancer, esophageal cancer, and stomach cancer [16–27]. Theoretically, specific immunotherapy should be more beneficial than nonspecific immunotherapy, but it is not yet available for clinical use. Nonspecific immunotherapy such as various immune potentiators or biologic response modifiers (BRM) are now commonly in use.

Advantages of postoperative immunochemotherapy have been described in terms of prolonged remission and survival, improved bone marrow tolerance, delayed recurrence, and possible prevention of recurrence. Suga et al. [34] reported prolonged survival for patients treated for advanced gastric cancer with MFC and picibanil compared to those treated with MFC alone. In these studies, the treatment procedure consisted of two components. First, radical gastrectomy was performed as thoroughly as possible and regional lymph nodes including adjacent tissues were removed in an en bloc fashion. Then, early postoperative immunochemotherapy as a second treatment modality was performed to achieve the destruction of residual tumor cells including micrometastases, with the tumor burden being minimal.

According to the data presented in this study, it is evident that the 5-year survival rate of patients receiving surgery with early postoperative immunochemotherapy is better than that of the chemotherapy or control group. Immune status data also show improved reactivity in the immunochemotherapy group.

Surgery, as the means of achieving a complete removal of visible tumor mass, is of primary importance for multimodality therapy. Both types of therapy, however, should be practiced almost simultaneously to prolong the survival of gastric cancer patients.

Gastric carcinoma, including the advanced forms, will probably be curable with active immunochemosurgery in the near future. To reach this goal, further prospective randomized controlled clinical studies on immunochemosurgery should be initiated. Additionally, measures for local control, such as intraoperative radiation therapy and intraperitoneal chemotherapy, should be considered.

Conclusions

1. Real radical curative resection of gastric cancer together with complete systematic lymph node dissection is the most important primary treatment.
2. Retrocolic gastrojejunostomy after subtotal gastrectomy is highly recommended. In addition, after total gastrectomy, ligation of the afferent limb is an effective modification of loop esophagojejunostomy with a Braun anastomosis to prevent alkaline reflux.
3. Immunochemosurgery entailing early postoperative immunochemotherapy is the best multimodality treatment for advanced gastric cancer.
4. To kill the micrometastatic and residual small numbers of cancer cells, postoperative immunochemotherapy should be started in an early postoperative period. Hopefully immunotherapy should be started from the 4th or 5th postoperative day and chemotherapy from the 8th to 10th postoperative day.
5. Postoperative immunotherapy may also revive the depressed immunity of the patient with advanced cancer and may alleviate the adverse effect of postoperative chemotherapy.

References

1. Ministry of Health and Social Affairs Republic of Korea (1991) Report of central cancer registry programme in Korea July 1, 1989-June 30, 1990 (in Korean with English abstract). 3:1–134
2. Lee SK, Chi JG, Kim SI, et al (1979) Malignant tumors among Koreans. Relative frequency study on 7363 cancers during 1968 to 1977 (in Korean with English abstract). Korean J Pathol 13:3–20
3. Central Cancer Registry, Ministry of Health, Republic of Korea (1984) Three years' report on the cancer register programme in the Republic of Korea. July 1980-June 1983 (in Korean with English abstract). J Korean Cancer Res Assoc 16:73–217
4. Kim JP, Park JG (1983) The end results of surgical treatment of gastric cancer (in Korean with English abstract). J Korean Med Assoc 26:637–642
5. Buchholtz TW, Welch CE, Malt RA (1978) Clinical correlates of resectability and survival in gastric carcinoma. An Surg 188:711–715
6. The Gastrointestinal Tumor Study Group (1982) A comparative clinical assessment of combination chemotherapy in the management of advanced gastric carcinoma. Cancer 49:1362–1366
7. Kennedy BJ (1970) TNM classification for stomach cancer. Cancer 26:971–983

8. Weed JE, Nuessle W, Ochsner A (1981) Carcinoma of the stomach. Why are we failing to improve survival? Ann Surg 193:407–413

9. The Japanese Gastric Cancer Study Group (1981) Gastric cancer registry in Japan—5-year survival rate of cases between 1963 and 1966. Jpn J Cancer Clin 27:543–563

10. Japanese Research Society for Gastric Cancer (1981) General rules for gastric cancer study in surgery and pathology. Jpn J Surg 11

11. Kim KK, Kim BS, Kim SW, Lee KU, Kim JP, Chung JK, Lee MC (1988) The effect of proximal loop ligation in loop esophagojejunostomy after total gastrectomy on esophageal reflux (in Korean with English abstract). J Korean Gastroenterol Dis Soc 20:243–253

12. Taguchi T, Mattori T, Inoue K, et al (1979) Multihospital randomized study on adjuvant chemotherapy with mitomycin ± futraful for gastric cancer. In: Jones SE, Salmon SE (eds) Adjuvant therapy of cancer II. Grune and Stratton, New York, pp 581–586

13. MacDonald JS, Wooley PV, Smythe T, et al (1979) 5-fluorouracil, Adriamycin, and mitomycin-C (FAM) combination chemotherapy in the treatment of advanced gastric cancer. Cancer 44:42–47

14. Ota K, Kurita S, Nishimura M, et al (1972) Combination therapy with mitomycin-C, 5-fluorouracil and cytosine arabinoside for advanced cancer in man. Cancer Chemother 56:373–395

15. Moertel CG, Mittelman JA, Bakemeier RF (1976) Sequential and combination chemotherapy of advanced gastric cancer. Cancer 38:678–682

16. Mathé G (1971) Active immunotherapy. Adv Cancer Res 14:1–36

17. Morton DL, Eilber FR, Holmes EC, et al (1976) BCG Immunotherapy as a systemic adjunct to surgery in malignant melanoma. Med Clin North Am 60:431–439

18. Rosenberg SA (1985) Lymphokine-activated killer cells: A new approach to immunotherapy of cancer. J Natl Cancer Inst 7:595–616

19. Powles RO, Crowther D, Bateman CJT, et al (1973) Immunotherapy for acute myelogenous leukemia. Br J Cancer 28:365–376

20. Gutterman JU, Cardenas JO, Blumenschein GR, et al (1976) Chemoimmunotherapy of advanced breast cancer: Prolongation of remission and survival with BCG. Br Med J 2:1222–1225

21. Morton DL, Eilber FR, Malmgren RA, Wood WC (1970) Immunological factors which influence the response to immunotherapy in malignant melanoma. Surgery 68:158–164

22. Gutterman JU, Mavligit GM, Blumenshein G, et al (1976) Immunotherapy of human solid tumors with BCG: Prolongation of disease-free interval and survival in malignant melanoma, breast and colorectal cancer. Ann NY Acad Sci 277:135–157

23. Richman SP, Livingston RB, Gutterman JU, et al (1976) Chemotherapy versus chemoimmunotherapy of head and neck cancer: Report of a randomized study. Cancer Treat Rep 60:353–385

24. Wanebo HJ, Thaler HT, Hansen JA, et al (1978) Immunologic reactivity in patients with primary operable breast cancer. Cancer 41:84–94

25. Alberts DS (1977) Adjuvant immunotherapy with BCG of advanced ovarian cancer: A preliminary report. In: Salmon SE, Jones SE (eds) Adjuvant therapy of cancer. Proceedings in the International Conference on the Adjuvant Therapy of Cancer, Amsterdam, North Holland, pp 327–334

26. Hattori T, Mori A, Hirata K, Ito I (1972) Five-year survival rate of gastric cancer patients treated by gastrectomy, large dose of mitomycin-C and/or allogeneic bone marrow transplantation. Gann 63:517–522

27. Okudaira Y, Sugimachi K, Inokuchi K, et al (1982) Postoperative long-term immuno-chemotherapy for esophageal carcinoma. Jpn J Surg 12:249–268
28. Kim JP, Yoo IH (1978) Relationship between the advance of stomach cancer and the change in immunity (in Korean with English abstract). J Korean Surg Soc 20:195–204
29. Chun SH, Yoo IH, Kim JP (1984) The significance of the measurement of immuno-suppressive acid protein (IAP) in various cancer patients (in Korean with English abstract). Korean J Immunol 6:31–42
30. Orita K, Miwa H, Fukuda H, et al (1976) Preoperative cell-mediated immune status of gastric cancer patients. Cancer 38:2343–2348
31. Kim JP, Choi WJ (1986) A study on histologic type of gastric carcinoma: Analysis of clinicopathologic characterization and its implication as a prognostic factor (in Korean with English abstract). J Korean Cancer Res Assoc 18:194–213
32. Kim JP, Jung SE (1986) Staging patients with gastric cancer and their prognosis (in Korean with English abstract). J Korean Cancer Res Assoc 18:9–13
33. Nissen-Meyer R, Kjellgren K, Malmio K, et al (1978) Surgical adjuvant chemo-therapy: Results with one short course with cyclophosphamide after mastectomy for breast cancer. Cancer 41:2088–2098
34. Suga S, Tsunekawa H, Washino M (1977) Treatment of gastric cancer, with special reference to the survivals of the cancer patients treated with multiple combina-tion MFC therapy or immunochemotherapy of MFC plus OK 432 (NSC B116209). Gastroenterol Jpn 12:20–46

Palliative Treatment from the Surgical Point of View

J.R. Siewert, K. Böttcher, J.D. Roder, and U. Fink[1]

Key words. Gastric cancer—Palliative treatment

Introduction

While the published literature usually discriminates between curative and palliative resection of gastric carcinoma, these terms are frequently not defined, although the so-called R-classification established by the International Union Against Cancer (UICC) in 1987 [1] provides a good basis for defining the result of the surgical procedure:

Each kind of surgical procedure not resulting in complete local excision of the tumor, that is, complete extirpation of the primary tumor in all three dimensions (oral, aboral, and depth of tumor) and in the area of lymphatic drainage is, according to the UICC classification of 1987, an R1- or R2-resection (i.e., a resection leaving a residual microscopic or macroscopic tumor) and must be considered a palliative resection (Table 1 [2]).

The palliative character of R1- and R2-resections is clearly demonstrated by the 5-year survival rates in patients with gastric carcinoma (Fig. 1). The median survival time of these patients is only 9 months.

Table 1. Residual tumor (R)-classification according to the UICC (1987)*: The degree of residual tumor after treatment.

R0	no residual tumor
R1	microscopic residual tumor
R2	macroscopic residual tumor

UICC, International Union Against Cancer
* From [2]

[1]Chirurgische Klinik und Poliklinik, Technische Universität München, Klinikum rechts der Isar, Ismaninger Str. 22, 81675 Munich 80, Germany

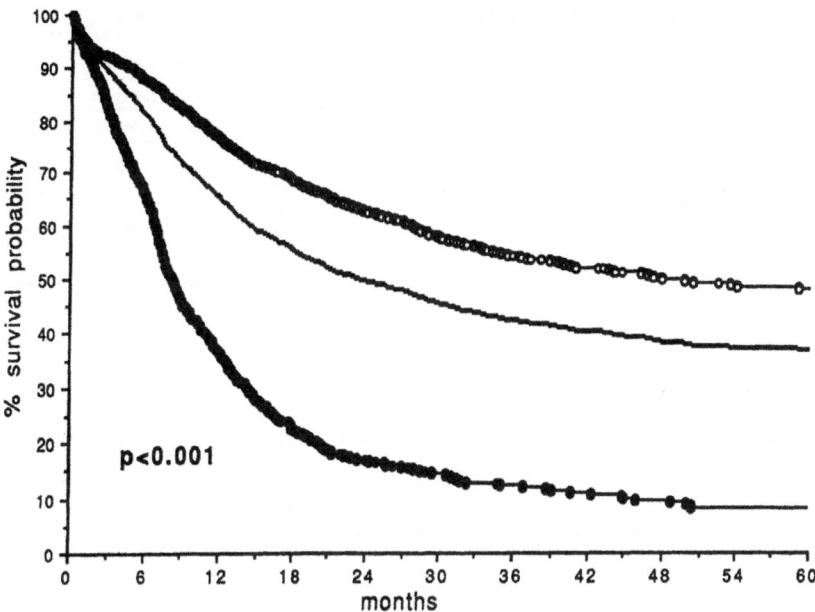

Fig. 1. Results of the German Gastric Carcinoma Study (GGCS) [2]: Survival probability of 1654 patients resected for gastric cancer according to residual tumor stage. *Open circles*, UICC R0-Resection (*n* = 1182). *Closed circles* UICC R1, 2-Resection (*n* = 472). *Solid line*, total (*n* = 1654)

This means that, in addition to leaving the entire tumor in situ, any type of surgery leaving a residual macroscopic or microscopic tumor at the resection margin, tumor bed, or in the lymphatic drainage must also be considered a palliative procedure.

Surgical Epidemiology

Due to the unclear definition given in the published literature, the rate of palliative procedures performed in patients with gastric carcinoma cannot be determined accurately. Based on our survey of the literature (Table 2), the rate of palliative procedures is estimated to be on the order of 25%. This figure corresponds to the rate of palliative resections (28%) which was extrapolated in 1992 by the German Gastric Carcinoma Study (GGCS) [3] and the results of a survey of the patient population of the Technical University (TU) of Munich, carried out in 1992 and based on diligent intraoperative evaluation and postoperative histopathologic documentation [4].

Obviously, there is a close correlation between the tumor stage and the degree of local tumor eradication that can be achieved by surgical resection. The rate of

Table 2. Resection rate in gastric carcinoma: A survey of the literature.

Study	Date	Total Number	Diagnostic laparotomy, gastroenterostomy		Resection rate					
					Total		Curative resection		Palliative resection	
			Number	Percent	Number	Percent	Number	Percent	Number	Percent
Ekbom [5]	1980	144	20	13.9	124	86.1	69	55.6	55	44.4
Gall [6]	1982	1419	413	29.1	996	70.9	814	81.7	182	18.3
Yap [7]	1982	465	182	39.4	283	60.6	235	83.0	48	17.0
Boddie [8]	1983	219	23	10.5	196	89.5	151	77.0	45	23.0
Nier [9]	1984	268	106	37.0	162	63.0	99	61.1	63	38.9
Yan [10]	1984	196	43	21.9	153	78.1	87	56.9	66	43.1
Scott [11]	1985	180	43	23.9	137	76.1	80	58.4	57	41.6
Bozzetti [12]	1987	837	185	22.1	652	77.9	591	93.6	61	6.4
Lindahl [13]	1988	264	93	35.2	171	64.8	140	81.9	31	18.1
*Allum [14]	1989	17565	8318	47.4	9247	52.6	6588	71.2	2659	28.8
*Haugvedst [15]	1989	1008	243	24.1	765	75.9	583	76.2	182	23.8
*Rohde [16]	1989	1278	325	25.4	953	74.6	621	65.2	332	34.8
*GGCS [3]	1992	1999	345	17.3	1654	82.7	1182	71.5	475	28.5
TU Munich [4]	1992	795	93	11.7	702	88.3	509	72.5	193	27.5

* Multicenter studies.

GGCS, German Gastric Carcinoma Study; TU, Technical University.

resection resulting in zero residual tumor (R0-resection rate) in patients with tumor stages I, II, and IIIB is surprisingly high, being on the order of 80%. Only in patients with tumor stage IV does the rate of R0-resection drop to under 40%. In quantitative terms, palliative surgery plays the largest role in these patients (Table 3 [1, 3, 4]). In multivariate analysis, the rate of R2-resections was independently influenced solely by a Karnofsky Index of less than 70, and not by age or concomitant disease.

Preoperative Diagnostics

Until very recently, complete resectability of a tumor could only be decided intraoperatively. Today, with the significant improvement in diagnostic imaging techniques, nonresectable tumors can be diagnosed with an accuracy of 75%–80% (see below). Consequently, the decision in favor of a palliative or curative resection can now be made preoperatively in the majority of patients.

The spectrum of diagnostic techniques to identify patients for palliative surgical therapy is large. It includes:

1. *Endoscopy*, which allows identification of macroscopic tumor types according to the Borrmann classification
2. *Endoluminal ultrasound*, which permits definitive establishment of the T-category, that is, the depth of invasion of the tumor
3. *Biopsies*, which allow tumor grading and growth pattern determination (intestinal and nonintestinal types are distinguished according to the Laurén classification)

Table 3. Rate of R0 resections according to UICC tumor stages for gastric carcinomas: A comparison of two studies.

UICC [1] (1987) Stage	TU Munich [4] (1992)						GGCS [3] (1992)					
	Total		R0		R1,2		Total		R0		R1,2	
	Number	Percent	Number	Percent	Number	Percent	Number	Percent	Number	Percent	Number	Percent
I A	101	14.4	101	100	—	—	229	13.8	226	98.7	3	1.3
I B	81	11.5	78	96.3	3	3.7	221	13.4	210	95.0	11	5.0
II	88	12.5	81	92.0	7	8.0	230	13.9	205	89.3	25	10.7
III A	111	15.8	93	83.8	18	16.2	262	15.8	211	80.5	51	19.5
III B	84	12.0	65	77.4	19	22.6	204	12.3	160	78.4	44	21.6
IV	237	33.8	91	38.4	146	61.6	508	30.7	170	33.5	338	66.5
Total	702	100	509	72.5	193	100	1654	100	1182	71.5	472	100

4. *Computer tomography and percutaneous ultrasound*, for the diagnosis of distant metastases
5. *Calculation of the tumor stage* according to these parameters using the Maruyama computer program
6. *Diagnostic video-laparoscopy* in patients with advanced tumors (T3, T4) with
   a) Intraperitoneal lavage to identify free tumor cells in the peritoneal cavity
   b) Intraabdominal laparoscopic ultrasound of the liver
   c) Inspection of the bursa omentalis and biopsy of lymph nodes at the celiac axis
7. *Preoperative risk analysis* to identify the risk of surgical resection

Therapeutic Options

If the detailed preoperative diagnostic workup indicates that the patient has an advanced tumor and that local tumor eradication cannot be achieved by surgical resection alone, there are three palliative therapeutic options:

1. *Preoperative chemotherapy* with subsequent surgical resection in those who respond to chemotherapy. A prerequisite for preoperative chemotherapy is a risk analysis showing that the patient can be operated on with a reasonable surgical risk
2. *Palliative tumor reduction* (the so-called debulking operation) aiming to remove as much tumor as possible and to improve the patient's quality of life for a short period (see below). With this approach it is hoped that residual macroscopic and microscopic tumors can be treated by postoperative chemotherapy
3. *Therapy of tumor complications* to improve the patient's quality of life temporarily only, e.g., therapy of gastric outlet obstruction by gastro-enterostomy, therapy of dysphagia by tumor pertubation in patients with proximal tumors, or therapy of bleeding from the tumor

Choice of Procedure

Preoperative Chemotherapy

As mentioned above, preoperative chemotherapy requires exact risk analysis. Patients who are enrolled in a protocol for preoperative chemotherapy should be able to tolerate an extensive surgical procedure, that is, a gastrectomy. In our experience, this requires a Karnofsky Index of over 70, an age of under 70 years, and adequate cardiopulmonary, renal, and hepatic functions. Our experience shows that the response rate to preoperative chemotherapy is better in patients with locally advanced tumors than in patients with regional tumors. Response to chemotherapy is poor in those patients with distant metastases and particularly those who have peritoneal tumor spread. As a rule, patients who will probably not respond to chemotherapy, that is, patients with peritoneal carcinosis, should be excluded from such an approach. Preoperative laparoscopy should therefore be performed in all patients with advanced tumor stages confirmed by endoscopic ultrasonography.

The aim of preoperative chemotherapy is to achieve a downstaging of the gastric carcinoma which would allow complete local tumor resection. The aggressive chemotherapy required to achieve this aim, however, is associated with a substantial risk.

The risk associated with surgical resection is not increased by preoperative chemotherapy. However, assessment of response to chemotherapy is difficult even intraoperatively because vital tumor tissue frequently cannot be differentiated macroscopically from scar tissue. Surgical resection in patients who had preoperative chemotherapy must consequently be performed according to the same radical principles as in patients without preoperative therapy. This is because the patients' prognosis is determined by the extent of lymphadenectomy even after preoperative chemotherapy.

Chemotherapy Regimen

The effect of a combination of adriamycin ($20\,mg/m^2$ i.v. on days 1 and 7), cisplatinum ($40\,mg/m^2$ i.v. on days 2 and 8), and etoposid ($120\,mg/m^2$ i.v. on days 4, 5, and 6) is stage-dependent, with a higher rate of responses and clinical complete remission occurring in patients with advanced tumor stages (who are on the etoposide/adriamycin/cisplatinum [EAP] regimen). This protocol is therefore suitable for preoperative use in patients with locally advanced tumor stages who do not have peritoneal carcinosis. Depending on the individual response, three to four cycles of chemotherapy are given. Prior to each new therapy cycle, progression of the disease must be excluded. Patients who respond to preoperative chemotherapy after 90–102 days undergo resection once the peripheral blood count has normalized. Because of markedly increased toxicity, postoperative adjuvant or additive chemotherapy is not given independently of the resection status (Fig. 2).

Own Results

In our own study we treated 30 patients (22 males, 8 females) whose mean age was 51.8 years (range: 23–68 years) with preoperative EAP. Tumor stages (according to the UICC classification of 1987 [1]) were: stage IIIA 8 (26.7%), stage IIIB 12 (40%), and stage IV 10 (33.3%). The primary tumor was located at the cardia or proximal third of the stomach in 18 patients (60%) and in the corpus or antrum in 10 patients (33%). Two patients (6.7%) had a linitis plastica. Sixty percent of the tumors had a nonintestinal pattern of growth, according to the Laurén classification. After an average of three cycles of chemotherapy, 8 patients

Locally advanced carcinoma of the stomach

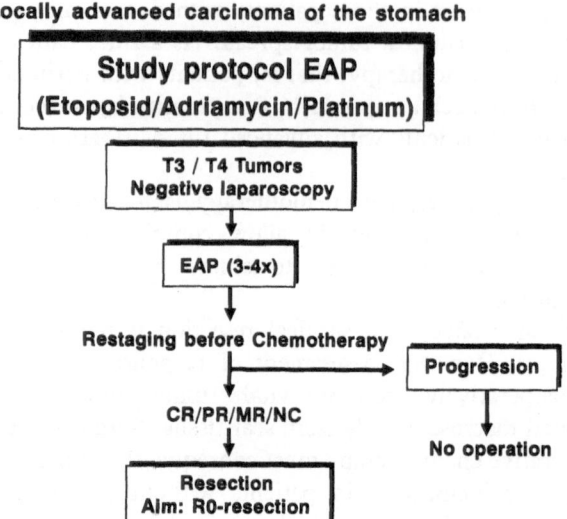

Fig. 2. The EAP (etoposid/adriamycin/cisplatinum) chemotherapy regimen. *CR*, complete response; *PR*, partial response; *MR*, minor response; *NC*, no change

(29.6%) showed complete endoscopic tumor regression, and another 9 patients (33%) displayed a marked reduction of tumor mass. Progression of the tumor was observed in 1 patient (3.7%) only. Chemotherapy was associated with a high rate of myelotoxicity (leucocytopenia WHO grade III in 40% and WHO grade IV in 16.7% of the patients; thrombocytopenia WHO grade III in 20% and WHO grade IV in 26.7% of the patients) which could be managed by early substitution (application of hematopoietic growth factors [rhG-CSF] for leucocytes at ≤15 000/μl and substitution of thrombocytes for a thrombocyte count of <30 000/μl).

Out of the total of 30 patients, 27 underwent resection after preoperative chemotherapy, which corresponds to a resection rate of 90%. Complete tumor resection, that is, an RO-resection according to the UICC 1987 definition [1] was possible in 24 of the patients, that is, 80% of all patients included in the study or 88.9% of those undergoing resection. One of the patients underwent subtotal gastrectomy, 8 had total gastrectomies, and 18 patients underwent extended total gastrectomies. All patients had a radical lymphadenectomy (D2-lymphadenectomy) with removal of an average of 53 lymph nodes. Despite the aggressive surgical approach, perioperative morbidity was not increased and there was no postoperative mortality. After a median follow-up of 24 months, 13 patients were alive without tumor recurrence, and 16 patients had died. The median survival time was 17 months in all 13 patients included in the study and 23 months in those who had complete tumor resection.

These preliminary data show that preoperative chemotherapy in patients with locally advanced gastric carcinoma is a reasonable approach if complete tumor resection is possible in those who respond to chemotherapy. In patients with locally advanced nonresectable gastric carcinoma (UICC stage IV), preoperative chemotherapy is a reasonable therapeutic option.

Debulking Operations

A debulking operation requires an exact preoperative risk analysis. The aim of a debulking operation is to reduce tumor mass in hopes of being able to treat the residual tumor with postoperative chemotherapy.

The advantage of a debulking operation is that its indications are broader in range than those for preoperative chemotherapy, e.g., there is no age limit.

Our research experience confirms the results of the German Gastric Carcinoma Study [3], in that it shows that palliative resection can be performed with acceptable morbidity and mortality rates (Tables 4a and b). Nevertheless, the morbidity rate of over 30% must be considered prior to initiation of the surgical procedure. In general, this is of particular importance when the expected survival time is short and postoperative morbidity requires prolonged hospitalization. The influence of the surgeon's experience on the rate of postoperative complications is illustrated in Tables 4a and b, which compare the results obtained at a single center with a large number of gastrectomies and those of a multicenter study. These results provide further evidence that, even in a palliative setting, standardized procedures yield the best results, while deviation from standardized procedures toward atypical resections are associated with a significantly higher complication rate. Radical lymph node dissection has no place in palliative procedures. Furthermore, resections of the tail of the pancreas should also be avoided in palliative procedures, because they are frequently associated with local and regional septic complications.

Available data from Europe and North America indicate that the concept of debulking operations with subsequent chemotherapy in patients with gastric carcinoma must be considered as having failed. None of the publications from the Western world shows postoperative chemotherapy as having had any effect in this situation. In contrast, several Japanese studies have demonstrated a beneficial effect resulting from postoperative chemotherapy. A possible explanation for this phenomenon could lie in the fact that, in the postoperative course reported in the Japanese literature, chemotherapy had been initiated at an earlier point of time. Japanese authors frequently start postoperative chemotherapy on the third postoperative day. In the Western world, the increased postoperative morbidity frequently precludes early use of postoperative chemotherapy. The timing of the initiation of postoperative chemotherapy may be an essential factor of its effectivity.

Palliative Procedures for the Treatment of Complications

The aim of these procedures, which can be performed at a reasonable risk (Table 5), is exclusively to treat acute complications without attempting to achieve tumor

Table 4a. Morbidity following palliative resection for gastric cancer: Results from the Technical University (TU) of Munich (Department of Surgery)*.

Complications	Subtotal gastrectomy (n = 41)		Total gastrectomy (n = 62)		Extended gastrectomy (n = 79)		Others (n = 11)		Total (n = 193)	
	Number	Percent	Number	Percent	Number	Percent	Number	Percent	Number	Percent
Anastomotic insufficiency	0	—	6	9.7	9	11.4	2	18.2	17	8.8
Bleeding	3	7.3	1	1.6	4	5.1	1	9.1	9	4.7
Wound infection	1	2.4	3	4.8	3	3.8	0	—	7	3.6
Abscess	3	7.3	3	4.8	7	8.9	0	—	13	6.7
Cardiopulmonary	2	4.9	4	6.5	4	5.1	0	—	10	5.2
Others	3	7.3	1	1.6	1	1.3	0	—	5	2.6
Total	12	29.3	18	29.0	28	35.4	3	27.3	61	31.6
30-day-mortality	2	4.9	2	3.2	1	1.3	0	—	5	2.6
Hospital mortality	2	4.9	3	4.8	4	5.1	0	—	9	4.7

* From [4]

Table 4b. Morbidity following palliative resection: Results of the German Gastric Carcinoma Study (GGCS)*.

Complications	Subtotal gastrectomy (n = 104)		Total gastrectomy (n = 205)		Extended gastrectomy (n = 134)		Others (n = 29)		Total (n = 472)	
	Number	Percent	Number	Percent	Number	Percent	Number	Percent	Number	Percent
Anastomotic insufficiency	2	1.9	11	5.4	18	13.4	6	20.7	37	7.8
Bleeding	2	1.9	6	2.9	1	0.8	1	3.4	10	2.1
Wound infection	2	1.9	2	1.0	7	5.2	1	3.4	12	2.5
Abscess	3	2.9	11	5.4	6	4.5	1	3.4	21	4.4
Cardiopulmonary	7	6.7	18	8.8	15	11.2	2	6.9	42	8.9
Others	2	1.9	5	2.4	5	3.7	1	3.4	13	2.8
Total	18	17.3	53	25.9	52	38.8	12	41.2	135	28.5
30-day-mortality	9	8.7	12	5.9	8	6.0	3	5.7	32	6.8
90-day-mortality	16	15.4	34	16.6	27	20.1	8	15.1	85	18.0

* From [3]

Table 5. Mortality following palliative treatment of gastric carcinoma: A survey of the literature.

Study	Date	Period	No resection		Resections			
			Diagnostic laparotomy	Gastro-enterostomy	Subtotal gastrectomy	Total gastrectomy	Extended gastrectomy	Proximal gastrectomy
Haugstvedt [15] (Norge Multicenter-study)	1989	1982–1984	9.0% (n = 156)	24.0% (n = 70)	18.0% (n = 34)	12.0% (n = 64)	—	14.0% (n = 14)
Kirchner [17] (TNM-study)	1992	1982–1984	8.8% (n = 223)	22.5% (n = 77)	(n = 126)	14.5% (n = 175)	—	(n = 31)
GGCS [3]	1992	1986–1989						
30-day-mortality			13.0%		8.7%	5.9%	6.0%	6.9%
90-day-mortality			35.7%		15.4%	16.6%	20.1%	20.7%
Hospital mortality			4.6%		6.7%	7.3%	8.3%	10.3%
			(n = 345)		(n = 104)	(n = 205)	(n = 134)	(n = 29)

TNM, tumor node metastasis

reduction. In patients with a bleeding complication, laser coagulation or endoscopic injection can be used. In patients with obstructions at the level of the cardia or the proximal third of the stomach, laser therapy for tumor vaporization is useful. In rare cases, implantation of a tube may be indicated. Surgical means of treating obstructions of the proximal third of the stomach should be avoided if possible, because they are risky and of uncertain outcome.

In patients with obstructions in the distal or middle third of the stomach, a gastroenterostomy is generally performed. Since the draining function of a gastroenterostomy is insufficient, however, it usually works only in patients with a complete obstruction. In our experience, the postoperative function is best with so-called cross-section gastroenterostomy. In this procedure, the stomach is divided above the tumor, the tumor is left behind, and the gastric remnant is anastomosed to a jejunal loop at its most distal end.

A very difficult problem is presented by small-bowel or large-bowel ileus in patients with diffuse peritoneal tumor spread. In these prognostically dismal situations, a surgical approach of acceptable risk is no longer possible, except in patients with isolated small-bowel or large-bowel stenosis. Total parenteral nutrition via a completely subcutaneously implanted central venous access system is the last resort for these patients.

Results

The survival time after palliative surgery is extremely short (Table 6). The median survival times after palliative—i.e., bypass or other—procedures were a mere 3–4 months in the German Gastric Carcinoma Study [3] and in our own experience [4]. In patients who had a palliative debulking resection, the survival time was only 8–10 months. This, however, does not indicate that debulking procedures prolong survival. Rather, the longer survival times following debulking procedures reflect earlier tumor stages in these patients. Consequently, survival time alone cannot be a criterium for the selection of a surgical procedure in the setting of palliation.

Preoperative chemotherapy is the only approach resulting in a markedly prolonged survival time in patients who respond to treatment. In our patient population, the median survival time in these patients was 23 months. Preoperative chemotherapy consequently appears to be the best option in patients with locally advanced gastric carcinoma. However, only the patients who respond to treatment benefit from this cost-intensive and risky option. Because the concept of debulking operations and postoperative chemotherapy must be considered as having failed, the identification of patients who might benefit from preoperative chemotherapy is of utmost importance.

Palliative Therapy: A Practical Approach

Therapeutic decisions can be made according to the following guidelines (Fig. 3):

Table 6. Median survival (in months) following palliative treatment of gastric carcinoma: A survey of the literature.

Study	Date	No. resection		Resections			
		Diagnostic laparotomy	Gastro- enterostomy	Subtotal gastrectomy	Total gastrectomy	Extended gastrectomy	proximal gastrectomy
Lawrence [18]	1958	4.6 (n = 239)	3.9 (n = 27)	9.5 (n = 67)	8.2 (n = 41)	—	
Buchholtz [19]	1978	2.6 (n = 51)	3.5 (n = 77)	—	—	—	—
Leinster [20]	1980	3.7 (n = 4)	7.1 (n = 8)	—		17.2 (n = 13)	
Gall [6]	1982	3.0 (n = 351)	2.5 (n = 20)	6.5 (n = 60)	4.0 (n = 53)		7.0 (n = 39)
Boddie [8]	1983	—	3.6 (n = 21)	—		10.4 (n = 45)	
Scott [11]	1985	4.6 (n = 32)	3.2 (n = 43)			6.1 (n = 57)	
Yan [10]	1985					9.3 (n = 66)	
Kirchner (TNM-study) [17]	1992	4.0 (n = 180)	3.5 (n = 77)	8.6 (n = 126)	8.5 (n = 175)	—	13.0 (n = 31)
GGCS [3]	1992	4.4 (n = 236)	4.6 (n = 49)	8.5 (n = 104)	7.9 (n = 205)	7.6 (n = 134)	9.0 (n = 29)
TU München [4]	1992	3.5 (n = 66)	4.5 (n = 22)	8.6 (n = 41)	9.5 (n = 62)	7.8 (n = 79)	8.3 (n = 14)

– If the preoperative diagnostic workup shows that an R0-resection is possible, primary resection should be performed
– If the preoperative diagnostic workup shows that, with a high degree of probability, local tumor eradication cannot be achieved by surgical resection, the

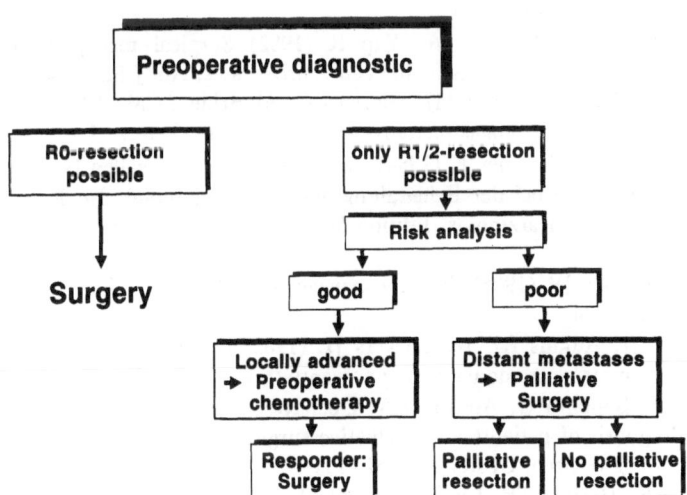

Fig. 3. Decisionmaking in palliative treatment of gastric carcinoma

patient's risk analysis is an essential basis for further decisions. Preoperative chemotherapy can only be recommended in patients with locally advanced tumors but no major risk factors. In patients with risk factors and/or distant metastases, a palliative surgical procedure may be indicated. Whether a palliative procedure can be performed with reasonable risk and low postoperative morbidity must be decided on the basis of the patient's individual situation. If a palliative resection is impossible, surgical procedures treating the individual complication should be performed

– For patients with peritoneal tumor spread, there is currently no reasonable therapy available. The present therapeutic options, including intraperitoneal chemotherapy in its various forms, must all be considered experimental

References

1. Hermanek P, Sobin LH (eds) (1987) UICC TNM classification of malignant tumours. 4th ed Springer, Berlin Heidelberg New York 39–46
2. Siewert JR, Fink U (1992) Multimodale Therapiekonzepte bei Tumoren des Gastrointestinaltraktes. Chirurg 63:242–250
3. Böttcher K, Roder JD, Busch R, Fink U, Siewert JR, Hermanek P und Meyer HJ für die Deutsche Magenkarzinom-Studiengruppe (1993) Epidemiologie des Magenkarzinoms aus chirurgischer Sicht—Ergebnisse der Deutschen Magenkarzinom-Studie 1992. Dtsch med Wschr 118:729–736
4. Böttcher K, Becker K, Busch R, Roder JD, Siewert JR (1992) Prognosefaktoren beim Magenkarzinom—Ergebnisse einer uni- und multivariaten Analyse. Chirurg 63:656–661
5. Ekbom GA, Gleysteen JJ (1980) Gastric malignancy: Resection for palliation. Surgery 88:476–481
6. Gall FP (1982) Operative Methodenwahl bei Palliativeingriffen. Langenbecks Arch Chir 358 (proceedings):85–90
7. Yap P, Pantangco E, Yap A, Yap R (1982) Surgical management of gastric carcinoma—Follow-up results in 465 consecutive cases. Am J Surg 143:284–287
8. Boddie AW Jr, McMurtrey MJ, Giacco GG, McBride ACM (1983) Palliative total gastrectomy and esophagogastrectomy—A reevaluation. Cancer 51:1195–1200
9. Nier H, Ulrich B, Kremer K (1984) Zur Frage der prinzipiellen Gastrektomie oder partiellen Resektion bei der Behandlung des Magenkarzinoms. In: R Häring (Hrsg) Therapie des Magencarzinoms. Edition Medizin, Weinheim, Deerfield Beach, Basel, pp 147–156
10. Yan C-J, Brooks JR (1985) Surgical management of gastric adenocarcinoma. Am J Surg 149:771–774
11. Scott HW Jr, Adkins RB Jr, Sawyers JL (1985) Results of an aggressive surgical approach to gastric carcinoma during a twenty-three-year period. Surgery 97:55–59
12. Bozzetti F, Bonfanti G, Audisio RA, Doci R, Dossena G, Gennari L, Andreola S (1987) Prognosis of patients after palliative surgical procedures for carcinoma of the stomach. Surg Gynecol Obstet 164:151–154
13. Lindahl AK, Harbitz TB, Liavag I (1988) The surgical treatment of gastric cancer: a retrospective study with special reference to total gastrectomy. Eur J Surg Oncol 14:55–62

14. Allum WH, Powell DJ, McConkey CC, Fielding JWL (1989) Gastric cancer: A 25-year review. Br J Surg 76:535–540
15. Haugstvedt R, Viste A, Eide GE, Söreide O, and participants in the Norwegian Stomach Cancer Trial (1989) The survival benefit of resection in patients with advanced stomach cancer: The Norwegian Multicenter Experience. World J Surg 13:617–622
16. Rohde H, Bauer P, Stützer H, Heimann K, Gebbensleben B, German Gastric Cancer TNM Study Group (1991) Proximal compared with distal adenocarcinoma of the stomach: Differences and consequences. Br J Surg 78:1242–1248
17. Kirchner R, Stützer H, Farthmann EH (1992) Palliative Eingriffe. Langenbecks Archiv Chir Supp (proceedings):142–146
18. Lawrence W Jr, McNeer G (1958) The effectiveness of surgery for palliation of incurable gastric cancer. Cancer 11:28–32
19. Buchholtz TW, Welch CE, Malt RA (1978) Clinical correlates of resectability and survival in gastric carcinoma. Ann Surg 188:711–715
20. Leinster SJ, Hughes LE (1980) The role of resection in advanced gastric carcinoma. Clin Oncol 6:55–61

Endoscopic Treatment of Early Gastric Cancer

Yoshiki Hiki[1]

Key words. Endoscopic resection—Laser irradiation—Early gastric cancer—Protruted type—Depressed type—Lymph node metastasis

Introduction

Progress in diagnostic techniques for gastric cancer has resulted in detection of microscopic lesions. We have reported that the surgical treatment of early gastric cancers shows satisfactory results. The 5-year relative cumulative survival rate for carcinoma in situ is 105.3%, and the 10-year rate is 101.9%, indicating that there are no cancer deaths. Thus, a surgical procedure is the treatment of first choice for gastric cancer. Although the types of candidates for surgery have increased because of the advancement of anesthesiology and postoperative management, there are still inoperable patients for reasons of severe complications or advanced age. As non-operative procedures, various types of endoscopic treatments are available for gastric cancers and have produced favorable results in some cases [1].

Types and Technical Procedures of Non-Operative Treatment for Gastric Cancer

There are three major methods: cauterization of lesions [2, 3], local injection of drugs into lesions, and local resection of early gastric cancers using endoscopy (Table 1). Local resection is one of the most focused upon procedures at present.

---

[1] Department of Surgery and Endoscopy, Kitasato University Hospital, 2-1-1 Asamizodai, Sagamihara, Kanagawa, 228 Japan

Table 1. Types of endoscopic therapy in gastric
cancer.

Endoscopic mucosectomy
Endoscopic coagulation
Laser irradiation
Nd-YAG
Ar
Ar-dye
Kr
N_2-dye
Cryosurgery
Microwave coagulation
Local injection

Endoscopic Resection

We now use endoscopic resection as the procedure of first choice, because it allows recovery of the tissue for histological determination of the depth of cancer invasion. To resect a lesion completely in a single operation, the maximum diameter of the resectable lesion will be 1 cm, in view of the technological limits of endoscopic therapy. The steps of carrying out this method are as follows. First, the extent of the lesion is confirmed. After marking the periphery, physiological saline is injected using an endoscopic needle into the submucosal layer to cause the lesion to protrude. The snare is opened through a channel of a two-channel scope for treatment, and a clasp forceps is introduced into the other channel. After the lesion is clasped and raised, the snare is closed to transect and remove the lesion under a high frequency electric current as is done in polypectomy (Figs. 1, 2). The resected specimen should be carefully handled (Figs. 3, 4). It is spread on a cork board using pins, and is cut along its entirety at 2-mm intervals.

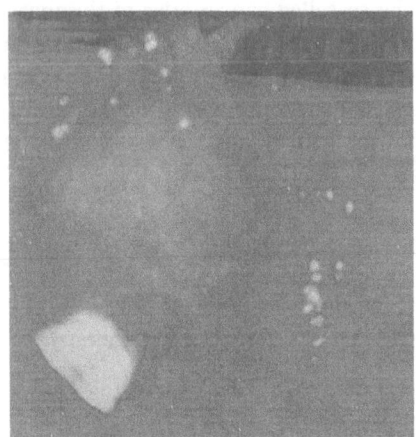

Fig. 1. Physiological saline is injected into the submucosal layer using an endoscopic needle

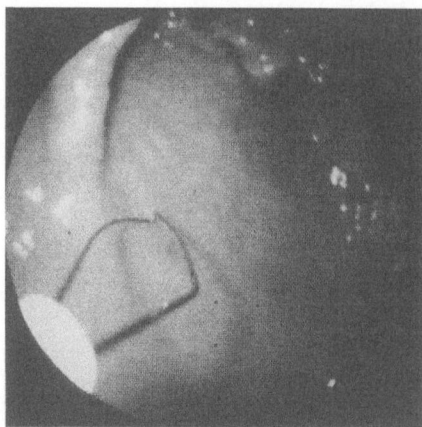

Fig. 2. The snare is opened through a channel of a two-channel scope

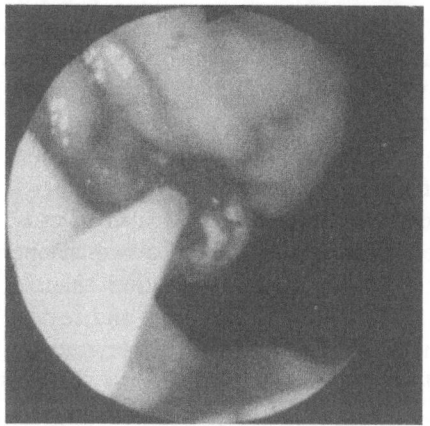

Fig. 3. The snare is closed to transect and remove the lesion under a high frequency electric current

The so-called cancer atlas of the focal region is drawn, based on histological findings, to determine the presence or absence of any residual lesion. The necessity of an additional laparotomy is determined on the basis of the depth of cancer invasion and the status of vascular invasion. It is our current policy to select radical surgery after laparotomy if the carcer has reached a level deeper than the submucosal layer.

Laser

There are two types of laser therapy, high-output thermal energy therapy and low-output photochemical therapy.

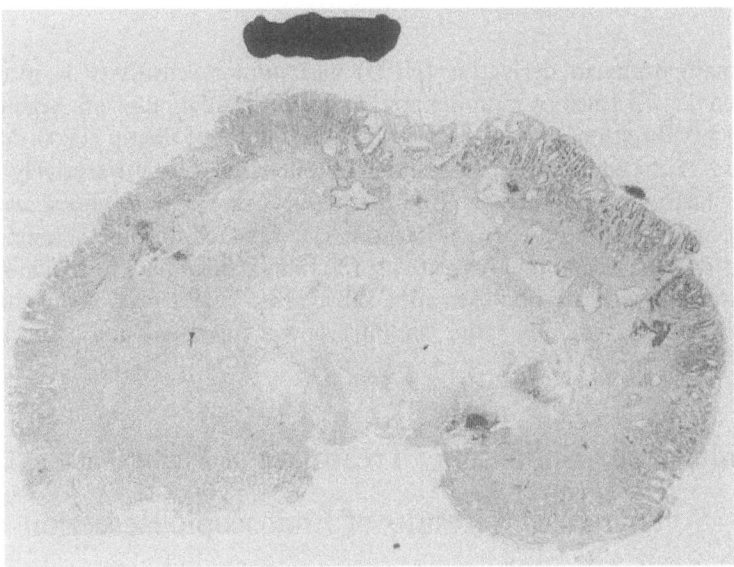

Fig. 4. The so-called cancer atlas of the focal region is drawn based on histological findings

High Output Laser

An Nd-YAG laser is intermittently irradiated at intervals of 0.5–1 s with a wavelength of 1064 nm and an output of 40–80 W. The laser tip is changed depending on whether or not it is to be in contact with the lesion during irradiation. Tips of various forms are available for the contact type. This type ensures irradiation at an output of 10–25 W with an efficacy equal to that of the non-contact type, which requires an output of 80 W. However, the non-contact type is more suitable for large lesions, because the irradiated field in the contact type is an aggregate of spots, rather than a plane (Fig. 5).

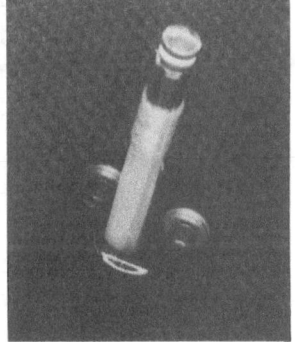

Fig. 5. Tips of various forms are available for the contact type apparatus

Low Output Laser

A hematoporphyrin derivative (HPD) with tumor sensitivity is intravenously injected 48–72 h before radiotherapy, and spot irradiation of an Argon-dye laser with a wavelength of 630 nm is given [5]. The output of the tip is 200–500 W, and because of the low output, the tumor is cauterized nearly selectively with only slight changes in the peripheral normal tissue. Among early gastric cancers, the superficial type with obscure demarcation is well suited for this therapy. Attention should be paid to any photosensitivity reaction, a side effect of hematoporphyrin derivatives, which are photosensitive substances. Direct rays of the sun must be avoided for 1–3 months after an intravenous injection, and this can pose a problem.

Results of the Endoscopic Treatment of Early Gastric Cancers

Therapeutic Results of Endoscopic Resection

In the 43 patients treated by endoscopic resection, with the exceptions of 2 in whom the cancers were located near the pylorus, all early cancers less than 1 cm in diameter disappeared after the initial treatment. It is our policy to opt for surgery for operable patients in whom cancers remain after the initial treatment. Surgery poses no problem because informed consent is routinely obtained from the patient and his/her family. Inoperable patients underwent laser therapy from the second treatment, which resulted in complete disappearance of the cancers.

Results of Laser Therapy

Endoscopic therapy involves less invasion than does surgical therapy and can be repeated. While this therapy is recommended after careful consideration of the possibility of lymph node metastasis, its technical limitations should be considered.

The following are the results of the initial treatment by laser irradiation at our hospital. Determination of the presence or absence of residual cancer following the initial laser irradiation in the 44 patients revealed a high residual rate among the lesions which were 4 cm or more in diameter. All these residual lesions completely disappeared after repeated treatments. Postoperative follow-ups with endoscopic biopsy are important. We carried out a biopsy at intervals of 1–3 months, and none of the patients has shown recurrence of the cancer.

Results of the Surgical Treatment of Early Gastric Cancers

The following are the relative survival rates among 1328 patients undergoing surgery for gastric cancer according to the presence or absence of lymph node metastasis. The group without lymph node metastasis (N_0) showed highly favor-

Table 2. The relative survival rates according to the presence or absence of lymph node metastasis.

Lymph node metastasis by histological examination	Cumulative survival rates	
	5-Year survival rate	10-Year survival rate
N0	98.0%	97.6%
N1	67.2%	66.1%
>N2	42.1%	38.7%

able results, with a 5-year survival rate of 98% and a 10-year rate of 97.6%. In contrast, the group showing involvement (N_1+) of the lymph nodes closest to the focal region (1st station) showed a 5-year survival rate of 67.2% and a 10-year rate of 66.1%. These survival rates indicate that cancer can be radically cured by surgical resection of the local lesion in the absence of lymph node metastasis (Table 2).

Lymph Node Metastasis of Early Gastric Cancer

There is a question of whether or not peripheral lymphadenectomy at a site remote from the primary focus is necessary in the surgical treatment of early gastric cancer. We think that exclusive dissection of the lymph nodes closest to the primary focus may be sufficient, or that no lymph nodes may need to be dissected. Of the 2072 patients who underwent surgery for gastric cancer at our hospital during the last 19 years, 788 had early cancers. We examined the incidence of lymph node metastasis of early gastric cancer to clarify the indications for endoscopic therapy. Of the 788 patients with early gastric cancer, 631 had single cancers, the rest having multiple cancers. The relationships of lymph node metastasis to the macroscopic type, histological type, and the presence or absence of an associated ulcer were examined in the 4-cm or smaller lesions (Table 3).

Table 3. Frequency of lymph node metastasis (631 cases, 1971–1990, Kitasato University).

Type	Size (mm)							Total (%)
	1–5	6–10	11–15	16–20	21–25	26–30	>31	
Protruded	0/1	0/2	0/6	0/7	0/5	1/12	5/35	6/68 (8.8)
Depressed Ul–	0/13	0/33	0/44	0/23	1/17	1/11	5/41	7/182 (3.8)
Ul+	0/2	1/17	1/27	2/24	1/37	3/33	31/160	39/300 (13.0)
Mixed		0/3	0/4	2/10	3/10	0/12	10/42	15/81 (18.5)
Total (%)	0/16 (0.0)	1/55 (1.8)	1/81 (1.2)	4/64 (6.3)	5/69 (7.2)	5/68 (7.4)	51/278 (18.3)	67/631 (10.6)

Ul, Ulcer, ±, with, =, without

Relationship Between the Macroscopic Type and Lymph Node Metastasis

The major diameter of the early gastric cancers was divided at 5-mm intervals for examination of its relationship with lymph node metastasis. None of the 2.5-cm or smaller protruding lesions showed lymph node metastasis. No metastasis was found among the 2-cm or smaller depressed lesions containing no ulcer or ulcer scar. In contrast, a patient in the group which had from 6 to 10-mm lesions with ulcer or ulcer scar showed metastasis. This is an important factor in deciding the indications for endoscopic therapy in gastric cancers of the depressed type.

Relationship Between the Histological Type and Lymph Node Metastasis

Comparison between the well-differentiated and undifferentiated types showed that the incidence of metastasis among the undifferentiated cancers increased with the diameter [6]. The undifferentiated type should not be considered suitable, because it frequently shows deep infiltration in the fundic area of the stomach and a high metastatic rate for lymph nodes.

Relationship Between the Presence of Ulcerative Lesions Including Scars in the Cancer Focus and Lymph Node Metastasis

Histopathological analysis of the surgical specimens obtained from the 631 patients with a single cancer revealed the absence of lymph node metastasis in the group having 2-cm or smaller lesions containing no ulcer or ulcer scar [Ul(−)]. This is a very important finding for deciding the suitability for endoscopic therapy.

Endoscopic Therapeutic Policy for Early Gastric Cancers

In view of the history of endoscopic therapy, the indications of early gastric cancer for this therapy can be divided into the absolute and the relative categories. The absolute category exclusively includes early gastric cancers without lymph node metastasis which were classified by statistical analysis of the patients with early gastric cancer who underwent surgical resection. In view of the technical limitations of endoscopic therapy, this category should also be limited to the size of lesions that can be completely eliminated in the initial treatment. The absolute indications are (1) 1-cm or smaller protruding-type lesions, and (2) 1-cm or smaller depressed-type lesions with no ulcer or ulcer scar.

While cancers of the other type have been regarded as being relative indications, there should be only a very small number of patients of this type. The relative indications involve high risks for surgery because of advanced age and severe complications, as determined after careful assessment by several physicians including an internist, surgeon, and anesthetist.

Selection of an Endoscopic Therapeutic Procedure

We first select endoscopic resection for patients showing the absolute indications when specimens are obtained. If the cancer remains, we usually perform gastrectomy, a conventional surgical procedure, after obtaining informed consent. If informed consent cannot be obtained, or if the general condition does not permit surgery, laser therapy is carried out to coagulate and necrotize the tumor. Laser therapy is effective for patients showing the relative indications based on the size and macroscopic type. A combination of endoscopic resection and laser therapy is used in some cases.

Problems of Surgical Procedures and the Future Development of Endoscopic Therapy

In order to replace the successful conventional surgical therapy with endoscopic therapy, the indications should be clearly defined. In addition, it is necessary to accumulate data during the subsequent 10 years to confirm that early gastric cancer can be completely healed by endoscopic therapy. Surgical death and postoperative complications are the primary problems inherent to conventional surgical operation which should be taken into consideration. In 1988, Watanabe et al. [7] summarized the findings of a questionnaire survey concerning endoscopic therapy. They reported that the surgical mortality rate for carcinoma in situ of the stomach was 0.58%. According to the report on the 1983 nationwide investigation of cancer registrations, the rate of direct surgical deaths among all patients with gastric cancer was 0.84%. Whether or not surgical results can be evaluated on the basis of the rate of cancer recurrence alone is at issue, because a long-term follow-up of postoperative complaints revealed a high rate of rehospitalization due to gastrectomy syndrome and intestinal adhesion, and also in view of the incidence of postoperative metabolic disorders. This problem is more serious in elderly patients [8]. Accidents and complications associated with endoscopic therapy should be investigated in detail for comparison between surgical results and the outcomes of endoscopic therapy.

Laparoscopic Wedge Resection of the Stomach for Early Gastric Cancer by the Lesion-Lifting Method of Ohgami-Kitajima

Endoscopic resection is a minimally invasive option for the treatment of mucosal gastric cancer. However, even if the selected cancer lesion has little possibility of lymph node metastasis, the indication for performing is limited in its depending

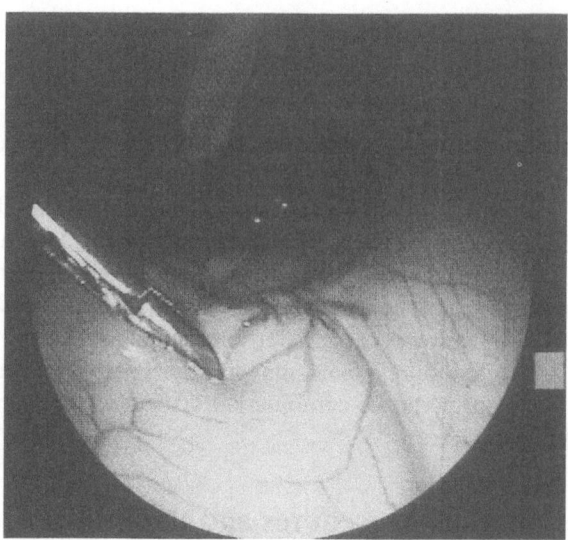

Fig. 6. The location of the cancer lesion is confirmed from outside of the stomach laparoscopically with the guidance of a gastroscope

on the size and the location of the lesion. Ohgami et al. have developed another innovative, minimally invasive method, the laparoscopic wedge resection, for early gastric cancer [9].

The entire surgical procedure is performed laparoscopically under general anesthesia. A laparoscope is inserted through the trocar at the umbilicus. Three or four additional trocars are inserted at the upper abdomen. The location of the cancerous lesion is confirmed from outside of the stomach with the guidance of a gastroscope (Fig. 6). If the lesion is in the greater curvature or in the posterior wall of the stomach, the gastric wall of the lesion should be exposed laparoscopically. The gastric wall in the vicinity of the lesion is pierced with a catheter which has a built-in straight needle, and is introduced through the working channel of the gastroscope (Fig. 7.a). The needle and the catheter are pulled to outside of the gastric wall. A small metal rod is connected by string to the end of the catheter, and is introduced into the stomach. Finally, raising by the string, the lesion is lifted upward with the support of the metal rod (lesion-lifting method) (Fig. 7.b). Wedge resection of the stomach is carried out using a stapling device, an ENDO GIA (US Surgical Corporation Conn.) (Fig. 7c,d). During the resection, the absence of any severe deformity or severe stenosis of the stomach is confirmed by gastroscopy. If there is enough distance between the metal rod and the stapling line, the surgical margin should be of sufficient distance from the cancerous lesion. The resected specimen is retrieved through the umbilical trocar wound (Fig. 8).

If necessary, perigastric lymph nodes can also be dissected laparoscopically in an en bloc fashion. However, because complete lymph node dissection by this

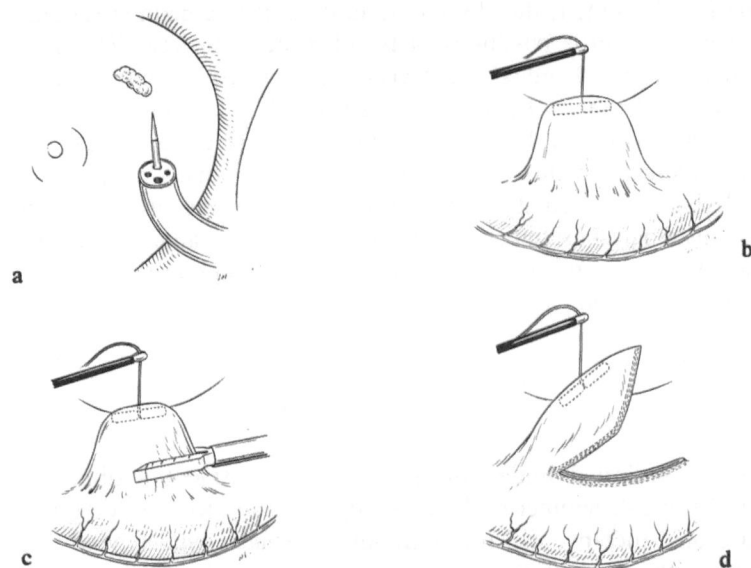

Fig. 7a–d. a The gastric wall in the vicinity of the lesion is pierced with a catheter, which has a built-in straight needle, and is introduced through the working channel of the gastroscope. **b** The cancerous lesion is lifted up with the support of a small metal rod (lesion-lifting method). **c** Wedge resection of the stomach is carried out using a stapling device, an ENDO GIA. **d** Water-tightness of the stapling line is secured. During the resection, the absence of any severe deformity or severe stenosis of the stomach is confirmed by gastroscopy

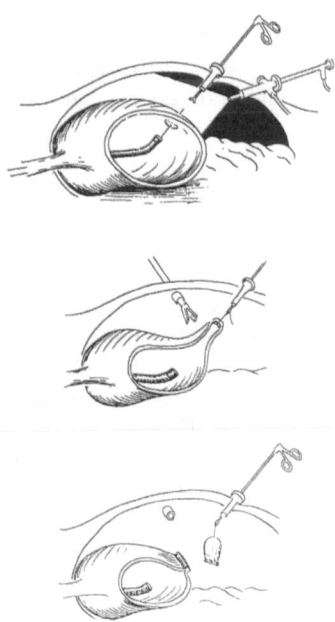

Fig. 8. Three-dimentional view of the lesion-lifting method described in Fig. 7

method is still limited, the absolute indication of this method should be for the lesion which has little possibility of lymph node metastasis. The indications for this procedure are: (1) mucosal cancer, (2) an elevated lesion (so-called Stage II a) < 25 mm or a depressed lesion (so-called Stage II c) < 15 mm and Ul (−), and (3) a lesion which is not at the lesser curvature nor near to the cardia or pylorus.

The advantages of this method are: (1) it is minimally invasive, (2) the cancerous lesion is resected at a sufficient distance from any surgical margin, and (3) detailed histological examination is feasible. The disadvantages are that it requires general anesthesia, and there is the limitation of its application depending on the location of the lesion.

Conclusions

Within the indicated limits, the laparascopic treatment outlined here should provide a valuable adjunct to the endoscopic therapy we have described.

Endoscopic therapy, which can eliminate lesions completely without surgery, can replace the conventional surgical therapy for early gastric cancers provided that the following two requirements are met. First, cancers should be at a very early stage without lymph node metastasis: the diagnostic technique should be improved to detect such cancers accurately. Secondly, physicians must attain technical proficiency in performing endoscopy to be able to remove cancers without any residue. The minimum requirement is to be able to obtain a biopsy endoscopically at any site in the stomach. A physician who meets this requirement should be able to eliminate early cancers endoscopically without surgery. As a result, "endoscopic therapy" will become a radical method of local resection as a procedure more thorough than a modified operation, although more satisfactory surgical procedures are being specifically established for the early, middle, and late stages of gastric cancer.

References

1. Hiki Y, Sakakibara U, Shimao H (1991) Endoscopic treatment of gastric cancer. Surg Endosc 5:11–13
2. Hiki Y (1984) Endoscopic laser therapy for gastrointestinal tumors. In: Okabe H, Honda T, Ohshiba S (eds) Endoscopic surgery. Excerpta Medica International Congress Series 638 Excerpta Medica, Amsterdam, pp 127–136
3. Nagai Y, Katsumi S, Tabuse K, et al (1986) Evaluation of endoscopic microwave coagulation therapy against early stomach cancer (in Japanese). Gastroenterol Endosc 28:1511–1517
4. Tada M, Shimada M, Takemato T (1984) The development of "strip biopsy", a new method for gastric biopsy (in Japanese). Stomach Intestine 19:1107
5. Dougherty TJ (1978) Photoradiation therapy for the treatment of malignant tumors. Cancer Res 38:2628–2635

6. Nakamura K (1991) "The triangle of stomach cancer": Radiographic diagnosis based on comparison of the site, gross morphology, and macroscopic findings. The depressed type not accompanied by ulcer (in Japanese). Stomach Intestine 26:15–25
7. Watanabe Y, et al (1988) Operative results and the therapeutic application of the endoscope: Questionnarie findings (in Japanese). Surg Diag Treatm 30:1206–1212
8. Hiki Y (1991) Present state of endoscopic treatments from a surgical viewpoint. Lecture by the President of the Japan Gastroenterological Endoscopy Society at its 41st Conference (in Japanese). Endoscopy 33:2285–2299
9. Ohgami M, Kumai K, Katajima M, et al (1993) Laparoscopic wedge resection of the stomach for early gastric cancer (lesion-lifting method) (in Japanese). Prog Dig Endos (in press)

Adjuvant and Neoadjuvant Chemotherapy in Gastric Cancer: A Review

Toshifusa Nakajima[1]

Key words. Gastric cancer—Adjuvant chemotherapy—Neoadjuvant chemotherapy—Minimum residual tumor—Dose intensity—Tumor burden—FLEP therapy

Introduction

In contrast to the negative reports from the Western world on the adjuvant chemotherapy of gastric cancer, many Japanese papers describe favorable results in limited subsets of the disease [1–3]. This beneficial outcome has led to the incorporation of adjuvant chemotherapy into routine multimodality therapy of locally advanced gastric cancer in Japan. Comparison of reports from Western countries and Japan might allow the pointing out of some differences in clinical stages of patients subjected to chemotherapy and in the selection of regimens. Reduced tumor burden, proper selection of patients, appropriate selection of drugs or regimens with enough dose intensity, and well-designed clinical protocol seem to be mandatory for the requisites of a successful adjuvant chemotherapy trial. In addition, a further improvement in the treatment results of advanced gastric cancer and establishment of the clinical significance of adjuvant chemotherapy require an alternate approach. The present paper deals with a brief review of adjuvant and neoadjuvant chemotherapy in gastric cancer and includes some discussion for future trials.

Treatment Results of Adjuvant Chemotherapy

Tables 1 and 2 summarize the main adjuvant chemotherapy regimens [4–24] in gastric cancer. Since the late 1950s, clinical trials of adjuvant chemotherapy started in the form of a phase III study (controlled randomized study). In

---

[1] Division of Gastrointestinal Tract Surgery, Cancer Institute Hospital, 1-37-1 Kamiikebukuro, Toshimaku, Tokyo, 170 Japan

404

Table 1. Surgical adjuvant chemotherapy in gastric cancer (1).

Reporters/year	Regimen	Number	5 ysr[a]
Longmire, Dixon [4]	TSPA high dose	82	24
(University Group)	Control	89	19
(1971)	TSPA low dose	177	24
	Control	182	24
Serlin et al. [6] (1977)	TSPA high dose	43	16
	Control	112	16
	TSPA low does	152	18
	Control	138	24
	FUDR	217	17
	Control	241	15
Blokhina et al. [7] (1972)	5FU	375	40[a]
	Control	402	37
Hugier et al. [11] (1980)	5FU, VBL, CPA	27	18
	Control	26	19
GITSG [8] (1982)	5FU, MeCCNU	71	45
	Control	71	32
VASOG [9] (1983)	5FU, MeCCUN	66	38[b]
	Control	68	39
ECOG [10] (1985)	5FU, MeCCNU	91	27
(Engstrom et al.)	Control	89	34
Schreml et al. [12] (1984)	5FU, BCNU	42	58
	Control	53	42

[a] 5 ysr, 5-Year survival rate
[b] 3-Year survival rate

the early days, triethylenethiophosphoramide (thio-TEPA) [4, 5], 5-fluoro-2-deoxyuridine (FUDR) [6], 5-fluorouracil (5FU) [7] or mitomycin C (MMC) [13–16] was employed as a single-drug regimen in the adjuvant setting. The former two drugs did not produce any survival benefit in the large scale clinical trials conducted in the United States [4–6] (Table 1).

5FU was proven to be active in the treatment of advanced gastrointestinal cancers and was used in the adjuvant setting with single or multidrug regimens (Table 2). Single 5FU administration did not reveal survival benefits in cases of curative resection, except for a temporary benefit in a small subset [7]. Conflicting results have been reported in terms of the combination chemotherapy with 5FU and Methyl-CCNU in the United State. The Gastrointestinal Tumor Study Group (GITSG) [8] reported a clinical benefit of combination chemotherapy with 5FU and Methyl-CCNU, although two other concurrent studies [Veterans Administration Surgical Oncology Group (VASOG) an Eastern Cooperative Oncology Group (ECOG)] [9, 10] reported no benefit in comparison with surgery alone. The regimens employed by the three groups were identical, although there was a difference in the selection of patients: GITSG selected curative cases as the subjects of chemotherapy, while the other two groups had no limitations. A combination of 5FU, vinblastin (VBL) and cyclophosphamide (CPM), or 5FU and 1,3-bis(2-chloroethyl)-1-nitrosourea (BCNU) also showed no benefit [11, 12].

Table 2. Surgical adjuvant chemotherapy (2).

Reporters/year	Regimen	Number	5 ysr
Imanaga, Nakazato [13]	MMC, moderate dose	242	68
(1977)	Control	283	54
Nakajima et al. [14] (1978)	MMC, moderate dose	207	52
	Control	223	44
Hattori et al. [15] (1972)	MMC, large dose	146	37
	Control	278	50
Alcobenas et al. [16] (1983)	MMC, large dose	33	79
	Control	37	38
Nakajima et al. [18] (1980)	MMC, 5FU, CA	42	67
	Control	38	50
Nakajima et al. [19] (1984)	MMC, 5FU, CA →		
	5FU	81	68
	MMC, FT, CA → FT	83	63
	Control	79	51
Fielding et al. [20] (1983)	5FU, VCR, CP-M, MTX		
	then 5FU, MMC	140	60[a]
	5FU, MMC	141	66
	Control	130	57
Schein et al. [24] (1985)	5FU, ADM, MMC	156	76[b]
	Control	155	72
Allum et al. [25] (1989)	5FU, ADM, MMC	145	27
	Radiotherapy	153	20
	Control	145	24
Coombes et al. [26] (1990)	5FU, ADM, MMC	133	44
	Control	148	39
Krook et al. [27] (1991)	5FU, ADM	61	32
	Control	64	33

CA, Cytosine arabinoside; *VCR*, vincristine; *CPM*, cyclophosphamide; *MTX*, methotrexate; *ADM*, adriamycin
[a] 1-Year survival rate
[b] 2.5-year survival rate
5 ysr, 5-Year survival rate

Adjuvant MMC has been reported in Japan to have a potential of life pro-longation in a moderately locally advanced stage of the disease (Table 2). Single MMC was used in two ways: one was the regimen of moderate-dose delivery over a long term, in which 0.08 mg/kg MMC was administered i.v. twice a week for 5 weeks [13, 14], and the other was the large-dose administration in short term, in which 20 and 10 mg per body were given in only 2 consecutive days immediately after surgery [15]. These regimens produced no statistically significant survival benefit in the overall number of cases, but the former regimen yielded a 10%–20% increase in the 5-year survival rates of Stage II or III of the disease between the treated (curative surgery + adjuvant chemotherapy) and control (surgery alone) groups ($P < 0.05$). The latter regimen produced a survival benefit exclusively in Stage III. Another large-dose regimen also produced a similar result [16]. The three-drug combination chemotherapy (MFC Therapy) [17] of MMC, 5FU, and cytosine arabinoside, one of the beneficial regimens in advanced gastric cancer, produced a favorable result in the adjuvant setting [18]. Although the survival difference did not achieve statistical significance in the overall number of cases because of the small sample size, it was significant in the subsets of Stages II and III of the diseases. MFC therapy was superior to single MMC in terms of survival benefit. Encouraged by this result, our next study was designed to compare the combination of intravenous MFC and oral 5FU(F) (MFC+F) with that wherein 5FU was replaced by futrafur (F', a derivative of 5FU) (MF'C+F') in cases with curative surgery [19]. In spite of there being no statistical difference in the survival of the overall number of cases, a 17% difference in the 5-year survival rates between MFC+F and the control groups seems to be an encouraging result for the clinicians. MFC+F regimen was superior to the surgery alone in the subsets of Stages I–III of the diseases ($P < 0.05$). These early studies selected all stages of curative surgery as the target of adjuvant chemotherapy. Positive results were obtained ony in the moderately advanced diseases (Stages II and III) by subset analysis, which leads to no definite conclusions from the statistical point of view.

A British study group failed to prove the advantage of adjuvant chemotherapy with 5FU, MMC, and other drugs [20]. Induction by MMC, followed by oral futrafur was proven to have a survival benefit in a certain curative subset [21], compared with MMC alone. Furthermore, the three-drug combination of MMC, futrafur, and PSK (a biological response modifier) produced about 10% better survival rates than those in other two-drug combinations (MMC+F' or MMC+PSK) [22]. FAM therapy [23], a combination of 5FU, Adriamycin (ADM), and MMC, was the most common chemotherapy regimen in advanced gastric cancer. Many clinical trials of FAM therapy have been carried out in the adjuvant setting. Recent reports [24–26] seem unfavorable to adjuvant FAM therapy, although a beneficial potential was reported in the subset of T3 and T4 [26]. A combination of 5FU and ADM also failed to produce a survival benefit [27]. Modification of FAM therapy, FAM2 [28] or FAMTX [29], is under investigation by EORTC, but no clinical significance has yet been reported.

Neoadjuvant Chemotherapy in Gastric Cancer

Relatively few regimens of neoadjuvant chemotherapy have been tried in gastric cancer. However, among the reported regimens, EAP therapy [30, 31] attracted attention because its response rate was higher than 70% and there was high resectability. However, later studies [32–34], reported lesser response rates with more toxicity than the original (Table 3). A randomized controlled study revealed the superiority of FAMTX therapy to EAP therapy [34]. O'Connell [35] stated that EAP therapy, as well as FAM therapy, could not be the standard therapy for advanced gastric cancer. Preoperative combination chemotherapy of 5FU and MTX [36], which is supposed to be activated by the mechanism of biochemical

Table 3. Recent reports on EAP therapy.

First author	No. of patients	Response rate (%)	Toxic deaths (%)
Preusser [30]	67	64	0
Katz [31]	25	72	10
Taguchi [32]	29	44	10
Lerner [33]	22	43	14
Kelsen [34]	30	20	13

Table 4. Regimen of FLEP therapy[a].

5FU	$370mg/m^2$ i.v. days 1–5
Leucovorin	30 mg/body i.v. days 1–5
CDDP	70 mg/m^2, intraaortic, days 7 and 21
Etoposide	70mg/m^2, intraaortic, days 7 and 21

[a] Repeat two courses every 6 weeks

modulation, or preoperative FAMTX (5FU, ADM, and MTX), also contributed to the increase in resectability [37]. A combination of CDDP, MMC, UFT, and etoposide (PMUE) [38] achieved partial response in seven of eight advanced cases, among which five were subjected to gastrectomy. Based on the excellent results of biochemical modulation of 5FU with leucovorin (LCV), and also of the synergism between CDDP and etoposide, the author initiated a combination of systemic delivery of 5FU and LCV, and intra-aortic delivery of CDDP and etoposide through a catheter, the tip of which was placed at the level of the 9th vertebra. The dose schedule (FLEP) is shown in Table 4. A preliminary report [39] revealed that the response rate was 58.3% (7/12) in the unresectable gastric cancers, and all responders were subjected to gastrectomy. Survival benefit has not yet been established because of a relatively short-term observation, although a patient who had curative gastrectomy is still surviving after more than 2 years. Figure 1 shows the changes in the CT scan before and after chemotherapy of 57 males who had an extensive lymphatic metastasis along the aorta. Before chemotherapy (*arrow*), the vena cava was distorted and displaced by the huge mass of involved nodes, and this condition almost disappeared after chemotherapy. Laparotomy after two cycles of this regimen revealed marked shrinkage of the involved para-aortic nodes surrounded by dense scar tissues. The patient had undergone a total gastrectomy, including pancreatosplenectomy. Macroscopically, there was no postoperative residual tumor. Histological examination revealed a small amount of cancer cells remaining in the resected specimens (stomach and para-aortic nodes). The latest data suggest that the main targets of this chemotherapy include unresectable primary lesions, extensive lymphatic metastasis, and liver metastasis. The clinical significance of this regimen seems to

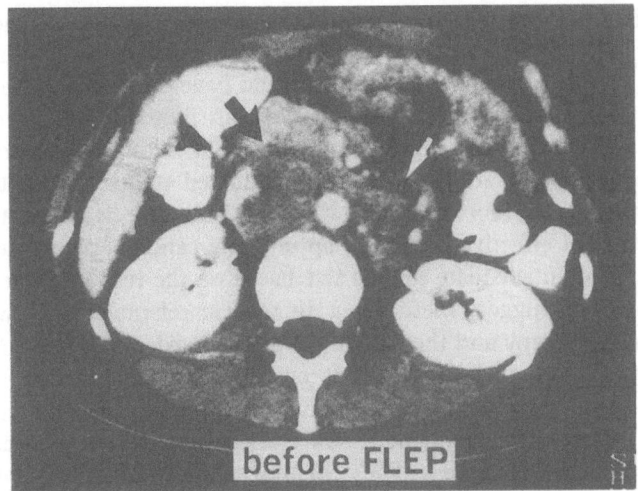

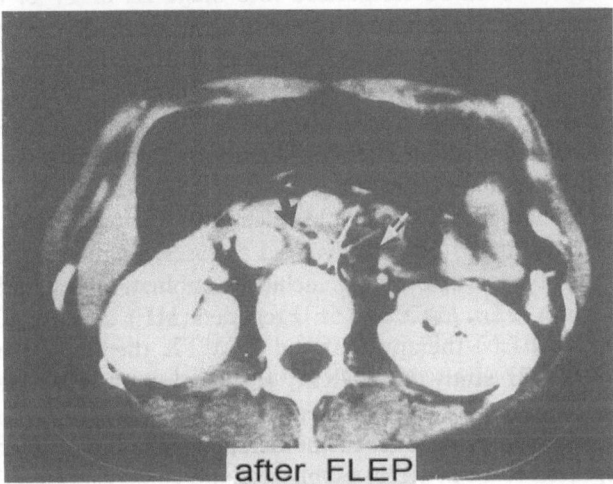

Fig. 1. A CT scan indicating the change in swelling of para-aorta lymph nodes before and after chemotherapy. *FLEP*, 5 FU, leucovorin, CDDP, etoposide (Table 1)

induce the down-staging of an unresectable tumor burden to a resectable state. Although our experience is rather limited, it seems promising as an alternate approach to far-advanced cases.

Future Trials of Adjuvant Chemotherapy in Gastric Cancer

Some Japanese trials have reported positive results which improved survivals of gastric cancer patients with curative gastrectomy and chemotherapy. Most of the favorable results did not achieve a statistical significance in the overall number of cases, but it did in certain subsets, i.e., moderately locally advanced diseases (Stage II or III). If chemotherapy were directed primarily to such subsets with enough of a sample size, favorable results would have been proved statistically. In other words, failure in a clinical study might be attributed to the improper design of the study. When the results are encouraging, but statistically not significant, a secondary confirmatory study should be conducted under the control of well-designed protocol. A thorough review of the literature is mandatory for the proper selection of effective regimens, appropriate candidates for chemotherapy, and estimation of an adequate sample size based on the response rate.

Preclinical trials suggest there being an inverse relationship between the response of chemotherapy and the amount of tumor burden. Tumor burden should be surgically reduced to be as small as possible to obtain a survival benefit of adjuvant chemotherapy. Comparing them with the relatively high survival rates of Japanese gastric cancer patients, 5-year survival rates range between 20% and 40% in the Western countries. These figures suggest that most of the patients subjected to surgery could be categorized into Stage III or IV of the diseases. Japanese trials also failed to improve the survivals of diseases in Stage IV. Early detection and extensive surgery might contribute to the reduction of the amount of residual tumors after surgery. Preoperative or intraoperative chemotherapy seems to have an alternate potential of survival benefit by down-staging and preventing intraoperative dissemination. These approaches may also be helpful for minimizing the residual tumor burden.

As adjuvant chemotherapy, we should select an effective regimen which has been proven by a phase II study in advanced diseases. Regimens which seem to have some potential in gastric cancer include combination chemotherapy with 5FU and Leucovorin (FL), MTX and 5FU regimen (MF), and FAMTX therapy. Etoposide and FL (ELF) therapy [40] and FAMTX therapy are under investigation in a phase III study by EORTC (Protocol # 40902). Moderate-dose MTX and 5FU therapy [41] has been reported to be effective in the control of diffuse-type gastric cancer. Immunochemotherapy, including interferon alpha-2a and 5FU, is reported to be active in esophageal and colon cancers [42–43]. This regimen deserves a clinical trial in gastric cancer. Intraperitoneal (i.p.) administration has attracted the attention of oncologists because of its potential of controlling intraoperative peritoneal dissemination [44–46]. Such administration may allow high-dose intensity in the peritoneal cavity as well as systemic distribution through the portal vein. The effect of i.p. administration should be evaluated by a randomized controlled study. A combination of hyperthermia with i.p. chemotherapy was reported to have a survival benefit in controlling peritoneal dissemination [47–49]. This combined modality may be worthy for the subject of a controlled study.

Extensive patient accumulation is mandatory for clinical trials of adjuvant chemotherapy. For achieving this purpose, a multi-institutional study should be conducted. Referring to the experiences of the United State and Europe, organization of a well-equipped data center is fundamental for controlling the quality of data derived from various institutions.

Conclusions

Although there are few beneficial regimens of adjuvant chemotherapy with any statistical significance, single MMC, combination therapy of 5-FU and Methyl-CCNU, MFC therapy, and FAM therapy seem to have a potential of survival benefit in the various groups of curative surgery. The clinical significance of long-term oral maintenance therapy still remains to be elucidated. Incorporation of new drugs into adjuvant or neo-adjuvant chemotherapy might open a new aspect of multi-modality therapy in gastric cancer.

References

1. Douglass, HO Jr (1988) Western surgical adjuvant trials in gastric cancer: Lessons from current trials to be applied to the future. In: Douglass HO (ed) Contemporary issues in clinical oncology, vol 8. Churchill Livingston, New York, pp 145–172
2. Nakajima T, Nishi M (1988) Adjuvant chemotherapy, immunochemotherapy, and neoadjuvant therapy for gastric cancer in Japan. In: Douglass HO (ed) Contemporary issues in clinical oncology, vol. 8: Gastric cancer. Churchill Livingston, New York, pp 125–143
3. Nakajima T (1990) Adjuvant chemotherapy for gastric cancer in Japan: Present status and suggestions for rational clinical trials. Jpn J Clin Oncol 20:30–42
4. Longmire WP Jr, Dixon WJ (1968) The use of triethylenethiophosphoramide as an adjuvant to the surgical treatment of gastric carcinoma. Ann Surg 167:293–312
5. Dixon WJ, Longmire WP Jr, Holden WD (1971) Use of triethylene-thiophosphoramide as an adjuvant to the surgical treatment of gastric and colorectal carcinoma. Ten-year follow-up. Ann Surg 173:26–39
6. Serlin O, Keehan RJ, Higgins GA Jr, et al (1969) Use of 5-fluorodeoxyuridine (FUDR) as an adjuvant to the surgical management of carcinoma of the stomach. Cancer 24:223–228
7. Blokhina NG, Garin AM, Moros LV, et al (1972) Treatment with 5-fluorouracil in prophylaxis of relapse and metastasis of stomach cancer. Neoplasma 19:351–356
8. Gastrointestinal Tumor Study Group (1982) Controlled trial of adjuvant chemotherapy following curative resection for gastric cancer. Cancer 49:1116–1122
9. Higgins GA, Amadeo JH, Smith DE, et al (1983) Efficacy of prolonged intermittent therapy with Combined 5-FU and methyl-CCNU following resection for gastric carcinoma. A Veterans Administration Surgical Oncology Group report. Cancer 52:1105–1112
10. Engstrom PF, Lavin PT, Douglass HO Jr, et al (1985) Postoperative adjuvant 5-fluorouracil plus methyl-CCNU therapy for gastric cancer patients. Cancer 55: 1868–1873
11. Hugier M, Destroyes J-P, Baschet C, et al (1980) Gastric carcinoma treated by chemotherapy after resection. A controlled study. Am J Surg 139:197–199
12. Schreml W, Schlag P, Herfarth C, et al (1984) In: Jones SE, Salmon SE (eds) Adjuvant therapy of cancer IV: Adjuvant 5-FU/BCNU in gastric carcinoma. Grune and Stratton, Orlando, pp 441–448
13. Imanaga H, Nakazato H (1977) Results of surgery for gastric cancer and effect of adjuvant mitomycin C on cancer recurrence. World J Surg 1:213–221

14. Nakajima T, Fukami A, Ohashi I, Kajitani T (1978) Long-term follow-up study of gastric cancer patients treated with surgery and adjuvant chemotherapy with mitomycin C. Int J Clin Pharmacol 16:209–216

15. Hattori T, Mori A, Hirata K, Ito I (1972) Five-year survival rate of gastric cancer patients treated by gastrectomy, large dose mitomycin C, and/or allogeneic bone marrow transplantation. Gann 63:517–522

16. Alcobenas F, Milla A, Estape J, Curto J, Pera C (1983) Mitomycin-C as adjuvant in resected gastric cancer. Ann Surg 198:13–17

17. Ota K, Kurita S, Nishimura M, Ogawa M, Kamei Y, Imai K, Ariyoshi Y, Kataoka K, Oyama A, Hoshino A, Amo H, Kato T (1972) Combination therapy with mitomycin C (NSC-26980), 5-fluorouracil (NSC-19893), and cytosine arabinoside (NSC-63878) for advanced cancer in man. Cancer Chemother Rep 56:373–385

18. Nakajima T, Fukami A, Takagi K, Kajitani T (1980) Adjuvant chemotherapy with mitomycin C, and with a multi-drug combination of mitomycin C, 5-fluorouracil and cytosine arabinoside after curative resection of gastric cancer. Jpn J Clin Oncol 10:187–194

19. Nakajima T, Takahashi T, Takagi K, Kuno K, Kajitani T (1984) Comparison of 5-fluorouracil with Futrafur in adjuvant chemotherapy with combined inductive and maintenance therapies for gastric cancer. J Clin Oncol 2:1366–1371

20. Fielding JWL, Jagg SL, Jones BG, et al (1983) An interim report of a prospective, randomized, controlled study of adjuvant chemotherapy in operable gastric cancer: British Stomach Cancer Group. World J Surg 7:390–399

21. Taguchi T, Hattori T, Kondo T, Itoh I, Kikuchi K, Sugie S, Inokuchi K (1981) Postoperative adjuvant chemotherapy with mitomycin C plus futrafur for gastric cancer. In: Salmon SE, Jones SE (eds) Adjuvant chemotherapy III. Grune and Stratton, New York, pp 511–518

22. Nakajima T, Inokuchi K, Hattori T, Inoue G, Taguchi T, Kondo T, Abe O, Kikuchi K, Tanabe T, Ogawa N (1989) Multi-institutional study on the postoperative adjuvant immunochemotherapy for gastric cancer. No. 3, on the five-year survival rate (in Japanese). Gan to Kagakuryoho 16:799–806

23. Macdonald JS, Woolley PV, Smythe T, et al (1979) 5-fluorouracil, adriamycin, and mitomycin C (FAM) combination chemotherapy in the treatment of advanced gastric cancer. Cancer 44:42–47

24. Schein PS, Coombes RC, Chilvers C (1985) For the International Adjuvant Trial in Gastric Cancer A controlled trial of FAM (5-FU, doxorubicin, and mitomycin-C) chemotherapy as adjuvant treatment for resected gastric carcinoma: An interim report. Proc Amer Soc Clin Oncol 5:79

25. Allum WH, Halliscey MT, Ward LC, Hockey MS (1989) A controlled prospective randomized trial of adjuvant chemotherapy or radiotherapy in resectable gastric cancer: Interim report. Br J Cancer 60:739–744

26. Coombes RC, Schein PS, Chilvers CED, et al (1990) A randomized trial comparing adjuvant fluorouracil, doxorubicin, and mitomycin with no treatment in operable gastric cancer. J Clin Oncol 8:1362–1369

27. Krook JE, O'Connell MJ, Wieand HR, et al (1991) A prospective, randomized evaluation of intensive course 5-fluorouracil plus doxorubicin as surgical adjuvant chemotherapy for resected gastric cancer. Cancer 67:2454–2458

28. Lise M, Nitti D, Buyse M, Marchet A, Fiorentino M, Guimaraes J, Dues N (1989) Adjuvant FAM2 in resectable gastric cancer. Anticancer Res 9:1017–1022

29. Klein HO, Wickrammanayake PD, Farrokh GR (1986) 5-fluorouraicl, adriamycin and methotrexate—a combination protocol (FAMtx) for treatment of metastasized stomach cancer. Proc Amer Soc Clin Oncol 5:84
30. Preusser P, Wilke H, Achterrath W, et al (1987) Phase-II-Studie mit Etoposid, Adriamycin, Cisplatin (EAP) beim primaer inoperablen, metastasierten Magenkarzinom. Tumor Diag Ther 8:43–48
31. Katz A, Gansl R, Simon S, et al (1989) Phase II trial of VP-16, Adriamycin, and cisplatinum in patients with advanced gastric cancer. Proc Am Soc Clin Oncol 8:98
32. Taguchi T (1989) Combination chemotherapy with etoposide (E), adriamycin (A), and cisplatin (P) (EAP) for advanced gastric cancer. Proc Amer Soc Clin Oncol 8:108
33. Lerner A, Steele GD, Mayer RJ (1990) Etoposide, doxorubicin, cisplatin (EAP) chemotherapy for advanced gastric adenocarcinoma: Results of a phase II trial. Proc Amer Soc Clin Oncol 8:103
34. Kelsen DK, Atig OT, Saltz L, et al (1992) FAMTX versus etoposide, doxorubicin, and cisplatin: A random assignment trial in gastric cancer. J Clin Oncol 10:541–548
35. O'Connell MJ (1992) Etoposide, doxorubicin, and cisplatin cheotherapy for advanced gastric cancer: An old lesson revisited. J Clin Oncol 10:515–516
36. Plukker JTh, Mulder NH, Sleijfer DTh, et al (1991) Chemotherapy and surgery for locally advanced cancer of the cardia and fundus: Phase II study with methotrexate and 5-fluorouracil. Br J Surg 78:955–958
37. Kremer B, Henne-Bruns D, Weh HJ, et al (1989) Advanced gastric cancer: A new combined surgical and oncological approach. Hepatogastroenterology 36:23–26
38. Kato S, Kinoshita K, Sawa T, et al (1990) Neoadjuvant chemotherapy in far advanced gastric carcinoma. Effect of preoperative chemotherapy with PMUE (CDDP, MMC, UFT, Etoposide) (in Japanese). Gan to Kagakuryoho 17:391–396
39. Nakajima T, Ishihara S, Ota K, et al (1992) Down-staging of inoperable gastric cancer with biaxial chemotherapy. Proc 45th Annual Cancer Symposium of The Society of Surgical Oncology. p 130
40. Stahl M, Wilke H, Preusser P, et al (1989) Etoposide (E), leucovorin (L), 5-FU (ELF) in advanced gastric carcinoma (GC)—final results of a phase II study. Abstr Eur Conf Clin Oncol, p 0695
41. Akazawa S, Yoshida S (1988) The role of thymidylate synthetase in sequential dose of MTX and 5-FU for the advanced scirrhous type gastric cancer (in Japanese). Gan to Kagakuryouhou 15:1273–1278
42. Kelsen D, Lovett D, Wong J, et al (1992) Interferon alfa-2a and fluorouracil in the treatment of patients with advanced esophageal cancer. J Clin Oncol 10:269–274
43. Wadler S, Lembersky B, Atkins M, et al (1991) Phase II trial of fluorouracil and recombinant interferon alfa-2a in patients with advanced colorectal carcinoma: An Eastern Cooperative Oncology Group Study. J Clin Oncol 9:1806–1810
44. Surbone A, Myers CE (1989) Regional therapies. In: Magrath I (ed) New directions in cancer treatment. Springer, Berlin, pp 166–190
45. Speyer JL (1985) The rationale behind intraperitoneal chemotherapy in gastrointestinal malignancies. Semin Oncol 12:3 [Suppl 4]:23–28
46. Sugarbaker PH, Cunliffe WJ, Belliveau J, et al (1989) Rationale for integrating early postoperative intraperitoneal chemotherapy into the surgical treatment of gastrointestinal cancer. Sem Oncol 16:83–97

47. Koga S, Hamazoe R, Maeta M, et al (1988) Prophylactic therapy for peritoneal recurrence of gastric cancer by continous hyperthermic peritoneal perfusion with mitomycin C. Cancer 61:232–237
48. Kaibara N, Hamazoe R, Iitsuka Y, et al (1989) Hyperthermic peritoneal perfusion combined with anticancer chemotherapy as prophylactic treatment of peritoneal recurrence of gastric cancer. Hepatogastroenterology 36:75–78
49. Fujimura T, Yonemura Y, Fuchida S, et al (1990) Continuous hyperthermic peritoneal perfusion for the treatment of peritoneal dissemination in gastric cancers and subsequent second-look operation. Cancer 65:65–71

New Systemic Chemotherapy

P. Preusser and H. Wilke[1]

Key words. Review article—Chemotherapy—Gastric cancer

Introduction

While the annual incidence of gastric cancer has been steadily declining in many Western countries, it remains a very frequent tumor in Japan and in most of Europe.

In spite of modern surgical procedures having improved the prognosis of at least the subsets of gastric cancer patients, the overall outcome remains poor. Especially the prognosis of patients with advanced disease—locally confined or metastasized—has not essentially changed during recent decades. The main reasons, therefore, are primarily irresectable tumors or the high frequency of local or distant recurrences even after so-called curative resections. The pattern of relapse and/or tumor spread in patients with advanced stages of gastric cancer clearly show that prognosis will not be changed by local treatment alone, but rather by systemic treatment given either alone or in combination with surgery and/or irradiation.

It was not long ago that most physicians regarded gastric cancer as a rather chemoinsensitive tumor. However, because of the recent successes being reported with newer and active combinations, this tumor has been established as being chemosensitive [1].

Single Agent Chemotherapy

In terms of only disease-orientated phase II trials with more than 14 previously untreated patients per trial which were conducted according to WHO criteria, objective remissions [complete (CR) plus partial (PR) remission] of $\geq 15\%$ were

[1] Klinik und Poliklinik für Allgemeine Chirurgie, Westfälische Wilhelms-Universität Münster, Jungeblodtplatz 1, 4400 Münster, Germany

Table 1. Single agent activity in patients without previous chemotherapy (>14 patients per trial). (From [2]).

Drug	Patients (n)	CR n (%)	CR + PR n (%)	mR (months)
5-Fluorouracil	54	1 (2)	11 (20)	4
Doxorubicin	124	10 (8)	21 (17)	4–6
Epirubicin	39	2 (5)	8 (21)	nr
Cisplatin	14	2 (14)	5 (36)	3–6
Etoposide	14	0	3 (21)	1–5
Mitomycin	211	nr	63 (30)	nr
BCNU	55	1 (2)	10 (18)	5

mR, Median remission duration; nr, not reported; CR, complete remission; PR, partial remission

induced by cisplatin, doxorubicin, 4-epidoxorubicin, 5-fluorouracil, mitomycin, BCNU, and etoposide (Table 1) [2]. Complete remission rates, observed with cisplatin (14%) and doxorubicin (8%) were higher in comparison to the other drugs [2] (Table 1).

Idarubicin, aclacinomycin, mitoxantrone, bisantrene, amsacrine, vindesine, razoxane, and carboplatin were inactive or only marginally active in gastric cancer (CR/PR rate less than 10%) [2–4]. In patients with gastric cancer refractory to combination chemotherapy, cisplatin, doxorubicin, methotrexate, and triazinate achieved more than 10% of CR/PR. After pretreatment with 5-fluorouracil (5-FU), doxorubicin, and mitomycin (FAM), cisplatin induced 20% of CR/PR [2]. After 5-FU/doxorubicin or 5-FU/nitrosoureas, CR/PR rates of 17%, 15%, and 11% were observed with doxorubicin, triazinate, and methotrexate, respectively [2]. Less than 10% of CR/PR or no remissions were seen with carboplatin, etoposide, razoxane, and mitoxantrone in pretreated patients [2].

Combination Chemotherapy

During the past two decades, numerous two-, three-, and four-drug combinations have been investigated in disease-orientated phase II and III trials [2].

Until recently, the combination of 5-FU, doxorubicin, and mitomycin (FAM) was regarded as the so-called standard chemotherapy of gastric cancer. However, FAM usually induced less than 30% of objective remissions, very infrequently complete remissions, and showed median survival times of only approximately 7 months. Substituting mitomycin in the FAM regimen by cisplatin, methyl-CCNU, or BCNU, or adding a fourth drug to this combination did not lead to better results when compared to FAM [2, 5–7] (Table 2).

Since the early 1980s, a number of new active combinations had been developed for the treatment of gastric cancer leading to a more optimistic attitude concerning the outcome of chemotherapy for this tumor (Table 3). Klein et al.

Table 2. Results of more frequently used 5-FU/doxorubicin-based combinations. (From [2, 6, 7]).

Combination	Patients (n)	CR n (%)	CR/PR n (%)	mR (Months)	mS (Months)
FAM	792	11 (1) (0–2)[a]	212 (27) (24–30)	5–10	6–9+
FAMe	83	10 (12) (5–19)[a]	20 (24) (15–33)[a]	5	6–8
FAB	117	10 (6) (3–9)[a]	50 (43) (36–50)[a]	7–9	6–8
FAP	187	9 (5) (2–8)[a]	68 (36) (29–43)[a]	5–7	6–13

[a] 95% Confidence limits
mR, Median remission duration; mS, median survival time; F, 5-FU; A, doxorubicin; Me, Methyl-CCNU, B, BCNU; FAM, 5-FU, doxorubicin and mitomycin; P, Cisplatin

Table 3. Newer active combinations for gastric cancer.

Combination	Patients (n)	CR n (%)	CR/PR n (%)	mR (Months)	mS (Months)	References
FAMTX	298	29 (10) (7–13)[a]	123 (41) (35–47)[a]	5–9	3–9.6	[5, 6, 8–10]
EAP	439	35 (9) (6–12)[a]	193 (44) (39–49)[a]	5–7	3–16	[5, 11–21]
ELF[b]	71	6 (8) (2–14)[a]	36 (51) (39–63)[a]	8	11.5	[22, 23]
Cisplatin/ 5 FU[b]	211	9 (4) (1–7)[a]	94 (45) (37–52)[a]	nr	7–17.5	[7, 24–26]
ECF	47	5 (10) (1–19)[a]	37 (83) (72–94)[a]	nr	nr	[27]

[a] 95% Confidence limits
[b] Partially pretreated
mR, Median remission duration; mS, median survival time; nr, not reported; FAMTX, 5-FU, doxorubicin, methotrexate; EAP, etoposide, doxorubicin, cisplatin; ELF, etoposide, folinic acid, 5-FU; ECF, 4-epidoxorubicin, cisplatin, 5-FU

reported more than 50% of objective remissions and more than 10% of clinically complete remissions with 5-FU, doxorubicin, methotrexate (FAMTX) in 100 patients with advanced disease [8]. Subsequent phase II–III studies revealed contradictory results [5, 6, 8–10] (Table 4). However, in a recently published phase III trial of the EORTC (European Organization for Research and Treatment of Cancer) with FAMTX versus FAM, FAMTX induced significantly higher remission rates (42% versus 9%) and a significantly longer median survival

Table 4. Results of FAMTX (≥14 patients per study).

First author [Reference]	Patients (n)	CR n (%)	CR/PR n (%)	mS (Months)
Klein [8]	100	12 (12)	59 (59)	8
Wils [10]	67	9 (13)	22 (33)	6
Herrmann [9]	20	0	0	3
Wils [6]	81[a]	5 (6)	33 (42)	9.6
Kelsen [5]	30[a]	3 (10)	9 (30)	7.4

[a] Randomized trial
mS, Median survival time

Table 5. EAP in advanced gastric cancer (>14 patients per study).

First author (Reference)	Patients (n)	CR/PR n (%)	CR n (%)	mS (Months)
Tagushi [11]	50	22 (44)	ns	5.1
Tokunaga [12]	14	4 (29)	1 (7)	nr
Katz [13]	29	21 (72)	4 (14)	7.2
Kim [14]	20	12 (60)	nr	8+
Wilke [15]	145	83 (57)	22 (15)	10–16
Lerner [16]	28	12 (43)	3 (11)	6
Raeth [17]	45	8 (18)	0	9
Villar [18]	16	1 (6)	3 (19)	nr
Haim [19]	17	6 (36)	1 (6)	nr
Bajetta [20]	26	10 (38)	3 (11)	nr
Kelsen [5]	30	6 (21)	0	6
Shimada [21]	19	8 (42)	0	7
Total	439	193/439 (44)	35/369 (9)	3–16

mS, Median survival time; nr, not reported

time (42 versus 29 weeks) than FAM [10]. Because to these results, FAMTX could be regarded as a new chemotherapeutic standard to which other investigational protocols should be compared.

High remission rates have also been reported with etoposide, doxorubicin, and cisplatin (EAP). More than 400 patients have been treated with this combination, mostly in phase II trials. An overall response rate of 44% (6%–72%) including 9% of complete remissions (part of which were histopathologically confirmed) and median survival times of up to 16 months (range 5–16 months) had been observed in disease-orientated phase II trials including ≥ 14 patients per trial [5, 11–21] (Table 5). Such a wide range of tumor responses and survival times are well known from gastric cancer trials with other combinations, and may be explained by patient populations with different chemotherapy-related prognostic factors. In nearly all EAP trials, a high percentage of WHO grade 3–4 myelotoxicity and clinically relevant infections including lethal septicemias were observed. Therefore, this intensive combination cannot be recommended when treatment intention is palliation at best (i.e., metastasized disease).

Another promising combination for the treatment of advanced gastric cancer is ELF (etoposide, folinic acid, 5-FU) which was investigated in two phase II studies [22, 23]. In 51 previously untreated patients who were either older than 65 years or who had cardiac risks and could therefore not be treated with anthracyclines, an objective remission rate of 53%, including 12% clinically complete remissions, and a median survival time of 11 months were achieved [22]. This combination was well tolerated and could be safely administered as an outpatient treatment. Similar results (PR 45%, median survival 11.5 months, low toxicity) were observed with ELF as a second line treatment after carboplatin [23]. Because of these results, the EORTC has recently initiated a randomized phase III trial comparing ELF versus FAMTX versus cisplatin/5-fluorouracil.

Objective remissions ranging between 40% and 50% were also induced by cisplatin/5-fluorouracil in 211 patients with locally advanced and metastasized disease [7, 24–26].

Also of note are the results of a phase II trial with a combination of 4-epidoxorubicin and cisplatin i.v. on day 1 and repeated every 21 days, plus 5-fluorouracil (ECF) as continuous infusion for 21 weeks [27]. In 47 previously untreated patients, 10% complete remissions and 72% partial remissions and good toleration to this regimen were reported. These extremely good results warrant further confirmation in randomized studies.

Postoperative (Adjuvant) Chemotherapy

Adjuvant chemotherapy trials geared to reduce the rate of local and systemic recurrences were carried out during the past two decades in patients who underwent complete tumor resection. In these trials, adjuvant treatment consisted of single agents and various (mostly 5-FU based) two- and three-drug combinations [2, 28, 29] (Table 6). Except for one Gastrointestinal Tumor Study Group (GITSG) trial with 5-FU/BCNU versus control [29] and one other trial with adjuvant chemotherapy versus adjuvant chemoimmunotherapy [30], all other trials failed to show any significant survival benefit with postoperative chemotherapy compared to the surgical control groups. However, the results of these trials should not lead to the conclusion that adjuvant chemotherapy is generally ineffective in gastric cancer. No one would expect that only marginally active single agents or combinations that produce remission rates of less than 20%–30% could have a significant influence on survival when given as adjuvant treatment. Moreover, the majority of these studies entered patient numbers which were too small to detect a survival benefit with sufficient statistical value.

Adjuvant chemotherapy of gastric cancer remains an investigational approach, and its future role in the multidisciplinary management of gastric cancer has to be subjected to well-designed trials with newer and more active combinations.

Table 6. Results of adjuvant chemotherapy versus surgery.

Regimen	Patients (n)	Significant survival benefit for adjuvant chemotherapy	Reference
Thiotepa	194	No	[2]
FUdr	397	No	[2]
5-FU/MeCCNU	156	No	[2]
5-FU/MeCCNU	142	$P < 0.03$	[30]
5-FU/MeCCNU	160	No	[2]
Mitomycin/Thiotepa	209	No	[2]
Mitomycin/cyclophosphamide/ cromomycin A3	350	No	[2]
Mitomycin/5FU	460	No	[2]
5-FU/Mitomycin	411	No	[2]
FAM	281	No	[28]

FUdr, Fluorouridine

Table 7. Results of preoperative chemotherapy in locally advanced stages of gastric cancer.

Author (Reference)	Patients	CR/PR (%)	R0-Resection rate (%)	mS (Months)
Mahjoubi [24]	26	61	62	17.5
Verschueren [38]	17	nr	41	nr[a]
Wilke [39]	35	72	46	16[b]

[a] Four patients alive and disease-free from 11+ to 24 months
[b] 20% Disease-free long-term survival after 40 months
mS, Median survival time

Preopeative (Neoadjuvant) Chemotherapy

The experience with preoperative chemotherapy of gastric cancer is still limited to a few trials in patients with either clinically resectable tumors [31–37] or with locally advanced disease [24, 38, 39]. The possible impact of this neoadjuvant approach on resectability and survival cannot be answered by those trials, which used preoperative chemotherapy in clinically resectable stages.

The well-known difficulties of staging of gastric cancer by clinical means do not allow a proper definition of the stage and resectability prior to chemotherapy. For this reason and because most trials were nonrandomized without surgical controls, it remains unclear whether preoperative chemotherapy has contributed to the rather high 5-year survival rates in Stage III tumors [31–34]. In three phase II trials, preoperative chemotherapy was investigated in patients with locally advanced tumors (Table 7). With cisplatin/5-fluorouracil, Mahjoubi et al. achieved an objective remission rate of 52% in patients with locally far-advanced tumors (clinical/surgical staging) [24]. Sixty-two percent of the patients underwent curative surgery after chemotherapy. The median survival time was 17.5 months and the 2-year survival rate was 45%.

Methotrexate, 5-fluorouracil was used by Verschueren et al. in 17 patients whose tumors were defined as being irresectable at explorative laparotomy [38]. After chemotherapy, curative resection of residual disease could be performed in seven (41%) of these patients and four of them were alive and disease-free from 11+ to 24+ months.

Prior to a planned second-look operation, EAP was administered to 35 patients who had technically irresectable gastric cancer as determined by explorative laparotomy [39]. The overall remission and complete remission rates of 72% and 23% were achieved, respectively. Twenty-one patients had second-look surgery. Six clinical complete remissions were pathohistologically confirmed, and ten patients had R0 resections while three others had R1 resections (no evidence of disease after consolidation chemotherapy). The median survival time for the whole group was 16 months and it was 24 months for patients who were disease-free after chemotherapy ± surgery. The long-term survival rate after 40 months was 20%.

These three trials clearly demonstrate that an active regimen of preoperative chemotherapy may render primarily irresectable gastric cancer resectable, thereby increasing the curative resection rates. They also show that this multimodal approach may result in disease-free long-term survival of patients who cannot be cured by surgery.

Conclusions and Future Perspectives

Gastric cancer is now being recognized as being a chemosensitive lesion and also as a tumor whose prognosis may be improved by interdisciplinary efforts. In a situation where more than two-thirds of the patients will die of locally uncontrolled or metastasized disease, an effective program of chemotherapy will become one of the cornerstones of multimodal treatment of this challenging malignancy.

The first steps towards achieving this goal have been taken. Objective remission rates of 40%–50%—in locally advanced disease even up to 70%—have been achieved with FAMTX, EAP, ELF, cisplatin/5-fluorouracil, ECF, and other newer protocols. Moreover, in one randomized trial, it could be shown that chemotherapy does not only induce "abstract" remissions but also significantly prolongs survival, compared to supportive care alone [40]. In the preoperative setting, chemotherapy has demonstrated its efficacy, at least in locally advanced disease where it may offer a chance for cure in patients with an otherwise fatal outcome [24, 38, 39].

Nevertheless, there is clearly an urgent need for the development of a still more effective program of chemotherapy. This might also lead to the use of hematopoietic growth factors (higher dose intensity, reduction of myelosuppression-related complications) and of immunomodulators as well as biochemical modulators. Moreover, there is also a need for the definition of

422 P. Preusser and H. Wilke

prognostic factors in order to pretherapeutically identify those patients who will benefit from cytostatic treatment.

In the perioperative treatment of locoregionally confined tumors, adjuvant trials with the newer, effective combinations should be undertaken on the basis of clearly defined surgical procedures and a pathohistologic work-up of the resected material. The first promising trials with preoperative chemotherapy in locally advanced disease should be extended, and randomized trials with surgery alone versus preoperative chemotherapy in T3-T4 N1-2 M0 tumors should be initiated.

References

1. Cunningham D (1988) Gastric cancer—the recognition of a chemosensitive tumour. Br J Cancer 58:695–699
2. Preusser P, Achterrath W, Wilke H, Lenaz L, Fink U, Heinicke H, Meyer J, Bünte H (1988) Chemotherapy of gastric cancer. Cancer Treat Rev 15:257–277
3. Preusser P, Wilke H, Achterrath W, Lenaz L, Stahl M, Casper J, Meyer HJ, Meyer J, Blum M, Schmoll HJ (1990) Phase II study of carboplatin in untreated inoperable advanced stomach cancer. Eur J Cancer 26:1108–1109
4. Beer M, Cavalli F, Kaye SB, Lev LM, Clavel M, Smyth J, van Glabbeke M, Renard J, Pinedo HM (1987) A phase II study of carboplatin in advanced or metastatic stomach cancer. Eur J Cancer Clin Oncol 23:1365–1367
5. Kelsen D, Atig O, Saltz L, Toomasi F, Trochanowski B, Niedzwiecki D (1991) FAMTX [fluorouracil (F), methotrexate (MTX), adriamycin (A)] is as effective and less toxic than EAP [etoposide (E), A, cisplatin (P)]: A random-assigned trial in gastric cancer (GC) (abstract). Proc Am Soc Clin Oncol 10:137
6. Wils JA, Klein HO, Wagener DJT, Bleiberg H, Reis H, Korsten F, Conroy T, Fickers M, Leyvraz S, Buyse M, Duesz N (1991) Sequential high-dose methotrexate and fluorouracil combined with doxorubicin— a step ahead in the treatment of advanced gastric cancer. A trial of the European Organization for Research and Treatment of Cancer Gastrointestinal Tract Cooperative Group. J Clin Oncol 9:872–831
7. Kim NK, Park YS, Suh CI, Kan WK, Kim HT, Heo DS, Bang YJ (1991) Phase III randomized comparison of 5-FU vs FAM (5-FU/ADRIA/MMC) vs FP (5-FU/Cisplatin) in patients with advanced gastric carcinoma (AGC) (abstract). Proc Am Soc Clin Oncol 10:144
8. Klein HO, Wickramanayake D, Farrokh GH (1986) 5-Fluorouracil (5-FU), Adriamycin (ADM) and methotrexate (MTX)—a combination protocol (FAMTX) for treatment of metastasized stomach cancer (abstract). Proc Am Soc Clin Oncol 5:84
9. Herrmann R, Fritze D, Queißer W, Flechtner H, Ho AD, Schlag P, König H (1984) Chemotherapie des Magenkarzinoms. DMW 109:1704
10. Wils J, Bleiberg H, Blijham G (1986) An EORTC gastrointestinal group evaluation of the combination of sequential methotrexate (MTX) and 5-fluorouracil (F), combined with Adriamycin (A) (FAMTX) in advanced measurable gastric cancer. J Clin Oncol 4:1799–1803
11. Taguchi T, Ohta J, Orino M, Oshiba S, Yamada S, Okazima K, Ohtani T, Hurukawa H, Iwanaga T, Numata N (1990) Combination chemotherapy with etoposide, ADM, CDDP (EAP) for advanced gastric cancer. Gan To Kagaku Ryoho 17(11):2191–2196

12. Tokunaga A, Onda M, Mizutani T, Miyamoto M, Nomura T, Hayashi H, Kiyama T, Umehara M, Nishi K, Andoh T (1989) Combination chemotherapy with etoposide, adriamycin and cisplatin in advanced primary and recurrent gastric cancer. Gan To Kagaku Ryoho 16(12):3713–3718

13. Katz A, Gansl RC, Simon SD, Gama-Rodrigues J, Waitzberg D, Bresciani CJ, Pinotti HW (1991) Phase II trial of etoposide (V), adriamycin (A), and cisplatinum (P) in patients with metastatic gastric cancer. Am J Clin Oncol 14(4):357–358

14. Kim SY, Song MH, Park CS, Lee HY, Kim YK, Lee BH, An BJ (1989) Etoposide, adriamycin, and cisplatin (EAP) combination chemotherapy for advanced gastric cancer (abstract). Blut 59:257

15. Wilke H, Preusser P, Fink U, Achterrath W, Meyer HJ, Stahl M, Lenaz L, Meyer J, Siewert JR, Geerlings H, Köhne-Wömpner CH, Harstrick A, Schmoll HJ (1990) New developments in the treatment of gastric cancer. Semin Oncol 17 [Suppl 2]:61–70

16. Lerner A, Steele GD, Meyer RJ (1990) Etoposide, doxorubicin, cisplatin (EAP) chemotherapy for advanced gastric adenocarcinoma: Results of a phase II trial (abstract). Proc Am Soc Clin Oncol 9:103

17. Raeth U, Flechtner H, Selbach J, Harjung H, Manegold C, Kabelitz K, Trux FA, Edler L, Schlag P, Queißer W (1990) Etoposide, adriamycin, and cisplatinum (EAP) combination chemotherapy for advanced gastric cancer. Onkologie 13:194–197

18. Villar-Grimalt A, Candel MT, Garcia J, Bernacer B, Jimeno J (1991) Combination of etoposide, adriamycin and cisplatin (EAP) in gastric cancer: Association with severe toxicity. Ann Oncol 2:310–311

19. Haim N, Robinson E (1991) Combination of etoposide, adriamycin and cisplatin (EAP) in gastric cancer: Association with severe toxicity. Ann Oncol 2:311–312

20. Bajetta E, Di Bartolomeo M, Buzzoni R, Lambiase A, Biganzoli I (1991) Doxorubicin, VP-16, CDDP (EAP) in advanced gastric cancer (AGC): A study by the Italian Trials in Medical Oncology (ITMO) Group (abstract). Eur J Cancer 91 [Suppl 2]:79

21. Shimada Y, Yoshida S, Ohtsu A, Saito D, Miyamoto K, Yoshino M, Fujii T, Tajiri H, Yamaguchi H, Yoshino M, Yoshida T, Yishimori M, Ohkura H, Okazaki N (1990) A phase II study of combination chemotherapy with etoposide, adriamycin and cisplatin (EAP) for advanced gastric cancer in Japan (abstract). J Cancer Res Clin Oncol 116 [Suppl]:673

22. Stahl M, Wilke H, Preusser P, Fink U, Achterrath W, Schöber C, Köhne-Wömpner CH, Harstrick A, Meyer HJ, Meyer J, Lenaz L, Schmoll HJ (1991) Etoposide, leukovorin and 5-fluorouracil (ELF) in advanced gastric carcinoma—final results of a phase II study in elderly patients or patients with cardial risk. Onkologie 14:314–318

23. Wilke H, Preusser P, Stahl M, Harstrick A, Meyer HJ, Achterrath W, Schmoll HJ, Seeber S (1991) Etoposide, folinic acid, and 5-fluorouracil in carboplatin-pretreated patients with advanced gastric cancer. Cancer Chemother Pharmacol 29:83–84

24. Mahjoubi M, Rougier P, Oliviera J, Tigaud JM, Bognel C, Lasser P, Droz JP (1990) Phase II trial of combined 5-FU + CDDP in gastric cancer (GC) (abstract). J Cancer Res Clin Oncol (Suppl, part 1) 116:677

25. Yoshida S, Shimada Y, Saito D, Ohtsu A, Shirao K, Sugano K, Ohkura H, Yoshino M, Soshimori M (1991) Phase II trial of 5-fluorouracil (FU) and cisplatin (CDDP) in metastatic cancer, as second-line chemotherapy (abstract). Proc Am Soc Clin Oncol 10:160

26. Lacave AJ, Baron FJ, Anton LM, Estrada E, De Sande LMG, Palacio I, Esteban E, Gracia JM, Buesa JM, Fernandez OA, Baron MG (1991) Combination chemotherapy

with cisplatin and 5-fluorouracil 5-day infusion in the therapy of advanced gastric cancer: A phase II trial. Ann Oncol 2:751–754

27. Findlay M, Mansi JL, Ford HT, Nash AT, Cunningham D (1991) Epirubicin, cisplatin and 5-fluorouracil (ECF) is highly effective in advanced gastric cancer (abstract). Eur J Cancer [Suppl 2]:71

28. Coombes RC, Schein PS, Chilvers CED, Wils J, Beretta G, Bliss JM, Rutten A, Amadori D, Cortes-Funes H, Villar-Grimalt A, McArdle C, Rauschecker HF, Boven E, Vassilopoulos P, Welvaart K, Pinto Ferreira E, Wiig J, Gisselbrecht C, Rougier P, Woods EMA (1990) A randomized trial comparing adjuvant fluorouracil, doxorubicin, and mitomycin with no treatment in operable gastric cancer. J Clin Oncol 8:1362–1369

29. Gastrointestinal Tumor Study Group (1982) Controlled trial of adjuvant chemotherapy following curative resection for gastric cancer. Cancer 49:1116–1122

30. Kim BS, Chung CH, Roh JK, Park YJ, Koh EH, Kim JH, Min JS, Lee KS, Lee KB, Youn JK (1991) A controlled trial of 5-FU, doxorubicin (FA) chemotherapy vs FA-polyadenylic, polyuridylic acid (poly-AU) chemoimmunotherapy for locally advanced gastric cancer after curative resection: An interim report (abstract). Proc Am Soc Clin Oncol 10:134

31. Fujimoto S, Akao T, Ito B, Koshizuka I, Koyano K (1976) A study of survival in patients with stomach cancer treated by a combination of preoperative intra-arterial infusion thrapy and surgery. Cancer 37:1648–1654

32. Nishioka B, Ouchi T, Watanabe S, Umehara M, Yamane E, Yahata K, Muto F, Kojima O, Nomiyama S, Sakita M, Fujita Y, Majima S (1982) Follow-up study of preoperative oral administration of an antineoplastic agent as an adjuvant chemotherapy in stomach cancer. Gan To Kagaku Ryoho 9:1427–1430

33. Jinnai D, Higashi H (1976) Extended radical operation with preoperative chemotherapy for gastric cancer. In: Hirayama T (ed) Cancer in Asia. University Park Press, Baltimore

34. Stephens FO (1988) Management of gastric cancer with regional chemotherapy proceding gastrectomy—5-year survival results. Reg Cancer Treat 1:80–82

35. Ajani JA, Ota DM, Jessup JM, Ames FC, McBride C, Boddie A, Levin B, Jackson, DE, Roh M, Hohn D (1991) Resectable gastric carcinoma—An evaluation of preoperative and postoperative chemotherapy. Cancer 68:1501–1506

36. Leichman L, Silberman H, Leichman C, Laine L, Ramos H, Spears P, Jeffers S (1990) Neoadjuvant chemotherapy for gastric adenocarcinoma followed by postoperative intraperitoneal (IP) chemotherapy (abstract). Proc Am Soc Clin Oncol 9:109

37. Iaffaioli RV, Frasci G, Facchini G, Tortoriello A, Persico G, Canove G, Bianco AR (1991) Neoadjuvant immunochemotherapy (FEP-IFN) in locally advanced gastric cancer (abstract). Preliminary data. Eur J Cancer [Suppl 2]:77

38. Verschueren RJC, Willemse PHB, Sleijfer DTH, de Vries EGE, Mulder HH (1988) Combined chemotherapeutic-surgical approach of locally advanced gastric cancer (abstract). Proc Am Soc Clin Oncol 7:93

39. Wilke H, Preusser P, Fink U, Gunzer U, Meyer HJ, Meyer J, Siewert JR, Achterrath W, Lenaz L, Knipp H, Schmoll HJ (1989) Preoperative chemotherapy in locally advanced and nonresectable gastric cancer: A phase II study with etoposide, doxorubicin, and cisplatin. J Clin Oncol 7:1318–1326

40. Kuitunen T, Pyrhönen S (1991) A randomized phase III trial comparing fluorouracil, epidoxorubicin and methotrexate (FEMTX) with no treatment in nonresectable gastric cancer (abstract). Eur J Cancer [Suppl 2]:80

Chemotherapy in Gastric Cancer

Minoru Kurihara[1]

Key words. Chemotherapy—Gastric cancer—5'-DFUR—CDDP—Response criteria—Quality of life

Introduction

In any evaluation of systemic chemotherapy for gastric cancer, the subjects undergoing the various kinds of therapeutic regimens must be carefully analyzed. For intance, the subjects of EAP reported by Preusser were less than 60 years old and had a Performance Status (PS) of 0–2 [1]. On the other hand, 34.2% of the subjects receiving tegafur + MMC and UFT + MMC (in a well-controlled randomized trial involving 13 institutions throughout Japan) were more than 70 years old and 16% had a PS of 3 [2]. These kinds of data influence the most important factors determining the response rate of systemic chemotherapy. Moreover, the cancer volume in a patient's body affects both response rate and survival. If the target organ is limited to Virchow lymph node metastasis as a result of recurrence after gastric resection of advanced cancer, complete response (CR) is easily gained. For the patient with a large primary focus with multiple liver metastases (often with ascities), even partial response (PR) is seldom gained. In Japan, gastric cancer is often detected in elderly patients and has already metastasized by the time of detection, resulting in many inoperable cases. Therefore, many of the gastric cancer patients undergoing chemotherapy have intact primary foci at the time of treatment. In 1981, the median survival time of patients with gastric cancer treated with various forms of chemotherapy was 10 months for the abdominal localized type, 4.5 months for the liver metastatic type, 4.0 months for the ascitic type, and 3.0 months for the distant metastatic type [3].

---

[1] Department of Gastroenterology, Toyosu Hospital, Showa University, 4-1-18 Toyosu, Kouto-ku, Tokyo, 135 Japan

Because of great advances in diagnostic techniques of gastric cancer by radiology, endoscopy, US, and CT scan, evaluation of the chemotherapeutic effect has also been examined by these same methods in Japan. This also influences response rates. In fact, 75% of our patients had intact primary foci. Out of 109 patients undergoing chemotherapy for advanced gastric cancer, those achieving a tumor reduction of over 50%, as based on X-ray findings, amounted to only 7 (6.4%), while 8 of the 68 patients (62.4% of 109 patients) who had palpable intra-abdominal masses were evaluated as having a PR by palpation (an 11.8% response rate) [4].

The first Response Criteria of Gastric Cancer Chemotherapy by the Japanese Research Society for Gastric Cancer will be introduced and will be followed by a report on the recent results of a randomized controlled study and an especially most promising pilot study with 5'-DFUR plus Cisplatin.

Response Criteria of Gastric Cancer Chemotherapy by the Japanese Research Society for Gastric Cancer

It is extremely difficult to accurately measure the size of the primary foci in the majority of patients. The Japanese Research Society for Gastric Cancer took these circumstances into consideration, and devised a new evaluation method to provide an objective and precise way to assess the therapeutic efficacy of chemotherapy based on roentgenographic or endoscopic changes [5]. Generally, it is desirable for the efficacy of chemotherapy to be evaluated from X-ray and endoscopic findings, if a primary tumor is present.

The above-mentioned new criteria for the evaluation of chemotherapy for gastric cancer are easy to apply, and were designed in consideration of organ-specific properties, following the principles of the Japanese Criteria for the Evaluation of the Direct Effects of Cancer Chemotherapy for Solid Tumors [6]. The efficacy is evaluated on the basis of the rate of regression of measurable lesions, as is described in "Reporting of response" in the WHO Handbook for Reporting Results of Cancer Treatment (WHO offset publication no. 48 (1979) World Health Organization, Geneva).

The following is an introduction of the Evaluation Criteria for Cancer Chemotherapy on Gastric Cancer and our experience in evaluation of the primary foci in inoperable gastric cancer.

Response Criteria for Measurable Gastric Lesions (a)

Complete Response (aCR)

The lesion cannot be identified as cancer because of its complete disappearance on X-ray or endoscopic examination, and no new lesions appear for more than 4 weeks.

Partial Response (aPR)

This category consists of two types of lesions: (1) those which can be measured in two directions by roentgenography or endoscopy, show a more than 50% regression rate, and no new lesions appear for more than 4 weeks, and (2) those which can be measured in one direction by roentgenography or endoscopy, show a more than 30% regression rate, and no new lesions appear for more than 4 weeks.

No Change (aNC)

Lesions measurable in either one or two directions show less than 30% and 50% regression rates, respectively, or either of them enlarges by less than 25%, and no new lesions appear for more than 4 weeks.

Minor Response (aMR)

The two types of these lesions consist of (1) those measurable in one or two directions and are reduced in size by more than 30% or 50%, respectively, for less than 4 weeks, and (2) those measurable in two directions and are reduced in size by more than 25% but less than 50% for more than 4 weeks.

Progressive Disease (aPD)

There is 25% or more increase in the size of one or more measurable lesions, or the aggravation of other lesions and/or the appearance of new lesions.

Response Criteria for Gastric Lesions, Which are Difficult to Measure But Evaluable (b)

Complete Response (bCR)

The tumorous lesions all disappear on X-ray or endoscopic examination, and no new lesions appear for more than 4 weeks.

Partial Response (bPR)

X-ray or endoscopic findings clearly differ from pretreatment findings, e.g., showing marked regression and flattening of elevated or ulcerated lesions (an estimated decrease of more than 50%), and these changes are continuously observed for more than 4 weeks.

No Change (bNC)

X-ray or endoscopic examinations show no changes in comparison with pretreatment findings or no changes suitable to be categorized as PR (estimated decrease of less than 50%), and no new lesions appear for more than 4 weeks.

Minor Response (bMR)

These include (1) changes corresponding to the above-mentioned criteria for PR last for less than 4 weeks, and (2) changes such as marked regression and flattening of elevated or ulcerated lesions are less marked than those categorized as PR, but are continuously observed for more than 4 weeks.

Progressive Disease (bPD)

X-ray or endoscopic examinations show progression in comparison with pretreatment findings, or new lesions appear.

Response Criteria for Diffuse Infiltrating Gastric Lesions (c)

According to the criteria, the rate of enlargement of the affected region after treatment is calculated in comparison with its pretreatment area using the following procedure.

Calculation

X-ray films taken in the same position are used. As a general rule, each focus in a barium-filled stomach is measured in the standing position, and then the rate of enlargement is calculated using the formula described below. Since a posttreatment X-ray film is compared with a pretreatment film, these films should be taken in the same position using the same amount of contrast medium.

$$\text{Rate of enlargement (\%)} = \frac{\text{posttreatment area} - \text{pretreatment area}}{\text{pretreatment area}} \times 100$$

Degree of Efficacy

1. Complete response (cCR): the tumor lesions all disappear on X-ray or endoscopic examination, and no new lesions appear for more than 4 weeks.
2. Partial response (cPR): the affected area in the posttreatment X-ray film is enlarged by more than 50% in comparison with the pretreatment area, and endoscopic findings also confirm this effect. The continuation of an effect has to be certified for more than 4 weeks.
3. No change (cNC): the affected area is unchanged or enlarged by less than 50% for more than 4 weeks on X-ray examination in comparison with the pretreatment area.

    Minor response (cMR): Changes corresponding to those categorized as PR are observed for less than 4 weeks.
4. Progressive disease (cPD): the tumor lesion progresses on X-ray examination, or new lesions appear.

Using these criteria, 368 advanced gastric cancer patients with intact primary foci, who were treated with various anticancer agents over a 10-year period at ten

Table 1. Effect of chemotherapy on inoperable gastric cancer with intact primary foci.

Lesion	CR	PR	NC + PD (MR)	Response rate
a	4	8	68	12/ 80 (15%)
b	3	25	128(1)	28/156 (18%)
c	0	4	146(2)	4/150(2.7%)

CR, complete response; PR, partial response; NC, no change; PD, progressive disease; MR, minor response

institutions in Japan, were evaluated. Eligibility of these patients and efficacy were judged by an extramural review. As the one of authors was the head of this study, 18 cases from our institution were added to the survey. The distribution of types **a, b** and **c** gastric lesions is shown in Table 1. Of the 386 cases, 80 (20.7%) had type **a** lesions, 156 (38.9%) had **b** lesions, and 150 (40.4%) had **c** lesions. The response rate was 12/80 (15%) for **a** lesions, 28/156 (18%) for **b** lesions, and 4/150 (2.7%) for **c** lesions. It was possible to evaluate the actual efficacy of chemotherapy in gastric cancer patients when types **a, b,** and **c** lesions were judged separately.

Randomized Controlled Trials

Despite the many reports of chemotherapy for inoperable or recurrent gastric cancer in Japan, the results of various clinical trials with extramural review have not, unfortunately, met the international criteria for chemotherapy of gastric cancer. As of 10 years ago, we have been carrying out three multi-institutional randomized controlled trials with an extramural review by adhering strictly to the above-described response criteria (Table 2). Patients were stratified by tumor-spreading type into the following three groups before entry into the study: abdominal localized type, liver metastatic or ascitic type, and distant metastatic type [3]. They were randomly assigned by a central office to therapy regimens according to the tumor-spreading type. In the third trial of Table 2, a randomized controlled trial involving 13 institutions all over Japan was conducted in order to compare the efficacy of tegafur plus MMC with UFT (a combination of uracil and tegafur at the molar ratio of 4 to 1) plus MMC for patients with advanced gastric cancer who had not received any prior chemotherapy [2]. The overall response rate for tegafur plus MMC was 7.8% and that for UFT plus MMC was 25.3%, indicating that UFT plus MMC was superior to tegafur plus MMC with a significant difference (χ^2 test $P = 0.004$). When the survival rate for eligible cases, including the incomplete ones, was studied, the 50% survival time was 180 days for both Regimens A and B. This was partially attributable to the inclusion of cases with a poor performance status (Karnofsky's scale: 20%–40%). When we

Table 2. Three randomized controlled trials of inoperable gastric cancer.

Trial	Regimen	Dose	Route	Total (n)	CR	PR	NC (MR)	PD	Response rate (%)	50% Survival (days)
1[a]	UFT	375 mg/m² per day	p. o.	32	0	7	16 (1)	9	21.9	120
	MMC	5 mg/m² per 1–2 weeks	i. v.							
	UFT	375 mg/m² per day	p. o.	25	0	5	9 (1)	11	20.0	155
	ACNU	60 mg/m² per weeks × 2	i. v.							
2[a]	5′-DFUR	1400 mg/m² per day (day 1–4 week)	p. o.	38	0	4	18 (1)	15	10.5	133
	ACNU	60 mg/m² per weeks × 2	i. v.							
	5′-DFUR	1400 mg/m² per day (day 1–4 week)	p. o.	32	0	8	17 (1)	7	25.0	182
	ACNU	30 mg/m² per weeks × 2	i. v.							
	MMC	5 mg/m² per 8 week	i. v.							
3[a]	Futrafur	500 mg/m² per day	p. o.	90	0	7	53	30	7.8	180
	MMC	5 mg/m² per week	i. v.							
	UFT	375 mg/m² per day	p. o.	79	1	19	41	18	25.3	180
	MMC	5 mg/m² per week	i. v.							

[a] *Trials 1 and 2*, Advanced Gastric Cancer Chemotherapy Cooperative Study Group; *Trial 3*, details in [6]
UFT, Combined tegafur and uracil; *MMC*, mitomycin C; *5′-DFUR*, 5′-deoxy-5-fluorouridine; *ACNU*, nimustine hydrochloride

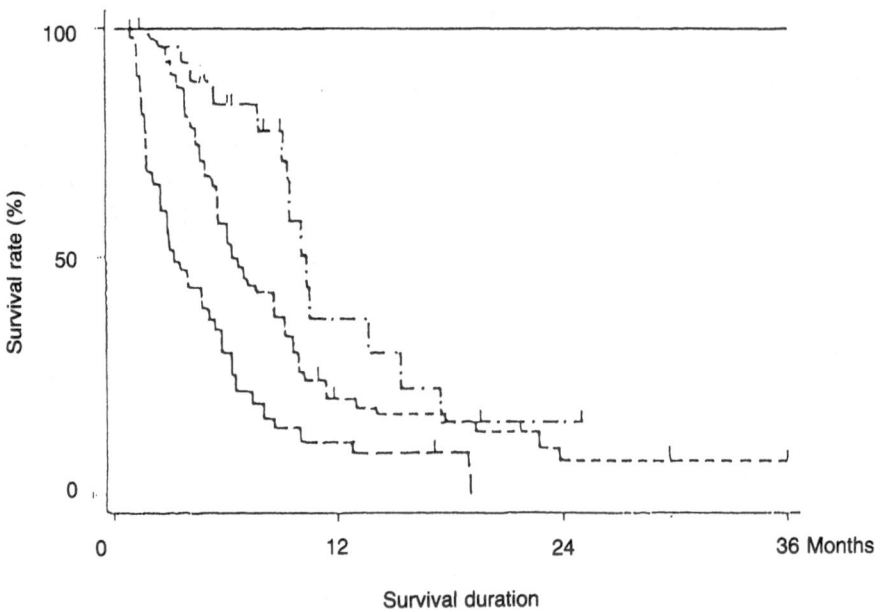

Fig. 1. Survival curves for patients by overall response rate. CR (——), PR (–·–·–), NC (----), PD (– – – –). Median survival period: PR, 312 days; NC, 198 days; PD, 97 days; PR vs NC $P = 0.01$, NC vs PD $P = 0.0001$ (generalized Wilcoxon test)

used the criterion of a longer duration, i.e., 1–1.5 years, the 1-year survival rate for Regimen A was 13.9%, and that for Regimen B was 22.4%, while the 1.5-year survival rate for Regimen A was 5.8%, and that for Regiman B was 14.8% (Log rank test: $P = 0.306$, generalized Wilcoxon test: $P = 0.4022$). Based on the proportional hazards model, eight background factors of the patients, including regimen, were analyzed. The differences in regimen ($P = 0.0398$), tumor-spreading type, lesion subtype, and performance status ($P < 0.0001$) were found to significantly affect survival; these results corresponded to our clinical experience. The survival durations for all patients according to efficacy were 312 days for patients with PR, 189 days for NC and 108 days for PD, showing a significant difference in antitumor effect (Fig. 1). Although WHO criteria have not been able to reveal any correlation between survival duration and PR and NC status, our study suggests that when the above-described new Japanese criteria are adopted, in other words, on the basis of a more difinitive evaluation of the outcome of chemotherapy than that used in the WHO criteria, there is a clear correlation between antitumor effect and survival duration. Additional studies to verify this are imprative.

Phase II Study of Combination Therapy with 5'-DFUR plus Cisplatin [7]

5-FU combined with cisplatin (CDDP) has been reported to have a synergic effect both in vitro [8, 9] and in clinical practice [10]. Recently, two or three combination thereapies including cisplatin with a high response rate was reported in gastric cancer chemotherapy [1, 11]. 5'-deoxy-5-fluorouridine (5'-DFUR, doxifluridine) has been developed as a prodrug for oral 5-fluorouracil (5-FU), which has been used clinically in Japan for the treatment of gastric, colorectal, and breast cancers [12, 13].

Therefore, a multicenter study to seek a more effective program of chemotherapy for gastric cancer was instituted by the Gastric Cancer Study Subgroup of the Cooperative Study Group for Multidisciplinary Therapy for Solid Tumors.

Patient Population and Eligibility

The patients in this study had adenocarcinoma which was histologically confirmed by biopsy, autopsy, or both. None had received chemotherapy prior to entering the present program. With 5 exceptions, 75 cases had an unresectable primary foci that had been evaluated by X-ray examination, endoscopy, or both, and also had metastatic lesions that had been confirmed by X-ray, CT scan, or palpation. The oldest patient was 75 years of age. The patients' performance status (PS) according to the WHO scale was 0–3. The results of the renal function tests were: creatinine clearance, 60 ml/min. or higher; BUN, less than 25 mg/dl; serum creatinine, less than 1.5 mg/dl. Liver function tests revealed: GOT or GPT of less than 100 U and total bilirubin of less than 3.0 mg/dl. Bone marrow functions exhibited: leukocytes, $4000/mm^3$ or more; thrombocytes, $100\,000/mm^3$ or more; hemoglobin, $10\,g/dl$ or more. All the participants had a minimum life expectancy of 2 months, were able to receive oral medications, and gave their informed consent.

Treatment Methods

In Regimen A, $1400\,mg/m^2$ per day of 5'-DFUR was orally administered from day 1 to day 4 in the same week, and $80\,mg/m^2$ per day of cisplatin was intravenously injected on day 5. Three weeks of this regimen corresponded to a course, which was repeated as long as possible. In Regimen B, the same dosage of 5'-DFUR was administered from day 1 to day 4 and day 15 to day 18, and the same dosage of cisplatin was intravenously administered on day 4. Four weeks of this regimen corresponded to a course. In both regimens, the patients were hydrated with normal saline for 24 h prior to CDDP injection (this was continued up to 24 h after therapy). When necessary, furosemide was administered to maintain a urine output of at least $100\,ml/h$. The therapy was repeated unless the lesion became aggravated or severe side effects developed. The dosages of these drugs were reduced by 80% for those subjects between 70 and 75 years of age.

Table 3. Background factors for eligible patients.

No. of Patients	Regimen A	Regimen B
Sex Male	19	31
Female	9	20
Mean age (years)	62.5	62
	(45–75)	(27–75)
PS o	4	7
1	12	26
2	8	12
3	4	6
Macroscopic type		
Borrmann I	1	0
II	5	8
III	12	24
IV	6	16
V	0	2
Primary focus (−)	4	1
Histology		
Differentiated	9	24
Undifferentiated	19	27
Tumor spreading type		
Abdominal localized	10	19
Liver metastatic or ascitic	14	24
Distant metastatic	4	8

Performance status (PS) should be in the grade range 1–3
[14]

Table 4. Mean doses and duration of administration.

	Regimen A	Regimen B
5'-DFUR	110.31 g	73.89 g
	(18–543.9 g)	(8–422.4 g)
	112.68 days	142.82 days
	(16–483 days)	(18–648 days)
CDDP	324.02 mg	357.59 mg
	(100–720 mg)	(100–1125 mg)
	2.92 times	3.23 times
	(1–6 times)	(1–9 times)

Response Criteria

The above-described criteria were used, with all determinations being made with strict adherence to the regulations set down by the extramural review.

Case Analysis and Background Factors

All the registered patients had been confirmed by a central office and 81 patients were considered to meet the eligibility criteria: two were excluded from the study as ineligible and 79 were considered as being eligible. Ten of the eligible cases were judged to be incomplete because of being discontinued (one case), being withdrawn (six cases), or incomplete observation (three cases) (these terms are defined in [14]). Thus, there were 69 evaluable patients (85.2%) consisting of 25 for Regimen A and 44 for regimen B.

Among the eligible patients, no differences in background factors were seen with regard to treatment regime (Table 3). For "complete" cases [13], the total administered doses in the treatment regimen were examined. The mean dose of CDDP in Regimen B was more than that given in Regimen A (Table 4). Because of severe side effects, the schedule of administration of 5'-DFUR and CDDP was modified more often in Regimen A than in Regimen B.

Antitumor Effect

The overall response rate for Regimen A was 40% [95% confidence interval (CI) 20.8%–59.2%] and that for Regimen B was 36.4% (95% CI 22.7%–50.1%) (Table 5).

When efficacy was assessed by target lesions, the response rates for the primary foci were 23.8% (5/21) in Regimen A and 32.6% (14/43) in Regimen B. The response rates for metastatic lesions involving the liver and abdominal lymph nodes were 36.4% (4/11) and 50.0% (4/8) in Regimen A, and 47.1% (8/17) and 30.8% (4/13) in Regimen B, respectively. The response rates for ascites were 100% (3/3) in Regimen A and 60% (3/5) in Regimen B.

Table 5. Antitumor effect.

	Regimen A					Regimen B				
	CR	PR	NC (MR)	PD	% Response rate (n)	CR	PR	NC (MR)	PD	% Response rate (n)
Overall	1	9	13(6)	2	40.0 (10/25) 95% C.I. 20.8%–59.2%		16	21	7	36.4 (16/44) 95% C.I. 22.7%–50.1%
Gastric lesion a		2	3(3)	1	33.3(2/6)		6	5		54.5(6/11)
b	1	2	7(2)		30.0(3/10)	1	6	9	1	41.2(7/17)
c			4(1)	1	(0/5)		1	12	2	7.1(1/15)
Liver		4	6	1	36.4(4/11)		8	5	4	47.1(8/17)
Abdominal lymph node	1	3	4		50.0(4/8)	1	3	8(1)	1	30.8(4/13)
Virchow lymph node				1	(0/1)			1	2	(0/3)
Others		1	3		25.0(1/4)	1		9(1)		10.0(1/10)

	Effective	No change	% Response rate (n)	Effective	No change	% Response rate (n)
Ascites	3	0	100(3/3)	3	2	60.0(3/5)

C.I., Confidence interval. Other abbreviations as in Table 1

The details of PR cases are shown in Tables 6 and 7. Two-year survival was actieved in two cases of Regimen A and five cases of Regimen B.

Prolongation of Survival

The median survival period was 273 days (9.1 months) in Regimen A and 274 days (9.1 months) in Regimen B (Table 8). The median survival periods by response or non-response to the chemotherapy were 292.5 days (9.8 months) and 273 days (9.1 months) in Regimen A, and 460 days (15.3 months) and 225.5 days (7.5 months) in Regimen B, respectively.

Toxicity

The major adverse effects of Regimen A were gastrointestinal disorders, bone marrow supression, and renal failure of WHO grade 3–4. In contrast, these adverse effects were markedly reduced in Regimen B (Table 9).

Quality of Life

The quality of life (QOL) of patients undergoing chemotherapy is an important clinical end point [15]. Changes with time of the QOL in patients who had undergone 5′-DFUR + CDDP for inoperable gastric cancers were investigated. The items studied included appetite, general feeling, sleep, fatigue, pain, under-

Table 6. The Details of PR cases in Regimen A.

No.	Sex	Age (years)	Performance status	Histology	Borrmann type	Primary lesion response	Metastatic lesion response	Response duration (days)	Survival period (days)
1	M	60	1	Tub$_2$	III	bMR	Liver PR	251	478
2	M	66	0	Por	III	bPR	Liver PR	50	873[a]
3	M	53	1	Sig			Abdominal lymph node PR	64	244
4	F	71	2	Por	III	bCR	Ascites disappeared	64	216
5	M	69	2	Tub$_1$	II	bPR	Liver PR	71	268
6	F	63	2	Por			Liver PR Abdominal lymph node CR	28	149
7	M	45	1	Sig	III	bNC	Abdominal lymph node PR	83	171
8	M	48	1	Por	IV	cNC	Abdominal lymph node PR	167	317
9	M	55	1	Por	III	aPR		36	318
10	M	71	0	Pap	III	aPR	Liver PR Lung PR	164	745[a]

tub$_1$, Well-differentiated tubular adenocarcinoma; *tub$_2$*, moderately differentiated tubular adenocarcinoma; *por*, poorly differentiated adenocarcinoma; *sig*, signet-ring cell carcinoma; *adeno*, adenocarcinoma. Other abbreviations as in Table 1
[a] Living now

Table 7. The Details of PR cases in Regimen B.

No.	Sex	Age (years)	Performance status	Histology	Borrmann type	Primary lesion response	Metastatic lesion response	Response duration (days)	Survival period (days)
1	M	74	1	Tub$_2$	3	bPR	Abdominal lymph node CR	642	944[a]
2	M	62	1	Tub$_1$	3	aPR	Abdominal lymph node PR	141	1020[a]
3	M	68	0	Tub$_1$	2	bCR	Liver PR	186	254
4	F	73	2	Tub$_1$	3	aPR	Liver PR	78	561
5	M	57	0	Tub$_1$	2	bPR	Liver PR	702	814
6	M	50	3	Por	3	aPR	Liver PR	171	460
7	F	67	1	Pap	3	bPR	Abdominal lymph node NC	125	523
8	M	66	2	Por	3	bPR	Liver PR Lung MR Abdominal lymph node MR	32	300
9	F	68	1	Por	3	aPR	Liver PR	81	195
10	M	70	1	Por	3	aPR	Liver PR	221	406
11	M	54	1	Tub$_1$	2	aNC	Liver PR	113	224
12	F	48	1	Sig	4	cPR	Large intestine CR	519	830[a]
13	M	52	1	Adeno	3	bPR	Abdominal lymph node PR	278	759[a]
14	F	71	0	Tub$_2$	2	aPR	Virchow NC	64	425
15	M	65	1	Por	3	bPR	Liver NC	28	190
16	F	48	1	Por	5	bNC	Abdominal lymph node PR	65	294

[a] Living now. Abbreviations as in Tables 1 and 6

Table 8. The median survival period.

Overall cases	Regimen A 273.0 days (25 patients)	Regimen B 274.0 days (44 patients)
Abdominal localized type	317.5 (10)	325.0 (16)
Ascitic type	216.0 (3)	209.5 (6)
Liver metastatic type	273.0 (9)	195.0 (15)
Distant metastatic type	147.0 (3)	314.0 (7)
CR	216.0 (1)	
PR	317.0 (9)	460.0 (16)
MR	493.5 (6)	
NC	258.0 (7)	267.0 (21)
PD	82.5 (2)	154.0 (7)
Response cases (CR + PR)	292.5 (10)	460.0 (16)
Non-response cases (MR+ NC + PD)	273.0 (15)	225.5 (28)

Abbreviations as in Table 1

Table 9. Toxicity (according to WHO criteria)[a].

	Regimen A					Regimen B				
	0	1	2	3	4	0	1	2	3	4
Diarrhea	13	2	3	6	3	35	8	2	1	
Anorexia	12	3	4	8		22	2	12	10	
Nausea, vomiting	9	3	7	8		26	8	13	9	
WBC	10	4	7	3	3	23	10	10	3	
PLT	23	1	2	1		44	2			
Anemia	21	1	4	1		38	1	3	4	
BUN	14	5	6		2	36	9			1
Creatinine	21	4	1	1		41	5			
Creatinine clearance	19	4	2	2		39	4	2	1	

PLT, Platelet count
[a] WHO offset publication no. 48 (1979) World Health Organization, Geneva

standing and cooperation in a familiar environment, association with friends and colleagues, anxiety concerning the disease, expectations of treatment, and activities of daily life [16]. There were ten items which were recorded from 2–4 weeks by the patients using five grades by a combination of the analog scale and category scale method. Moreover, an analog scale on "feeling", 10 cm in length, was also checked at the same time. We then could compare any change in responses to the QOL questionnaires between Regimens A and B. There were remarkable differences between the two groups in terms of appetite, general feeling, fatigue, expectations of treatment, and the analog scale on "feeling" as evaluated from the follow-up data (Fig. 2). From the viewpoint of QOL, the results indicated Regimen B to be much better than Regimen A.

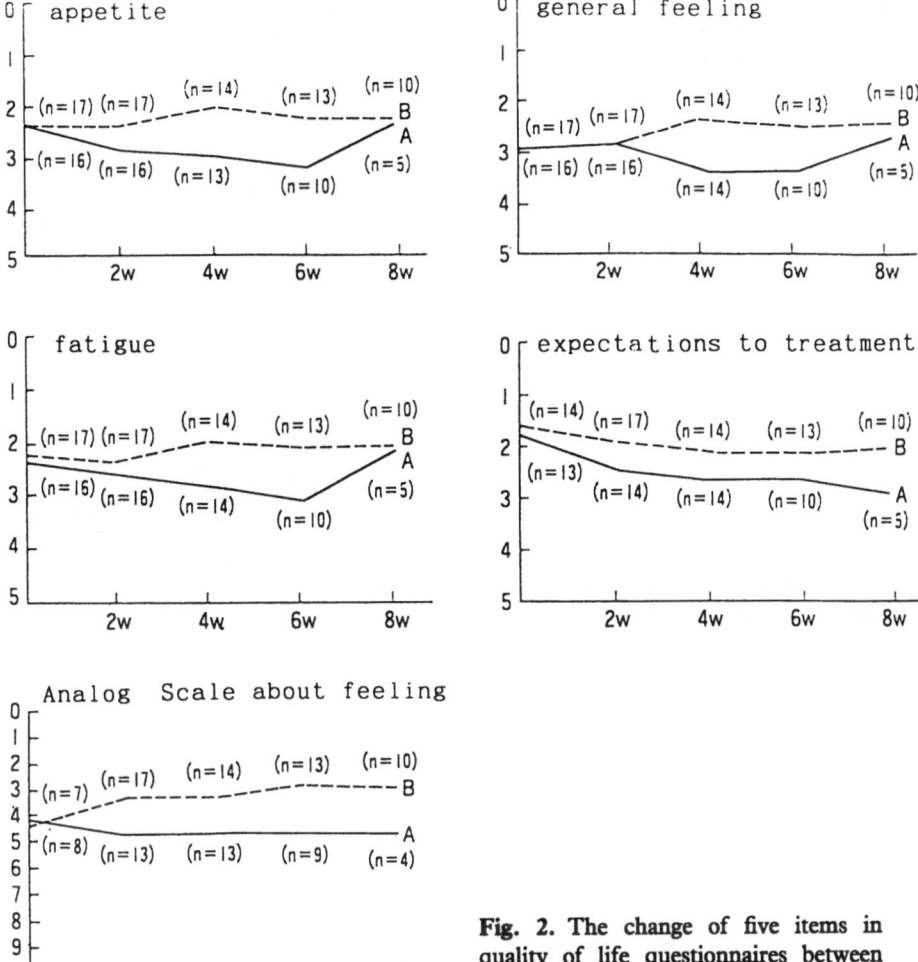

Fig. 2. The change of five items in quality of life questionnaires between Regimen A and Regimen B

Case Report: 48-Year-Old Female

The patient suffered from a stenotic feeling of cardia at the beginning of March, 1990. She was diagnosed by X-ray examination as having Borrmann type IV gastric cancer infiltrated to the transverse colon (Fig. 3). Therefore, 5'-DFUR 1800 mg/day was administered intermittently from April 7th. i.e., a 4-day administration followed by a 10-day period of withdrawal (q. 2W), and cisplatin 110 mg/body was intravenously administered on April 11th (q. 4W). In the X-ray films taken 1 month after the beginning of treatment, there was a marked improvement of pliability of the gastric wall in addition to expansion of the

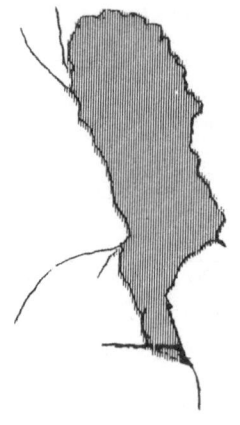

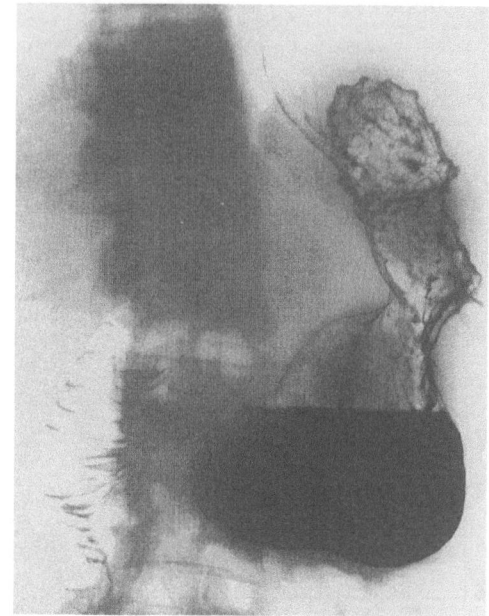

Fig. 3. Barium-filled stomach at pre-treatment (March 14, 1990)

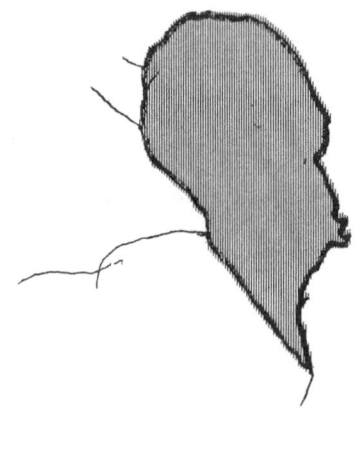

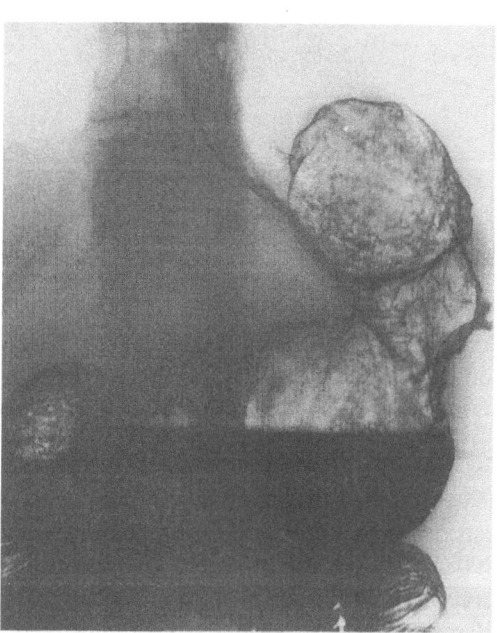

Fig. 4. Barium-filled stomach at 1 month after the beginning of treatment (May 12, 1990). Enlargement rate of affected area (74.9%)

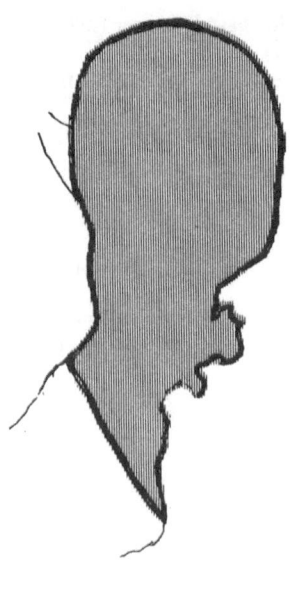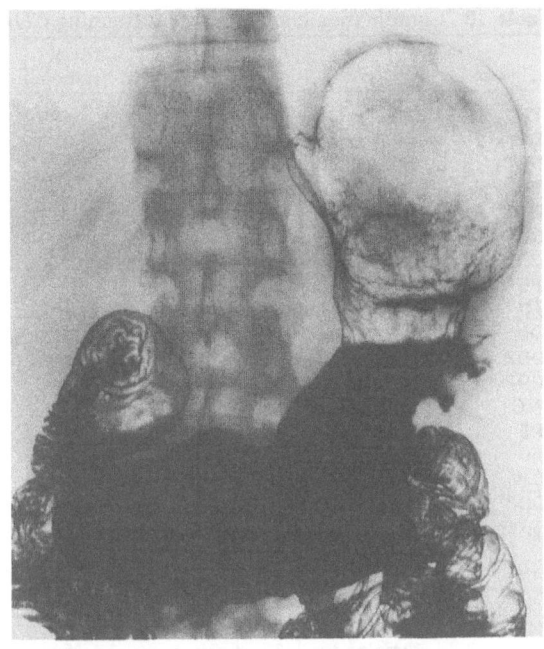

Fig. 5. Barium-filled stomach at 6.5 months after the beginning of treatment (October 31, 1990). Enlargement rate of a effected area (147.1%)

gastric lumen (an enlargement rate of 74.9%, Fig. 4). Colonic invasion had disappeared on X-ray films using a barium enema. It was initially evaluated as having a cPR effect. After four courses of therapy of 5'-DFUR, the cPR effect was confirmed by gastric X-ray films (with an enlargement rate of 147.1%, Fig. 5), because the cPR effect continued for more than 4 weeks. At this point in time, she was strongly persuaded to undergo an operation. Since she refused surgery, she was administered 5'-DFUR for more than 2 years. Except for visiting the outpatient clinic twice a month, she has enjoyed her usual activities of daily life, including doing aerobics, without any complaint. (She was treated at Dept. of Gastroenterol. Juntendo Univ. By the courtesy of Dr. T. Hamada).

Discussion

Cisplatin-based chemotherapy has most recently emerged as among the most active of combinations for patients with inoperable gastric cancer as reviewed by Leichman et al. [17]. FAP [18] and EAP [19] are the most prominent and have been followed in many institutions. Recent results of cisplatin-based chemotherapy are shown in Table 10. Lerner et al. [20] reported a response rate of 55% (no significant difference with FAM), but at the cost of treatment-related death

Table 10. Combination chemotherapy containing CDDP for gastric cancer ($\geq$25 cases).

Regimens			No. of patients	No. of responders	Response rate (%)	Investigators
5-FU ADM CDDP	600 mg/m^2 days 1, 8 40 mg/m^2 day 1 75 mg/m^2 day 1	q4w	35	10	28.6	Cazap et al. [26] (1986)
5-FU ADM CDDP	300 mg/m^2 days 1–5 40 mg/m^2 day 1 60 mg/m^2 day 1	q5w	26	13	50	Moertel et al. [18] (1986)
CDDP 5-FU	100 mg/m^2 day 1 1000 mg/m^2 day 1–5	q4w	31	14	45.2	Lacave et al. [27] (1987)
5-FU ADM CDDP	400 mg/m^2 days 1–3 50 mg/m^2 day 2 90 mg/m^2 day 2	q4w	32	11	34.4	Rougier et al. [28] (1987)
CDDP MMC UFT	75 mg/m^2 day 1 10 mg/body day 1 400 mg/day daily	q3w	37	11	29.7	Matsuki et al. [29] (1988)
5-FU ADM CDDP	300 mg/m^2 days 1, 8, 15, 22 30 mg/m^2 day 1 100 mg/m^2 day 1	q4w	30	6	20	GITS [30] (1988)
Etoposide ADM CDDP	120 mg/m^2 days 4, 5, 6 ($\geq$60y. 100 mg/m^2) 20 mg/m^2 days 1, 7 40 mg/m^2 days 2, 8	q4w	33	23	70	Preusser et al. [19] (1988)
Etoposide ADM CDDP	120 mg/m^2 days 4, 5, 6 20 mg/m^2 days 1, 7 40 mg/m^2 days 2, 8	q3w	25	18	72	Katz et al. [31] (1990)
5-FU Epirubicin CDDP	600 mg/m^2 day 1 60 mg/m^2 day 1 70 mg/m^2 day 1	q4w	52	19	36	Delfino et al. [32] (1990)
Etoposide ADM CDDP	100 mg/m^2 days 4, 5, 6 20 mg/m^2 days 1, 7 40 mg/m^2 days 2, 8	q3~4w	48	21	43.8	Taguchi et al. [21] (1989)
5-FU ADM CDDP	270~350 mg/m^2 days 1–5 25 mg/m^2 day 5 70 mg/m^2 day 1	q3w	32	6	19	Kikuchi et al. [33] (1990)
CDDP MMC UFT Etoposide	75 mg/m^2 day 1 10 mg/body day 1 400 mg/body daily 50 mg/body days 3–5	q3w	42	23	54.8	Sawa et al. [34] (1991)

(14%) and with a median survival of 6 months. Taguchi [21] also reported similar data. EAP regimen is considered to be adequate only for patients with locally advanced, surgically proved nonresectable gastric cancer, good PS ($\leq$ 2) and being less than 60 years old. In spite of strict evaluation methods, the 5'-DFUR plus cisplatin combination therapy produced response rates of more than 35%. The median survival of patients with primary foci (21/25 in Regimen A and 44/45 in Regimen B) and other metastatic sites was 9 months in both groups. The median survival of 16 PRs in Regimen B was 460 days with good QOL by patients' assessment. Currently, 5'-DFUR plus cisplatin and MMC for inoperable gastric cancer is under investigation. In the near future, randomized controlled studies with leucovorin plus 5-FU [22, 23] or FAMTX [24, 25] will be investigated.

References

1. Preusser P, Wilke H, Achterrath W, et al (1989) Phase II study with the combination etoposide, doxorubicin, and cisplatin in advanced measurable gastric cancer. J Clin Oncol 7:1310–1317
2. Kurihara M, Izumi T, Yoshida S, et al (1991) A cooperative randomized study on Tegafur plus Mitomycin C versus combined Tegafur and Uracil plus Mitomycin C in the treatment of advanced gastric cancer. Jpn J Cancer Res 82:613–620
3. Kurihara M (1981) Indication and prognostic factors. In: Kurihara M, Nakajima T (eds) Chemotherapy of gastric cancer (in Japanese). Shinkooigaku, Tokyo, pp 85–87
4. Kurihara M, Izumi T (1980) Chemotherapy of solid tumors: Evaluation of effects on gastric cancer (in Japanese), Jpn J Cancer Clin 26:652–658
5. Japanese Research Society for Gastric Cancer (1985) Evaluation of the effects of chemotherapy and radiotherapy on gastric cancer. In: The general rules for gastric cancer study, 11th edn (in Japanese). Kanehara, Tokyo, pp 108–125
6. Japan Society for Cancer Therapy (1986) Japanese criteria for the evaluation of the direct effects of cancer chemotherapy for solid tumors (in Japanese). J Jpn Soc Cancer Ther 21:931–942
7. Koizumi W, Kurihara M, Sasai T, et al (1993) A phase II study of combination therapy with 5'-DFUR and cisplatin in the treatment of advanced gastric cancer with primary foci. Cancer 72(3) (in press)
8. Schabel FM Jr, Trader MW, Laster WR Jr, et al (1979) Cis-dichlorodiammineplatinum (II): Combination chemotherapy and cross-resistance studies with tumors of mice. Cancer Treat Rep 63:1459–1473
9. Scanlon KJ, Newman EM, Lu Y, et al (1986) Biochemical basis for cisplatin and 5-fluorouracil synergism in human ovarian carcinoma cells. Proc Natl Acad Sci USA 83:8923–8925
10. Kish JA, Weaver A, Jabcobs J, et al (1984) Cisplatin and 5-fluorouracil infusion in patients with reccurent and disseminated epidermoid cancer of the head and neck. Cancer 53:1819–1824
11. Moertel CG, Rubin J, O'Connell MJ, et al (1986) A phase II study of combined 5-fluorouracil, doxorubicin, and cisplatin in the treatment of advanced upper gastrointestinal adenocarcinomas. J Clin Oncol 4:1053–1057
12. Wakui A: Phase II trial of 5'-deoxy-5-fluorouridine in the treatment of gastric cancer—a multicenter cooperative study. J Int Med Res 16 [Suppl 2]:17B–18B
13. Niitani H, Kimura K, Saito T, et al (1985) Phase II study of 5'-deoxy-5-fluorouridine (5'-DFUR) on patients with malignant cancer—multi-institutional cooperative study (in Japanese). Jpn J Cancer Chemother 12:2044–2051
14. Japan Society for Cancer Chemotherapy (1993) Criteria for the evaluation of the clinical effects of solid cancer chemotherapy. J Jpn Soc Cancer Ther 28(2):101–130
15. Johnson JR, Temple R (1985) Food and drug administration requirement of approval of new anticancer drugs. Cancer Treat Rep 69:1155–1157
16. Kurihara M, Izumi T, Denda T, et al (1990) Quality of life in gastrointestinal cancer chemotherapy (in Japanese). Jpn J Cancer Chemother 17(4):Part II, 887–894

17. Leichman L, Berry BT (1991) Cisplatin therapy for adenocarcinoma of stomach. Semin Oncol 18(1) [Suppl 3]:25–33
18. Moertel CG, Rubin J, O'Connell MJ, et al (1986) A phase II study of combined 5-fluorouracil, doxorubicin and cisplatin in the treatment of advanced upper gastro-intestinal adenocarcinomas. J Clin Oncol 4:1053
19. Preusser P, Wilke H, Achterrath W, et al (1989) Phase II study with the combination etoposide, doxorubicin, and cisplatin in advanced measurable gastric cancer. J Clin Oncol 7:1310–1317
20. Lerner A, Steele GD, Mayer RJ (1990) Etoposide, doxorubicin, cisplatin for advanced gastric adenocarcinoma: Results of a phase II trial (abstract). Proc Am Soc Clin Oncol 9:103
21. Taguchi T (1989) Combination chemotherapy with etoposide (E), Adriamycin (A) and cisplatin (P) (EAP) for advanced gastric cancer (abstract). Proc Am Soc Clin Oncol 8:108
22. Machover D, Goldschmid E, Chollet P, et al (1986) Treatment of advanced colorectal and gastric adenocarcinomas with 5-fluorouracil and high-dose folinic acid. J Clin Oncol 4:685–695
23. Louvet C, de Gramont A, Demuynck B, et al (1991) High-dose folinic acid, 5-fluorouracil bolus and continuous infusion in poor prognosis patients with advanced measurable gastric cancer. Ann Oncol 2:231–233
24. Wils J, Klein HO, Wagener DJTh, et al (1991) Sequential high dose methotrexate and 5-fluorouracil combined with doxorubicin: A step ahead in the treatment of advanced gastric cancer. A trial of the EORTC Gastrointestinal (GI) Tract Cooperative Group. J Clin Oncol 9:827–831
25. Kelsen D, Atiq O, Saltz L, et al (1991) FAMTX (fluorouracil [F], methotrexate [M], adriamycin [A]) is as effective and less toxic than EAP (etoposide [E], A, cisplatin [P]): A random assignment trial in gastric cancer (GC) (abstract). Proc Am Soc Clin Oncol 10:137
26. Cazap EL, Gisselbrecht C, Smith FP, et al (1986) Phase II trials of 5-FU, doxorubicin, and cisplatin in advanced, measurable adenocarcinoma of the lung and stomach. Cancer Treat Rep 70:781–783
27. Lacave AJ, Anton-Aparicio L, Gonzalez-Baron M, et al (1987) Cisplatin (CDDP) and 5 fluorouracil (5FU) 120-hr infusion for advanced gastric cancer (GC): A phase II multicenter study. Proc Am Soc Clin Oncol 7:91
28. Rougier P, Droz JP, Thedore C, et al (1987) Phase II trial of combined 5-Fluorouracil plus Doxorubicin plus Cisplatin (FAP regimen) in advanced gatric carcinoma. Cancer Treat Rep 71:1301–1302
29. Matsuki N, Sakuma H, Sawa T, et al (1988) Effect of PMU therapy (CDDP, MMC, and UFT) against terminal gastric carcinoma (in Japanese). Jpn J Cancer Chemother 15(4):Part I 655–659, April
30. Gastrointestinal Tumor Study Group (1988) Triazinate and platinum efficacy in combination with 5-fluorouracil and doxorubicin: Results of a three-arm randomized trial in metastatic gastric cancer. J Natl Cancer Inst 80:1011–1015
31. Katz A, Gansl R, Simon S, et al (1989) Phase II trial of VP-16 (V), Adriamycin(A), and cisplatinum(C) in patients with advanced gastric cancer (abstract). Proc Am Soc Clin Oncol 8:98
32. Delfino C, Caccia G, Alasino C, et al (1990) 5-Fluorouracil(F) + epirubicin(E) + cisplatin(C) in patients with advanced gastric cancer (abstract). Proc Am Soc Clin Oncol 9:123

33. Kikuchi K, Wakui A, Shimizu H, et al (1990) Randomized controlled study on chemotherapy with 5-FU, ADM plus CDDP for advanced gastric carcinoma (in Japanese). Jpn J Cancer Chemother 17(4): Part I, 655–662
34. Sawa T, Kinoshita K, Takekawa S, et al (1991) Effect of PMUE therapy (CDDP, MMC, UFT, Etoposide) for terminal gastric cancer (in Japanese). Jpn J Cancer Chemother 17(12):2381–2386

Index